NON-IMPACT AEROBICS

The NIA Technique®

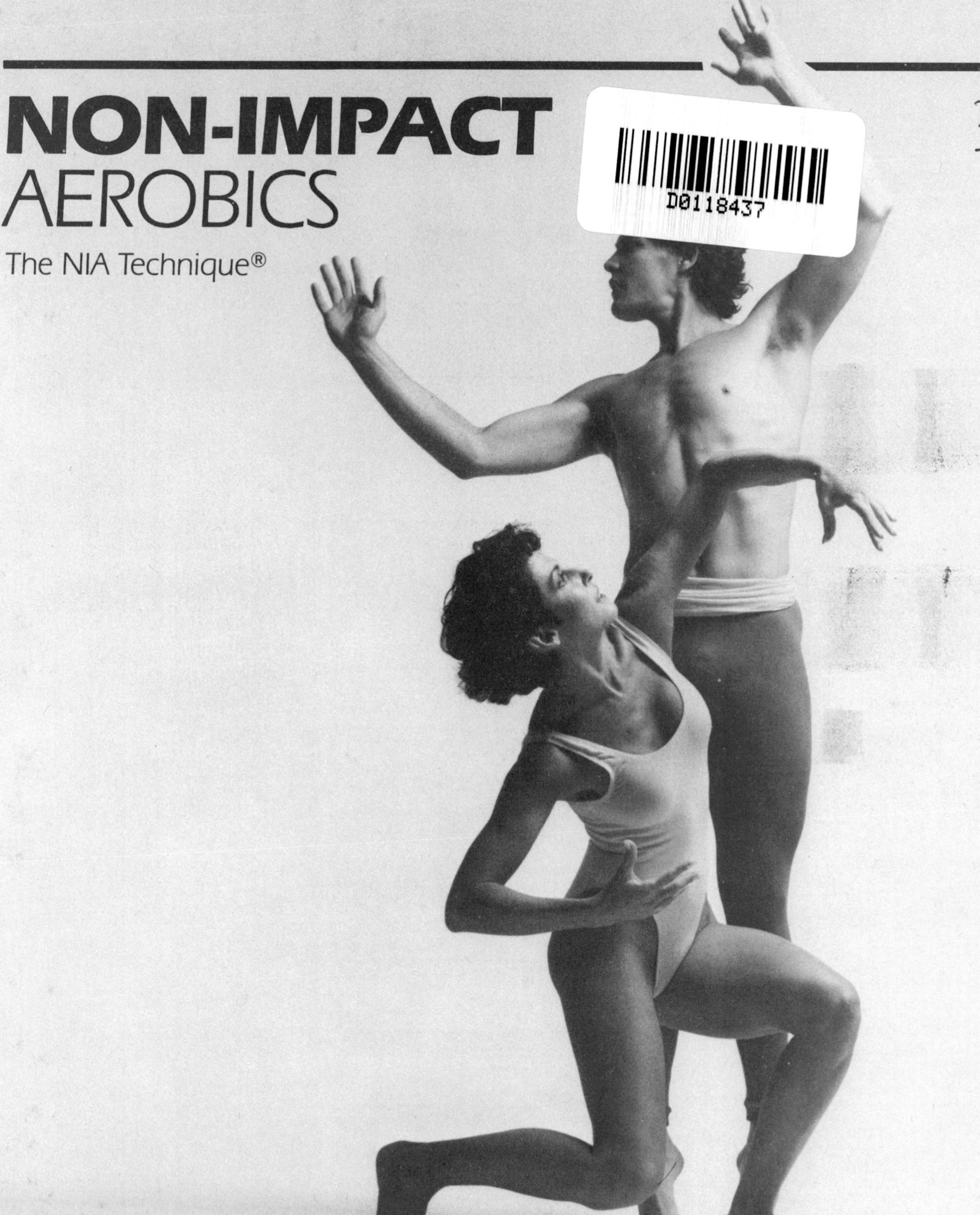

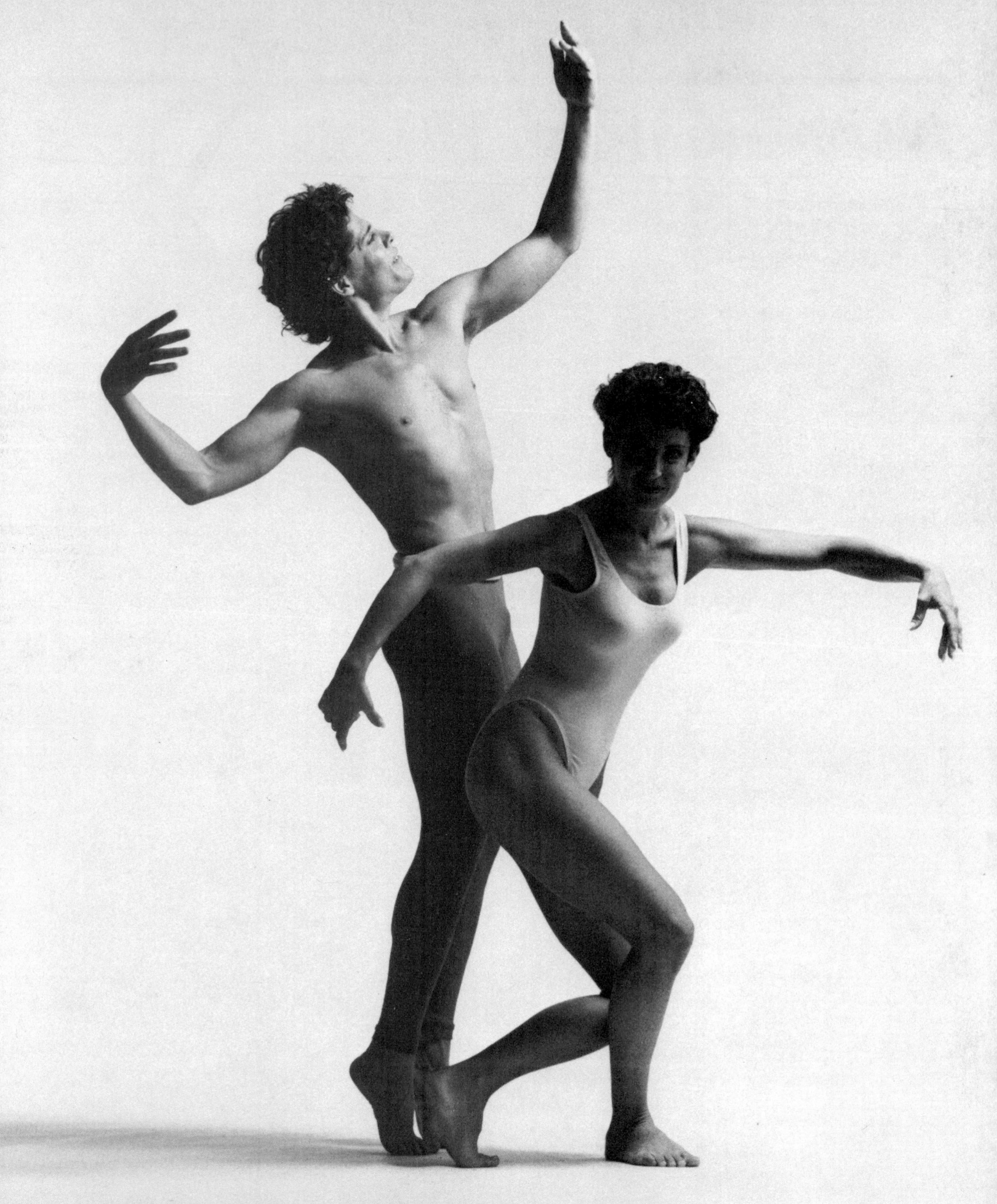

NON-IMPACT AEROBICS

The NIA Technique®

BY
DEBBIE & CARLOS ROSAS
WITH
KATHERINE MARTIN

Published in the United States by Villard Books, a division of Random House, Inc., New York, and simultaneously in Canada by Random House of Canada Limited, Toronto.

Designed by Aster Winslow Creative Inc.

Library of Congress Cataloging in Publication Data
Rosas, Debbie, 1951-
Non-impact aerobics.
1. Low impact aerobic exercises.
I. Rosas, Carlos. II. Martin, Katherine. III. Title.
RA781.15.R66 1987 613.7'1 86-40346
ISBN 0-394-55899-5

Manufactured in the United States of America
9 8 7 6 5 4 3 2

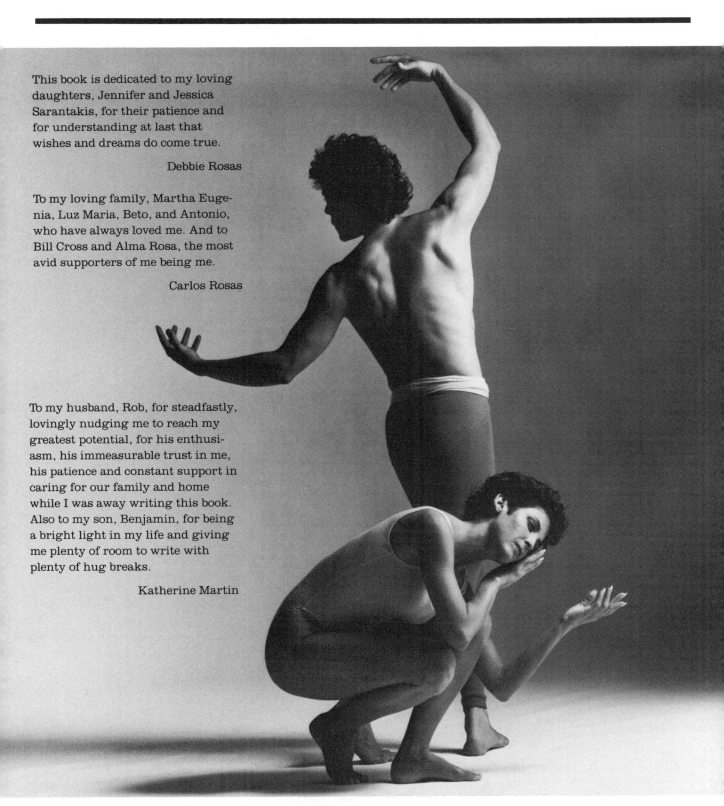

This book is dedicated to my loving daughters, Jennifer and Jessica Sarantakis, for their patience and for understanding at last that wishes and dreams do come true.

Debbie Rosas

To my loving family, Martha Eugenia, Luz Maria, Beto, and Antonio, who have always loved me. And to Bill Cross and Alma Rosa, the most avid supporters of me being me.

Carlos Rosas

To my husband, Rob, for steadfastly, lovingly nudging me to reach my greatest potential, for his enthusiasm, his immeasurable trust in me, his patience and constant support in caring for our family and home while I was away writing this book. Also to my son, Benjamin, for being a bright light in my life and giving me plenty of room to write with plenty of hug breaks.

Katherine Martin

ACKNOWLEDGMENTS

Our thanks to Jeanne and Arthur Bender for their much appreciated and needed support, faith, and trust; to Jennifer Fox for her never ending words of encouragement and belief in our dream; to the first Bod Squad staff of instructors, Karen Fazio, Deborah Walker, Tricia Tucker, Diane Singleton, Barbara Cocke, and Molly Nugent for their unending support, untiring cooperation, and meticulous tending to our business and classes while we were absent; to our Bod Squad class members for having the courage to change and grow with us and for trusting our vision; to photographer Lois Greenfield whose creative talent and sensitive vision of movement through photography made our book a work of art, and her assistant, Jack Deaso, for his talent and humor through the long, long hours of shooting in New York; to all the movement teachers who inspired our NIA dream, knowingly or unknowingly—Martha Graham, Mikhail Baryshnikov, Dan Millman, t'ai chi masters Al Huang and K. C. Mao, yogi B.K.S. Iyengar, jazz virtuosos David Jones and Ed Mock, and movement artist Joy Berta; to master sensei Gus Johnson of The Way of the Dragon for his guidance in the martial arts; to Robert Martin and Robert Adamich for bringing their joy and brilliant insights into our lives and business; to Diane Reverand, who recognized our vision and so energetically and brilliantly helped to bring it forth; to our agent, Connie Clausen, who eagerly and warmly trusted in our work and masterfully made it a reality; to Donna Gillien and Dr. James Garrick from the Center for Sports Medicine, St. Francis Hospital, San Francisco, who listened to what we had to say and responded with knowledge, sincerity, warmth, and encouragement; to Katherine Martin, our cowriter, for her sight, direction, inspiration, aliveness, patience, encouragement, and brilliant writing—without her, our book wouldn't be; and last of all, to each other for believing and never giving up and holding onto our greatest gift—our love for each other.

Debbie and Carlos Rosas

My thanks immeasurable to Lazaris for guiding this book on a smooth and easy course, to Peny for her treasured friendship and for steadfastly pointing out the greatest probabilities in life, to Jach and Michaell for endless inspiration and joy. To my parents, Ginny and Tate Lane, who raised me to believe that all things are always possible. To Connie Clausen and Diane Reverand for all of the above underscored with gratitude. To fellow writer and fitness explorer Keith Thompson who got me to my first NIA class. To the staff of Nautilus of Sausalito for the generous use of their facilities during the development of this book and to Susie and Rich and the folks at Winships and The Upstart Crow who plied me with food and drink during the lengthy editing of the manuscript. To Debbie and Carlos, who are truly two of the greatest people I know with the most genuine of hearts and most precious of gifts.

Katherine Martin

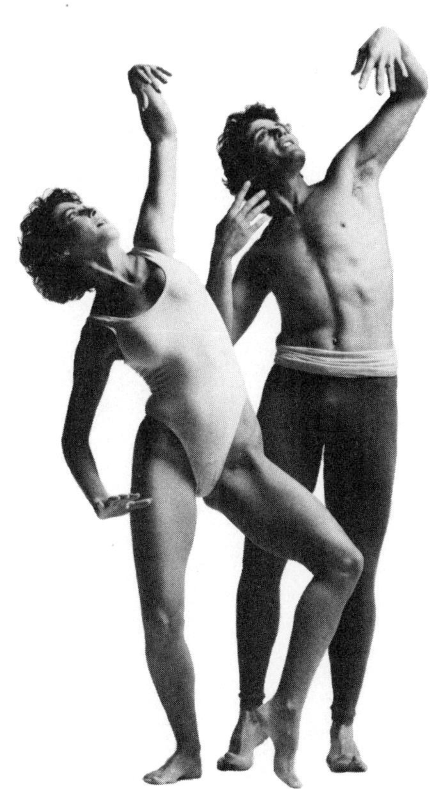

CONTENTS

PART I

THE DAWN OF A NEW AEROBIC ERA

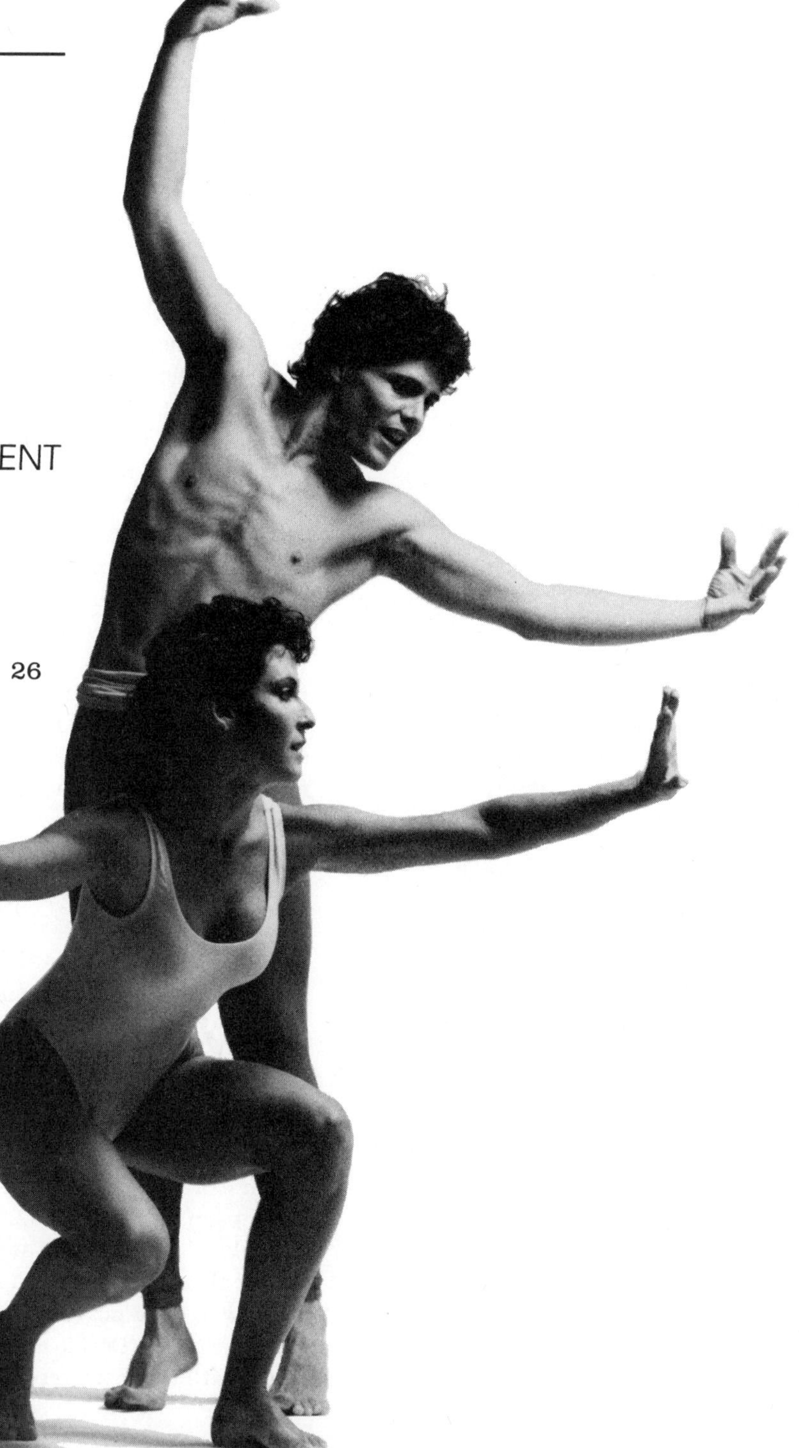

PART II

THE NIA TECHNIQUE® IN MOTION

3/ STARTING OUT RIGHT 31

PART III

THE NIA TECHNIQUE® WORKOUTS

4/ GET READY 61

5/ WORKOUT I 67

6/ WORKOUT II 125

PART IV

THE NIA TECHNIQUE® ON THE GO

7/ EVERYDAY NON-IMPACT AEROBICS 183

EPILOGUE 190

True fitness is not bred within the walls of health clubs or recreational centers, but in the way we live. It is not simply exercise, but an active embrace of life. Movement, ongoing movement, is the essence of fitness.

Of course, before beginning, you should check with your doctor to make certain the non-impact aerobic workout is right for you. Once you have begun, follow your instincts and intuitions to gear each and every workout to your very special and unique body.

Non-impact aerobics has become a generic term for a variety of "soft workouts." The NIA Technique®, taught exclusively through the Bod Squad, Inc., in San Rafael, California, was developed before *non-impact* became such a widely popularized term and is very unlike any other non-impact program.

AUTHORS' NOTE

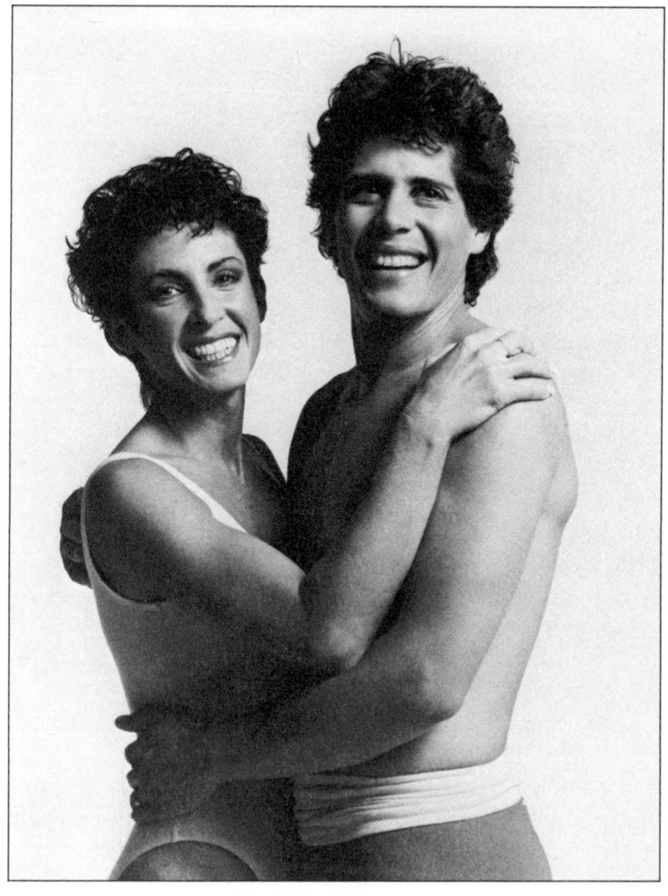

The NIA Technique is a revolutionary aerobic workout with absolutely *no* jumping, jogging, or jarring calisthenics. With the discovery of startlingly high injury rates among jump, or hard-impact, aerobic students and instructors, non-impact aerobics has been thrust to the forefront of a surging movement toward "soft workouts." We designed it to be safe. That was a given. But in searching for and creating the perfect workout, we were looking for much more.

Jump aerobics mobilized millions of Americans. We were part of that mobilization. It was great, but it was just a beginning. As years skipped by, we grew restless for something more than tedious donkey kicks and leg lifts. Bouncing through a spine-rattling hour made less and less sense. Most jump aerobic movements that weren't injurious simply weren't efficient, which meant we were putting in a good deal of grunt-and-groan effort for disproportionate paybacks. The cardiovascular conditioning was invaluable, but there had to be a better way to care for and refine the *whole* body—one that would caress the soul and stimulate the mind while sculpting the body.

Our search led us to the discovery of a far more efficient, effective way to tone the body comprehensively so that you get more for what you put in. That means a lot to busy people. You don't need to set aside time to work out on a Nautilus machine, another hour for a stretching class, a body-sculpting class, a yoga class, *plus* an aerobics class. You can get it *all* in just one non-impact aerobic workout.

The NIA Technique strengthens abdominals without sit-ups; defines muscles without external weights; increases lung capacity without "killer" aerobics that leave students gasping for air. Our technique provides flexibility without conventional stretching; positive postural changes; and a physical and emotional balance that puts the student back in charge of his or her own body.

The NIA Technique was built from the ground up, not adapted from a beginner's aerobics class. Unlike many low-impact classes, it provides full cardiovascular conditioning without any jumping, jogging, or hopping. The workout is chock full of innovative choreography to beat the boredom of dull, repetitious movements. We did an intensive study of Eastern and Western movement arts to design it. The development was exhilarating and exasperating at the same time, as you'll see in the first chapter of this book. We had little support for what we were doing and, in fact, became outcasts in the aerobic community when we stopped teaching jump-aerobics, which had been the mainstay of our careers. When we first tried to get across our concept of non-impact aerobics, people either stared at us blankly or laughed.

Today, however, the "soft aerobics" movement is in full swing. People are hungry for a safe, efficient way to get and stay fit. We've grown up around fitness. We're not so easily taken in by the hype and pipe dreams of looking like fitness celebrities. We want functional fitness for real people. That means using our heads, following our own common sense, and taking the time to build up gradually instead of chasing fast-fad fitness that leads to burnout and injury rates that have been registered at 76 percent for instructors and 44 percent for students. We're tired of the senseless "no pain, no gain" credo that pushes fitness beyond safety zones.

The crux of the NIA Technique is more gain with no pain, being comfortably inside your body while you work out, slowing down, keeping one foot on the floor at all times, and shifting body weight with fluid, purposeful placement. No more pounding motions that lead to shinsplints and an entire list of injuries to the foot, ankle, calf, knee, hip, and back. We use lyrical sinking movements set against the natural pull of gravity, extensions and contractions that allow muscle flex/release, and tensions/countertensions covering a full range of motion on different planes. We use more of the body, more creatively, and in so doing, get so much more from a single gourmet workout.

By taking the pounding out of aerobics, the NIA Technique has opened doors to people who couldn't tolerate the hard impact of traditional aerobics. One of our students, the mother of two young children, had to give up jump-aerobics after the birth of her second child because she'd lost enough bladder control that she couldn't get through a class without having to run to the bathroom. Nursing mothers and women with large breasts welcome the chance to get an aerobic workout without bouncing, as do new mothers looking for a gentle way to shed baby fat.

The NIA Technique has also given new hope to people with orthopedic and heart problems who can't take the stress of jump aerobics; people with high blood pressure and people battling the kind of overweight problems that can make jarring exercises a real threat to the musculoskeletal system; people recovering from injuries like stress fractures. One of our students recently threw away a knee brace that she'd had to wear whenever exercising because of surgery to remove cartilage from her knees; soon after starting our non-impact aerobic workout, another student shucked braces he'd worn on both knees for stability.

Perhaps most heartening, non-impact aerobics is finally drawing the "elite fit" who have the courage to begin anew, to stretch for something more. That includes people like professional athletes, dancers, weight lifters, and, yes, even traditional aerobics masters. To the millions of dedicated aerobicisers who have steadfastly worked toward greater levels of fitness, pushing out the boundaries that limited them, non-impact aerobics is a new frontier. Seizing the challenge, they gain new strength, endurance, and flexibility through our NIA Technique while utterly enjoying the delectable thrill of refined, efficient movement.

Over the past four years, we've limited our exercise exclusively to non-impact aerobics so that we can honestly see the effect it has on us. If we had continued biking, swimming, running, and weight lifting, we wouldn't have known which had caused what. So what you see in this book is what you can get: muscle definition and strength that come from the NIA Technique alone.

In many ways, the NIA Technique is our way of taking a new stand on fitness—one that calls for the kind of self-respect and self-determination that gives people back their inherent power to change, to take charge of their own well-being; one that honors the unique body structure of each of us and elicits the truest, most evocative expression of our emotional bodies moving in unison with our physical bodies. We ardently urge our students not to clone us, but to trust their own bodies and use what they have to take them elegantly to those thin thighs, flat abs, and firm buns; to be individually creative and expressive; to feel and emote, gaining more of themselves as people, physically and emotionally, even spiritually.

It's 1987, a new year, a new aerobic era. We're no longer looked at askance. The aerobics industry has, at last, embraced the concept of non-impact aerobics. National aerobics associations are actively encouraging instructors to develop low-impact programs to beat the escalating injuries, and although many are adaptations of beginners' jump-aerobics classes, the movement is firmly in place, a revolution under way.

As part of our revolution, we took off our shoes. It was one of the boldest things we did during the evolution of the NIA Technique. Working out barefooted was near heresy in a field that would give rise to a $177.5 million aerobic shoe business. The media was saturated with studies comparing a plethora of makes and models. People were aghast that we would dare to even consider the possibility of working out barefooted. We weaned ourselves carefully, at first trading our aerobic shoes for jazz shoes, then wrestling shoes, t'ai chi shoes, and finally gymnastics shoes, a transition we still recommend for students who don't take readily to the idea of bare feet. We made the final break from shoes when we'd gathered enough information to feel confident that for our kind of movement, shoes were not only unnecessary but, in fact, a hindrance. We do not, however, recommend this barefoot approach for people with structural foot problems or for students of any other aerobics classes.

We do non-impact aerobics on any smooth surface, with the exception of thick mats, which don't provide enough foot stability. The reason we can shed our shoes and not fret about sprung floors is the movement itself. The NIA Technique is based on non-impact movements, not low-impact or controlled-impact movements, which means that we've totally eliminated jumping, jogging, hopping, and leaping. Our technique is grounded mostly in natural heel-ball-toe movements that protect the thin metatarsal bones in the foot. During the hopping, jumping, and running in place of conventional aerobics, the metatarsals take a direct beating, and the tendons and ligaments of the ankle and foot can become inflamed or torn.

In the four years that we've been teaching the NIA Technique barefooted, we've had no reported foot injuries. The only complaint we've heard has come from students who worked out too long, too soon, and developed blisters. Otherwise, students report increased circulation, flexibility, and dexterity, decreased foot cramping, the disappearance of callouses, and even heightened arches, which runs counter to the theory that the arches will fall without the support of a shoe.

Testimonials about physical changes as a result of the NIA Technique have become almost a daily event. Every day we continue to learn and grow with the NIA Technique, and we'll never stop reaching for new horizons, new frontiers. Debbie is now teaching sixteen classes a week (jump-aerobics instructors usually burn out at ten), and she's always looking for the greatest efficiency, the fine line that divides building up and tearing down, honing her mind/body skills to help her monitor the edges of that line. Carlos is experimenting to see how much abdominal strength and definition he can get from breathing alone and is developing "abs-on-the-go" to see how many spontaneous, practical ways he can devise to strengthen abdominals throughout an ordinary day.

For us the NIA Technique is a way of life, our philosophy of mind, body, and spirit. We live it with singular dedication, spending endless evening hours designing new and better workouts in our living room, devoid now of any furniture but fully mirrored on one wall. The more the NIA Technique grows, the more we grow with it. Our exciting audio cassettes are available through local bookstores, as well as through NIA Techniques, Inc. (see page **191** for ordering); our *Non-Impact Aerobics* video is available through local video outlets; and certification and instructor-training programs in the NIA Technique are being conducted nationwide. As we travel to do guest workshops and trainings, we hope one day to meet you over that eloquent expression of the unique body and soul of each of us: movement, sweet, life-giving movement.

PART I: THE DAWN OF A NEW AEROBIC ERA

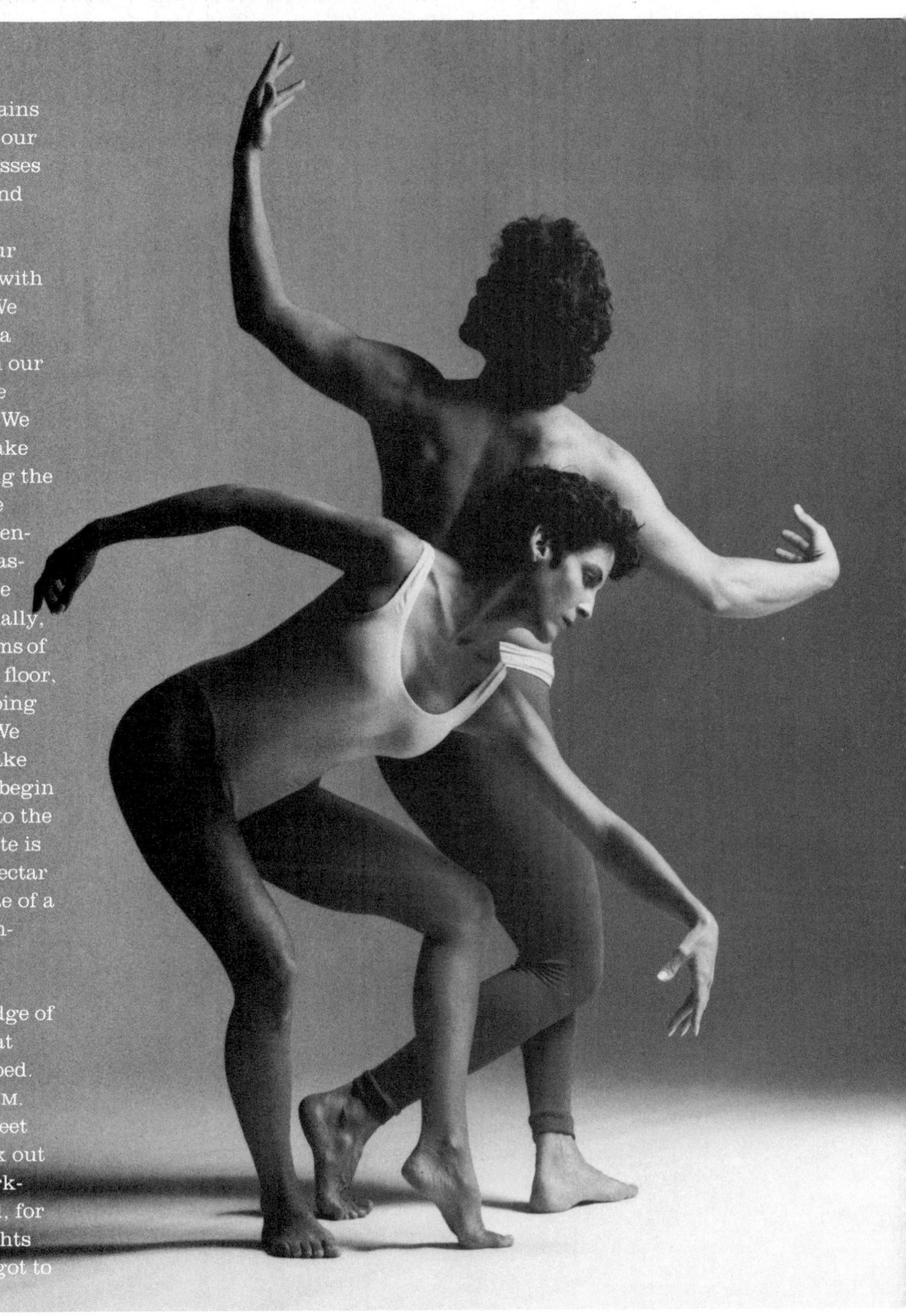

The Dream Classical strains fall like a gentle waterfall over our bodies. Mozart. The music caresses our minds. We close our eyes and feel the feathery touch of our breath, the steady beating of our hearts. We are at peace, at one with the life that moves within us. We smile at one another, and with a glint of nervous anticipation in our eyes, we take off our shoes. The carpet feels cool and receptive. We roll our feet back and forth, make circles around the edges, feeling the outline of our connection to the earth, our point of balance, listening to the crackle of joints releasing. It feels delicious. Slowly we begin to move, languidly, sensually, flowing with the natural rhythms of our bodies, sinking toward the floor, pushing away, our arms sweeping overhead, then circling close. We carve space with eloquence, make love to gravity. Beads of sweat begin to roll down our cheeks and into the corners of our mouths. The taste is not bitter, but sweet. It is the nectar of a dance of our souls, the taste of a future we will call the NIA Technique.

The Reality From the edge of a dream, a shrill scream tears at Mozart. We sit bolt upright in bed. The alarm clock flashes 5:30 A.M. Our classes start at 7:00. Our feet hit the floor. In silence we work out the kinks from yesterday's workouts. We look at each other and, for a poignant moment, our thoughts join in recognition. There has got to be a better way.

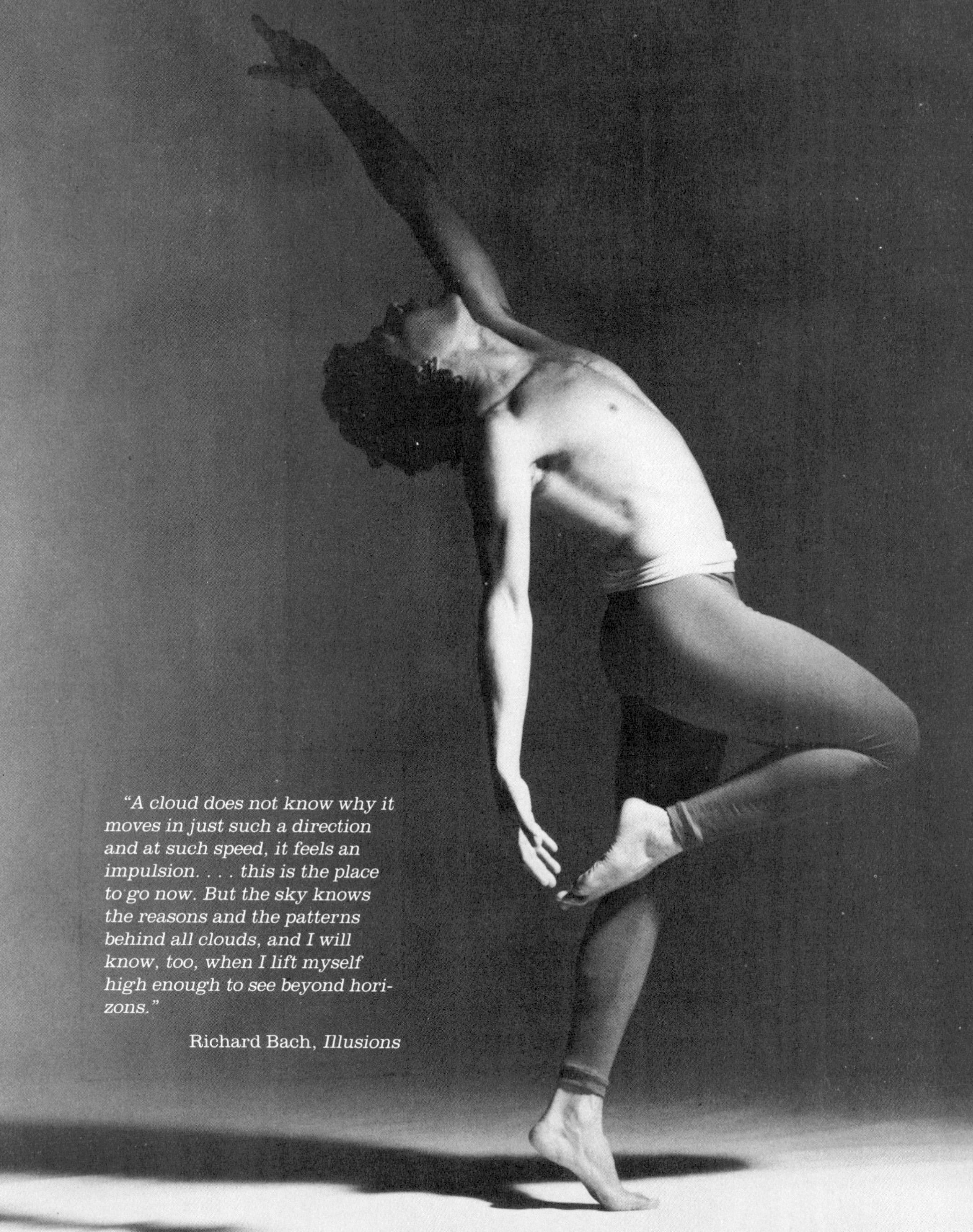

"*A cloud does not know why it moves in just such a direction and at such speed, it feels an impulsion. . . . this is the place to go now. But the sky knows the reasons and the patterns behind all clouds, and I will know, too, when I lift myself high enough to see beyond horizons.*"

Richard Bach, *Illusions*

1/THERE HAD TO BE A BETTER WAY . . .

It was 1981. Aerobics had really hit its stride, and no one, but no one, wanted to hear about the down side of this panacea for thin thighs, firm buttocks, and healthy hearts. Our own students were infatuated with status quo aerobics. We knew the feeling. It was hard to admit that anything could be wrong with a fitness program that got so many of us out of chairs and back into the vibrancy of life. We were still three years away from the startling research that would uncover a 76 percent injury rate among aerobics instructors, a 44 percent injury rate among students. Zealous aerobicisers were still working out with shinsplints, sore knees, back pain, not knowing, or not wanting to know, that their bodies were signaling injury ahead. A silent code of pain pervaded the aerobic community. We knew it intimately.

For five years we had been riding high on the great aerobic boom that was sweeping the country, mobilizing millions of Americans to shape up and trim down. Debbie had had her own personal catharsis through aerobics. After two children, she'd grown from a petite size 5 to a size 13. For someone who had prided herself on meticulous self-discipline, it was frightening. Her confidence hit rock bottom. Depressed and scared (life at twenty-four was not supposed to look like this), she had signed up for a local aerobics class. She didn't know it then, but it would be a turning point that would change the course of her life. Her career as a medical illustrator and commercial artist began to pale next to the excitement of fitness. In 1976 she made the break and, with typical zeal, founded what would become a highly successful aerobics business, The Bod Squad, Inc. In no time, she had parlayed her contagious enthusiasm into a six-figure business with fifty instructors teaching over a hundred classes a week throughout the San Francisco Bay area.

Meanwhile, Carlos was a tennis pro, teaching, competing in tournaments, and playing life on the edge of machismo. He might have gone on like that if it hadn't been for Richard Bach and *Illusions* and the faint longing for something more meaningful, something to give lyrical narration to movement. Lured to dance, yet loathe to trade his manly image for a ballet leotard, he geared up in sweats and took a Bod Squad class taught by Debbie. It was a match unlike anything he'd felt on a court. Despite the fact that he'd mapped out a bright future in tennis, he threw in the towel and signed up for Bod Squad's instructor-training program.

Bod Squad flourished, classes were jam-packed, and life should have been great. Except that Carlos was rolling out of bed every morning and grimacing through ten minutes of stretches to work out tendinitis, downing a cup of coffee and two aspirins before each class to rev up for the gung-ho hour that was murder on his shinsplints. And Debbie, although not injured, grew less and less tolerant of the discomfort of jump aerobics.

There had to be something more to fitness than routine exhaustion and stiffness, aches and pains. If we, well trained and robust, ached, what must students feel? What about the cadre of Bod Squad instructors? They'd been painstakingly trained in proper aerobic methodology. But, then, so had we.

Aerobic Rumblings

And so, together, we began to question the silent code of pain. Our probing wasn't particularly popular back then. We knew deep down that there had to be a better way, one that would be not only safe but more fulfilling, one that would more efficiently sculpt the body while conditioning the heart, one that would also enrich the mind and soul. Tedious donkey kicks and jumping jacks just couldn't be the end-all of fitness.

By 1983 the aerobic community was buzzing with talk of the need for better, well-cushioned aerobic shoes and resilient floorings, and faint rumblings could be heard about instructor certification. Later we would hear that a mere 10 percent of aerobic instructors were qualified to teach. Injury research was in the wings. One study would be conducted by two California podiatrists, Dr. Douglas Richie and Dr. Steven Kelso; another by the National Injury Prevention Foundation and San Diego State University, spearheaded by Dr. Peter Francis. Their findings would reveal shockingly high injury rates.

The Sports Medicine Center of Union Memorial Hospital in Baltimore would release statistics that confirmed our suspicions: 82 percent of aerobic dance injuries occur below the knee and are exacerbated by repetitive jumping movements. Topping the aerobic injury lists were shinsplints and foot problems. The Richie-Kelso study would rank injuries in order of decreasing frequency as those to the calf, low back, knee, ankle, neck, arm/shoulder, Achilles tendon, hip/pelvis, and thigh. Personal experience told us that those lists could have also included things like poor concentration, disturbed sleep, difficulty relaxing, and overall body stiffness.

While attention focused on shoes and floors and certification, we were convinced that the motion itself was the nut of the problem. A new understanding, a new experience of the body and the mind were far more important than a certificate, which eventually could be purchased for the fee of a weekend workshop. Improved floors and shoes, the latter becoming a multimillion-dollar industry, were simply bandages and, in an odd sort of way, relied on the threat of injury to keep business healthy. We believed the actual movements themselves could be designed to eliminate the cause of the problems instead of simply treating the symptoms.

The Search for a Better Way

We got our first glimpse of what we were looking for when we took a workshop given by a Japanese dancer who moved in the oddest way without saying a word, but with a smile spread across his face throughout the entire class. His dance looked deceptively simple, nothing fancy, but gentle, playful. And yet, moving in his wake, we dripped with sweat, our pulse rates rising steadily to our aerobic targets. It was a revelation, the first time we got cardiovascular conditioning unawares, without really having to *work* at it. Better yet, it was the first time we were deeply touched by movement. It was fluid, lyrical, softly luring open our tight aerobic muscles and joints. Slowly that smile crept over our own faces. We had the first whisper of an answer.

Our determination to find that answer was fueled when Debbie had her body fat and fitness level tested. With great anticipation, she stepped up for the aerobic testing, sure that the extra classes she'd added to her teaching schedule would put her well above her former fitness level. The results stunned her. Her aerobic capacity had decreased. She'd *lost* fitness.

That was it. We hit the library, did a computer search for studies, research, anything to validate what we suspected, but we came up empty-handed. If we were going to change, we'd have to do it on our own through trial and error, with only perseverance (and we would need a lot of it) to keep us going.

When we first publicly revealed our plans, we spoke of "muscle aerobics," afraid that the term *non-impact* would turn people away. Sure enough, when we got up the gumption to say what we really meant, people laughed and then, seeing that we were serious, made fast tracks for the "killer" aerobics across town. Some people didn't think it was so funny. Some were downright mad that we had the audacity to change, to take away their classes. One irate woman called us at home and hissed, "How dare you!"

Fortunately, we had each other for sanity checks and the kind of encouragement that kept us going as we turned our backs on aerobics and our aerobics friends turned their backs on us. We had to be nuts, they told us; ride the horse in the direction it's going. Well, we rode all right, but a horse that was definitely of a different color.

Starting Over

We gave up teaching jump aerobics and became students again, reaching out to the martial arts of karate, t'ai chi, and tae kwon do, to yoga and ballet, jazz, and modern dance. We were voracious, absorbing everything we could learn about Eastern and Western movement arts.

It was frightening to start over, humiliating to become beginners after all those years of applause for our aerobic aplomb. We missed our daily dose of compliments, the ego rush of forty people clapping wildly at the end of a class. We'd been consummate masters of aerobics and considered ourselves to be highly fit, strong, part of an elite fitness corps. The more we learned, however, the more we encountered our ignorance, our lack of awareness about our bodies. Next to dancers and black belts, we were weak, and veritable klutzes when it came to balance, grace, self-control. After all those donkey kicks and leg lifts, we couldn't hold a martial arts stance for more than ten seconds without our legs shaking.

Our first encounter with a martial arts dojo was, in retrospect only, laughable. A dojo is a place of learning where the revered sensei, or master, passes on his knowledge of the martial arts. It is not, we quickly discovered, anything like a fitness studio. We showed up in flashy designer leotards and leg warmers, snappy head and wrist bands—in short, bulls in a china shop. The first things to go were our forty-dollar aerobics shoes. We started to protest aerobic dancers never, never, never work out barefooted, but to no avail.

Feeling increasingly out of place, we padded inside, about to be stripped of more than our shoes. In the hushed quiet of a starkly plain room, we saw for the first time how much we relied on hard rock music to rev us up. Our master sensei was patient. "Please move," he said simply. We looked at him expectantly, waiting for him to finish. Move how? Flat back? Can-can kick? "Please move," he repeated. We looked at each other, embarrassed. What about music? We were naked without the hard drive of a rock beat, off balance without the familiar cushioning of our shoes, awkward as we pumped through one of our aerobic workouts like a silent version of Laurel and Hardy. Our sensei laughed, "You have fifteen seconds' worth of knowledge."

Methodically, he challenged our concepts of movement. He joked that he'd never get us to slow down our frenetic bump-and-grind aerobic pace, to grab hold of the very essence of movement. Gradually, very gradually, we discovered the power of controlled movement, learning to carve space subtly, yet profoundly, not bullishly. We came to know the true meaning of balance and harmony, that exercise must combine soft, slow movements with firm, fast ones to be efficient and effective.

The pulse of movement became not the hard beat of musical cues but the delicious discovery of our own inner rhythms. We learned how to move with those rhythms instead of throwing ourselves into postures, to work muscles from the inside out instead of riding momentum, to move in sync with the anatomical design of the body.

We gained a new appreciation for our feet and the natural heel-ball-toe movements that eliminate impact and cushion body weight. We developed a new relationship with gravity, a new awareness of the vast ranges and planes of movement, which offered rich possibilities for comprehensively and systemically toning the body. We began to grasp the totality of movement and space, to feel and perceive the body not simply as isolated parts but as a whole affected throughout by the most innocuous of movements.

By slowing down, we discovered muscles we'd never even felt in aerobics. We grunted "Hai!" more loudly with every karate kick and felt our breath working as a kind of kinetic sit-up that surprisingly tightened our abdominal muscles. We began to see new definition in our legs, hips, stomachs, and buttocks. Our photographer, who was recording our physical changes, was amazed and then peeved. We were getting "cuts," fine lines that define muscles, that she, as a weight lifter, envied and was pushing a lot of heavy metal and pain to try to get. We'd been nervous about not doing conventional floor work, afraid that our legs would go fat and flabby. And yet, ironically, we were getting svelte thighs and hips without boring donkey kicks that were murder on the lower back and numbing on the mind; stronger abdominals without any searing situps; firm buttocks without mindless leg lifts and bun squeezes. For the first time, it hit us. Conventional floor work could be replaced with something more efficient and a heck of a lot more fun.

Developing a New Choreography

We began to play with imagery, visual suggestions that would make the whole body respond naturally and spontaneously. Imagining the floor to be hot, we punctuated a tap out. Pretending to draw rainbows, we made more fluid, sweeping arcs with the arms. We tried out duck walks by flapping our arms, felt the sun on our chests, pulled bubble gum off our shoulders. Not only did the workout seem more like play, it more fully engaged the whole body. Stretching to touch the buttery soft petal of a lily that seemed to be just out of reach, we extended farther and used more muscles than by simply swinging our arms out to the sides. Pulling tight springs added just the right tension and utilization of the fingers and wrists to fully work the triceps and biceps.

Hand in hand with imagery came visualization, the neuromuscular programming athletes use to prepare mentally for competition. By visualizing the body in perfect motion, we used our minds to help our bodies follow. The more we imagined ourselves to be martial arts masters, the easier, more rapid, our progress became.

Our concept of fitness was irrevocably changed. Translating that new concept into workable form, however, was exasperating. Complicated movements had to be deciphered and broken down into easily learned parts. While Carlos could quickly grasp new rhythms, everything had to be tediously broken down for Debbie, who is slightly dyslexic. She became our guidepost for finding the simplest common denominator of each movement.

As we slowly evolved workouts, we argued, shouted, ranted, and raved. One day we would come home ecstatic, shouting "We've got it!" Three days would pass, and we'd lose it. We wanted to quit—often—to return to the comfort of all that was familiar and secure.

The new choreography was unbalanced, and we struggled to get the whole body fluidly involved. We kept probing, digging, making what seemed like thousands of minor changes in positioning, posture, sequence of movements. We couldn't just add a motion to fill space. We had to understand what it did to the body, how it affected the movement just before and after it.

Ballet added more artistry, grace, fluidity, and balance and taught us critical elements of positioning and postural alignment, the true meaning of strength and extension. Jazz got us loose, showed us the subtleties of isolation and the coordination of complex movements. Modern dance was lyrical and gave us a new understanding of our own individual expression of movement. Movement arts, we discovered, are not mere replication, but an eloquent reflection of the spirit, a mirror to the soul.

Our choreography was gelling, and yoga would give it the final depth. With slower, more controlled movements, we now had time to breathe deeply, to give our lungs time for the kind of expansion that can't happen when you're gasping for air. We learned to use breathing not only to oxygenate the brain for a wonderfully euphoric feeling, but to energize the entire body for increased staying power. We gained new flexibility from being aware of skeletal structure and paying attention to bone alignment and the posture of joints.

Clearly, we assured each other as the mainstream aerobic community bulged toward twenty million, we were on the verge of pioneering an elegant alternative to traditional aerobics—one that not only was safe but worked the heart more efficiently, more greatly increased lung capacity, more comprehensively toned muscles for greater definition in the legs, hips, buttocks, abdominals, and arms. Our new workout enticed the mind to play, the body to feel, the spirit to emote.

In a single workout we coalesced elements of six movement arts to create a cross-training effect, a concept that later would be greatly popularized in sports. Within one ultimately efficient class, we combined stretching, weight training, aerobic conditioning, body sculpting, and yoga. Better yet, by incorporating the basic fitness elements of strength, endurance, balance, relaxation, and flexibility within each movement, we developed a more systemic way to condition the entire body throughout an entire class. And we linked all those movement arts to the eloquence of the soul moving in harmonious reflection with the body and the mind. For people wanting the greatest payback from a workout, our technique was gold.

The NIA Technique was fun. It was passionate. It was everything we'd dreamed of in a perfect workout. We couldn't have asked for more, and yet, in those quiet, anticipatory, midnight hours on the eve of unveiling our completed work, we realized that we had, in fact, uncovered a sixth and a seventh element of fitness: passion and honor.

The Unveiling

With nervous anticipation, we unveiled the NIA Technique to our most loyal Bod Squad students. As we waited in the tomblike silence of the rec center on that Thursday night before the first students began to trickle in, our minds raced. What if they balked at taking off their shoes? At the classical music? At the utter absence of popping off the floor? What if their muscle memory was too firmly implanted with the staccato rhythm of jump aerobics? What if they thought all this lyrical stuff was a bore, the imagery hokey? Would they be disjointed without a hard rock beat to follow? Would their heart rates get up into their aerobic target zones as ours did? Could we get them to really let go with those "Yeet" grunts?

The reaction that night was mixed. It was hard to let go, to start over, to trust that this new, unfamiliar way of moving was really a better way to get fit. The aerobic mind-set, the "no pain, no gain" mentality, was hard to buck. Our students went through withdrawal in the beginning. We empathized. It hadn't been easy for us either.

Truth is, we'd had heated arguments about the issue of pain. We had grown accustomed to its being a benchmark of fitness, had actually set up goals based on how much pain we could endure. Without it, we were edgy. Was a workout really any good if we didn't work up the kind of muscle fatigue that left us feeling wiped out, if we didn't press through searing "burns" that we conquered by pounding the screaming muscle with a fist? Even after realizing that the answer was an unequivocal yes, we worried about convincing our students. Would they come back if they didn't have those familiar aches and pains they associated with fitness? Maybe we should leave in just a little hurt, just enough to convince them that this was bona fide exercise.

Gradually our own need for a hard aerobics "fix" had waned—and so did our students'. Hesitant at first, they removed their shoes. The thought that they could strengthen their ankles and feet by not relying on the support of a shoe did little to alleviate the awkwardness of naked ground contact. Having paid more attention to shoes than to the feet within, they encountered those marvelous sensors of stability for the first time.

The classical and soft blues music soon grew sweet, relaxing, calming, helping to melt tension and quiet their minds as they opened to a new awareness of their bodies, their internal energies, their feelings—all of which would help them move more efficiently, effectively, safely.

Slowly at first, one foot at a time, they stepped out, the heel extended, the toes drawn back, sinking and rolling through the flat of the foot. Moving rhythmically, back and forth, sinking and rising, becoming in sync . . . with the rhythm . . . of the body. Feeling the heat rising up from the feet, through the legs, into the hips, and now sweeping upward with arcing arms, fingers rippling the air, feathery, hands floating like leaves caught in an updraft, around and around . . . while the torso . . . lilted up and down . . . swaying side to side. Breathing steadily with the motion, like an undulating wave, a collective heart beat.

The memory of the hard yank of conventional, linear aerobics gave way to the soothing flow of circular movements that tone more muscles and take the strain off otherwise overused ones. Little by little, we could see them gaining new freedom of motion, their bodies becoming more flexible, responsive, agile. Inhibitions gave way to soft sensuality and a playful wriggling of fingertips, wrists, elbows, and shoulders, clear down to the toes, until the whole body was engaged. Reluctantly at first, they exposed their exhalations, working up to a full chorus of those karate "Yeet!" grunts that help protect the lower back and tighten abdominals.

At the end of class, one of our students who had been a devout jump-aerobics student likened the way she felt to the glow of a full-body massage. But, she asked, could something that felt so wonderful really be aerobic? Fortunately, the answer wasn't to be construed in a subjective sort of way. Pulse rates are inarguable. We now have to caution students that, because they work so many more muscle groups, they can easily slip over their aerobic target. That same student, who had also been running six miles a day during her jump-aerobics days, found she could get her heart rate higher and steadier with the NIA Technique without feeling that her body "had just taken a royal beating." Later, at the Center for Sports Medicine, St. Francis Hospital, San Francisco, we would test Carlos on an EKG to validate the NIA Technique conditioning on an already highly fit person and discover that his heart rate maintained at a steady aerobic target, whereas traditional aerobic dance rates can zigzag up and down.

Soon we were hearing a new language from our students. They spoke of internal strength, control, and power—mental as well as physical. They spoke of agility, grace, and increased range of motion. They spoke of groundedness and balance—emotional, as well as physical. They were relaxed even when working strenuously. Simple daily tasks like playing with the kids, cleaning the house, even turning around in the car, were becoming easier. Best of all, they began to equate fitness with movement, not simply isolated exercise, to see that fitness was not confined within the walls of a health club or rec center, not bound by the large hand of a clock. At its best, the NIA Technique was carrying them through the entire day with greater ease and grace.

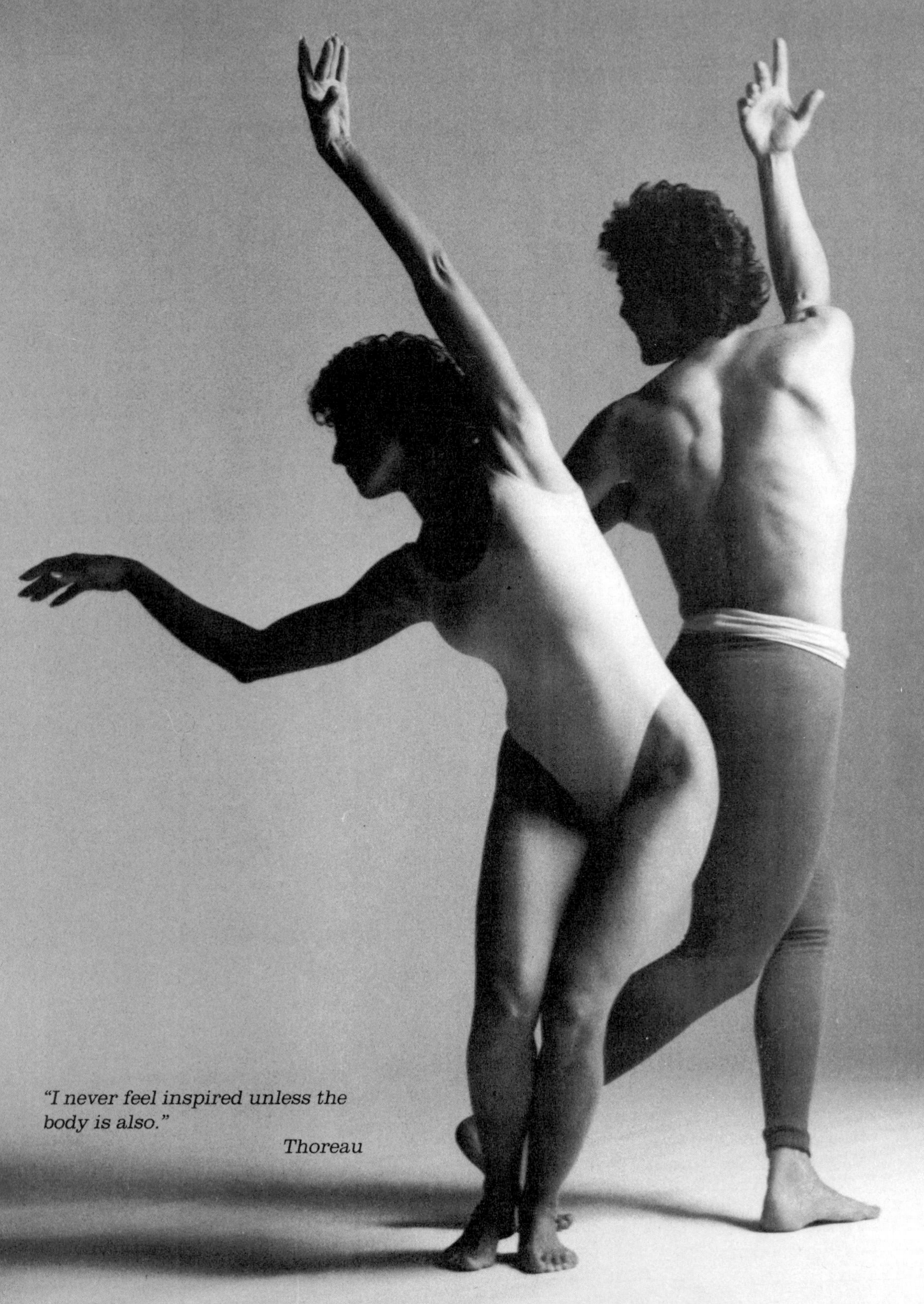

"I never feel inspired unless the body is also."

Thoreau

2/ GETTING TO KNOW MOVEMENT IN A BRAND NEW WAY

Catching on to Your Own Rhythm

At first glance, the NIA Technique may look intimidating if you're not a student of dance or the martial arts. Rest assured, it's simply because the choreography is unfamiliar and, like anything new, can appear more complicated than it really is. The NIA Technique isn't difficult. Honest. We've methodically broken down complex movements to accommodate Debbie's handicap. If she can do them, so can you.

We've seen exercise rookies begin to move like dancers after a few of our classes. It's just a matter of catching on to the rhyme and rhythm of the movements. Contrary to what you may think, rhythm is not the exclusive property of trained dancers. We all have a unique body rhythm, just as we all have a distinct voice tone and body mannerisms. We use that rhythm all day long as we walk, turn, reach, lower, lift. Strung together without stationary breaks, that rhythm can begin to look suspiciously like dance. Punch it up with a little music, a little umph behind the stroll, a little um-pa-pa behind the reach, and you're on your way to a cha-cha. There is dance lurking inside that body of yours. It just may take a little coaxing, a little luring to get it to play.

Let your own unique rhythm come out through the NIA Technique. Maybe you don't like to cha-cha.

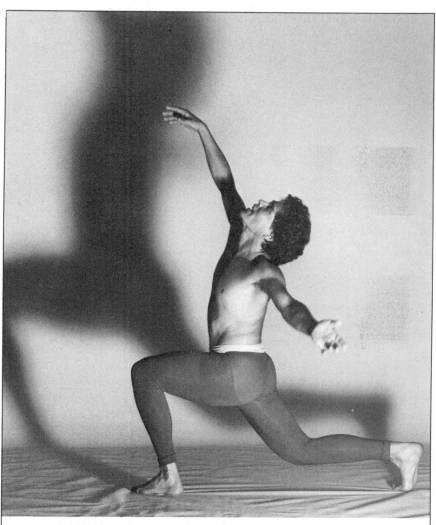

". . . nowhere on this planet can you find a people without music and dance . . .

"The truth of the matter is, the human animal was born a singer and dancer . . .

"At the root of all power and motion, at the burning center of existence itself, there is music and rhythm."

George Leonard, The Silent Pulse

Maybe you like to waltz, to jive. You can do the NIA Technique in whatever genre suits your mood, your style. Be jazzy, be lusciously lyrical, be snappy or sensually smooth, but most of all be passionately yourself. Don't stifle your rhythm, your beat, by trying to clone ours. This is your workout for your body and psyche, and it will look like you, not us. Since we're not inside your body, we can't tell you what that "look" should be; you alone know it, and the more you feel for it, the richer your workout will be. Your inner dance is a great fitness partner, helping to get you in shape faster, more playfully and safely.

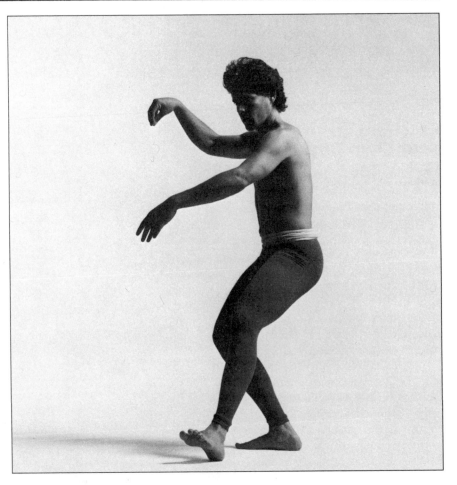

Maintaining Ground Contact

Taking the bump and grind out of aerobics can be like trying to break a wild horse. For jump-aerobics students, keeping the feet on the floor can be a real challenge. If you're new to aerobics, you have a definite edge in this regard. If you're accustomed to traditional aerobics, you may feel awkward without the propulsion of jumping. But don't give up. Once you're used to sinking and working with gravity, you'll feel the wonderful sensuality of moving fluidly, lyrically, and your body will thank you.

Sinking and Shifting vs. Jumping

Whenever you hop, jump, jog, or leap, your muscles stop working, albeit for a split second, but then down you come with an impact of three times your body weight. Watch one of those slow-motion movies of a runner's feet close up and you'll have a new appreciation for what that impact actually looks like. It's no small shakes to the ankles and feet, to say nothing of the shins, knees, hips, and lower back. Worse yet, running in place traumatizes the feet more than running forward because you don't utilize the natural forward propulsion.

Jump aerobics relies on jumping, jogging, and hopping to get the heart rate up into the aerobic zone for cardiovascular conditioning. More efficient and less injurious, however, is shifting the body weight slowly, deliberately, sinking and rising with controlled power and precision. It works more muscles more thoroughly, pumps your heart more efficiently and steadily, gently opens up flexibility through the joints, synthesizes mind/body effort for enhanced balance, and protects your lower extremities.

If you're worried that you won't be able to get your heart rate up into your aerobic zone from something so simple as sinking and shifting, you're about to be pleasantly surprised. Since the NIA Technique works so many more muscle groups, our students often have to gear down so they don't exceed their aerobic targets.

OEloel Braun is a third-generation dancer and teacher who grew up under the influence of her family's lifelong friend, Isadora Duncan, as well as other great dance pioneers like Martha Graham, José Limón, Charles Weidman, Doris Humphrey. Now in her sixties, OEleol has been studying with Debbie for two years and finds uncanny parallels between the NIA Technique and some of the more revolutionary dance methodologies that emerged during her lifetime.

"Isadora Duncan was the first dancer to rebel against the restrictions and artificiality of ballet. She discarded shoes and corsets and sought to develop the body within its own natural range of movement. She wanted to make it a strong, healthy instrument, free of distortion and thus not prone to injury. The NIA Technique is based on the same outlook and backed up with an excellent awareness and understanding of body mechanics.

"Ruth St. Denis also left ballet, and later three of her students left the Denis-Shawn Company to work out ideas of their own. Two were Doris Humphrey and Charles Weidman, who developed a technique based on 'breath-rhythm' and 'fall-recovery,' even analyzing walking as a series of tiny 'falls' and 'recoveries.' The NIA Technique reflects an awareness of these basic sources of movement and, at times, feels identical to a Humphrey-Weidman class.

"Martha Graham was the third St. Denis student to leave. Graham developed a technique based on 'contraction-release,' primarily of the torso. The NIA Technique uses contraction-release to find and use the natural aerobic center or core of movement, which is in the torso where one breathes. This is far more beneficial and effective than the separated arm and leg activity of conventional aerobics. In fact, it's the important secret of the NIA Technique. The response is much more direct, quicker, and safer than that achieved by jumping.

"José Limón took off from Humphrey-Weidman and developed 'isolations' as well as further refinements of 'fall-recovery' and 'breath-rhythm.' Again, the NIA Technique utilizes movements that recall a Limón class.

"The NIA Technique is not only beneficial for everyone, but an ideal therapy for dancers. By comparison, an average dance class is non-aerobic and tends to overuse some parts of the body while underusing others. The NIA Technique leaves the participant feeling 'massaged' all over. It has been making my sixty-year-old body feel over a decade younger, the most comfortable I can remember."

Systemic Movement

Did you know that you can—

- develop defined biceps without doing bicep curls?
- develop pectorals without doing conventional push-ups?
- tighten abdominals without doing sit-ups?
- create spine flexibility from breathing?
- define calf muscles by wiggling your toes and using your ankles?
- develop quadriceps by pushing your feet into the floor?
- create upper back strength by opening your chest?
- strengthen forearms by wiggling your fingers and using your hands?
- create neck flexibility by looking at your hands as you move?
- release tension in your lower back by letting your pelvis sway and circle?

The NIA Technique movements are designed as elegant whole-body motions, rich mixtures of comprehensive toning, strengthening, and stretching to work your body systemically as a complete unit instead of isolated parts, which means you get the very most out of what you put in. Generating movement from the undulating core of the body, we roll it down through the shoulders, picking up the elbows, rolling the wrists, wiggling the fingers. Staying loose and fluid through the spine, we ride the movement down through swishy hips, soft knees, flexible ankles, dexterous feet. The head gracefully joins in. The more of your body you use, the more you get in return. Using all of your body gives you a full-body massage, a full-body oxygen bath, a fully toned, symmetrically defined body.

By giving equal attention to opposing muscle groups, we achieve symmetry and balance, thus avoiding the kind of muscle imbalance that can lead to pulls and strains. Cross-training has become a popular way to create a well-rounded fitness program. That means varying your exercise to fill in benefit gaps in any one discipline. Weight lifting fills in strength, stretching class fills in flexibility, aerobics fills in cardiovascular conditioning and stamina, body-sculpting class fills in muscle definition, yoga fills in relaxation and balance. At its best, the NIA Technique is a self-contained cross-training program unto itself and gives you everything you need for a well-rounded fitness program.

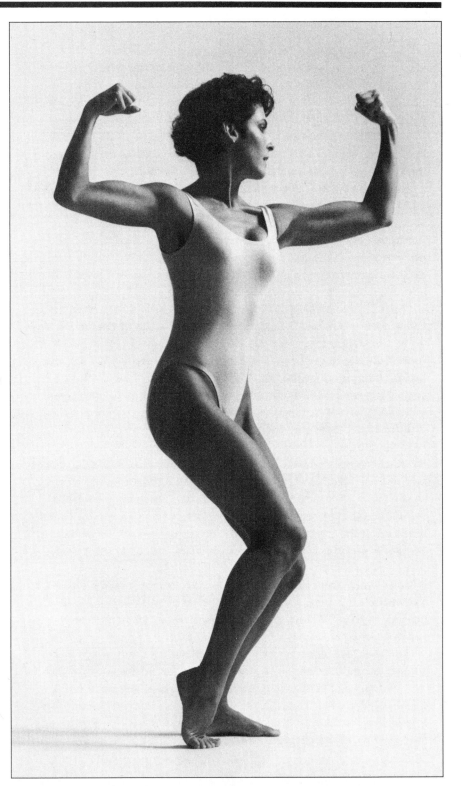

Ballistic Momentum vs. Deep Muscle Work

When momentum propels your movement, you lose the deep muscle work you could be getting by simply slowing down. To get an idea of what we mean, try this: Run around the room for a minute and then, for the same period of time, walk slowly, sinking deeply toward the floor with each step, rising up not quickly but as slowly as you lowered. Be aware of how your feet flex, how your toes stretch as you roll over the ball of your foot, how all the muscles along your calves and thigh contract and then stretch as your knees soften, as you press away from the floor, using the deep strength of your legs to carry the motion. That's using muscle instead of riding momentum.

Harnessing Self-Control

In the martial arts, the more self-control and inner awareness you achieve, the more power you gain. Throwing yourself haphazardly into movements is like throwing away gorgeous physical benefits and, worse, puts you at risk of injury. Instead of throwing yourself, place yourself with purpose and conscious will. For example, when you step out, feel for the stretch along the back of your leg, the extension through your heel, the flex of your ankle, the first delicious contact of flesh with the floor, the shifting of your weight and the strength of your supporting leg. Controlled and purposeful movement will make your workout more efficient and effective so that you get more for your effort.

Moving Fluidly and Fully

When you slow down, you have time to use more parts of your body more fully, to be fluid, lyrical, graceful—which means you'll tone more muscles for better overall definition, increase your flexibility, and demand more of your heart. For example, instead of swinging and pumping the arms in a jerky, *linear* manner, use a sweeping range of *circular* movements, leading at times with the elbow (to protect the shallow shoulder joint), the wrists, hands, even fingertips. It's surprising how, by simply wiggling your fingers, rolling your wrists, or changing the position of your arms so that the palm and back of your hand alternately face forward, you tone muscles of your forearm and upper arm that don't get worked if you simply swing your arms straight up and down. The art and subtleties of movement are quite extraordinary when you take the time to discover them.

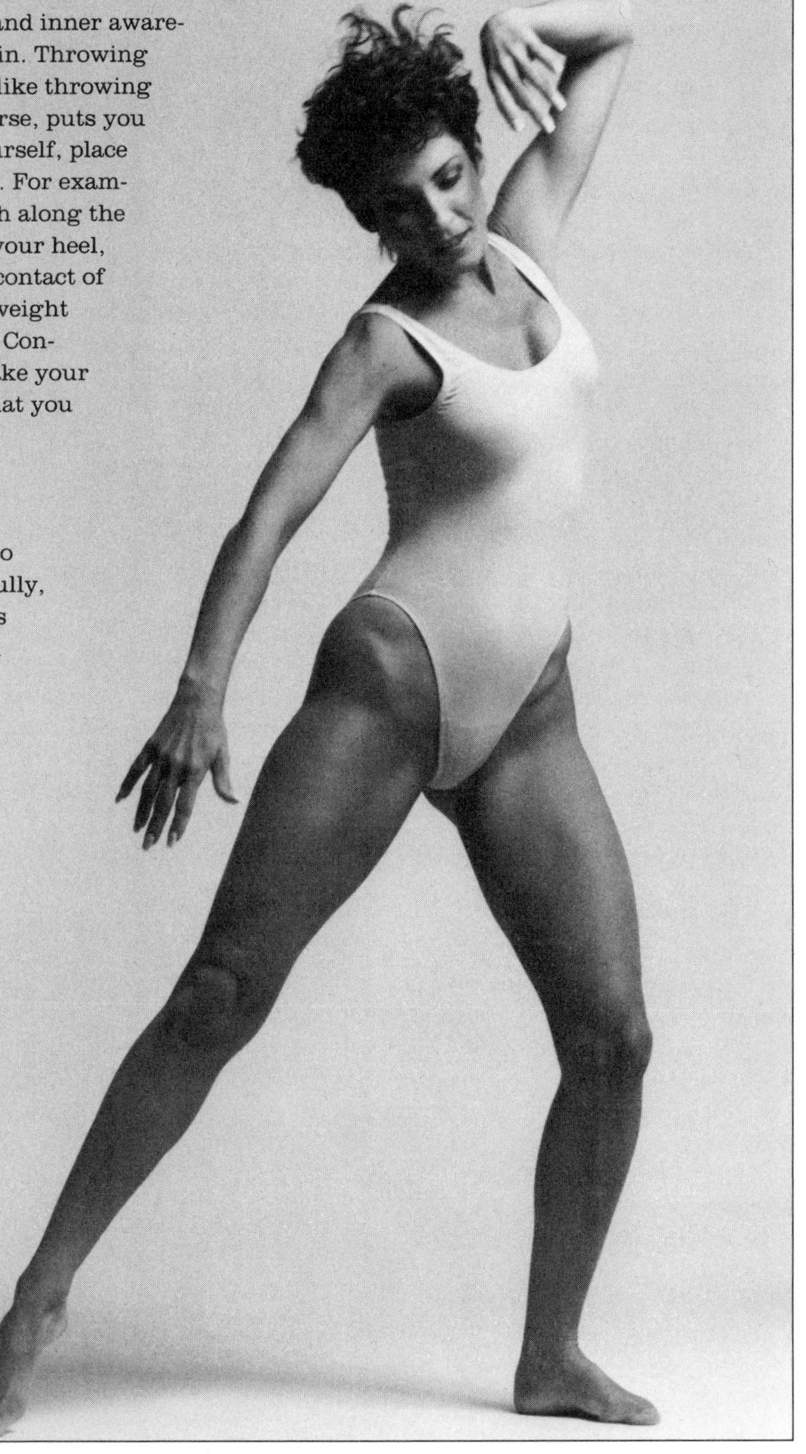

Moving with Imagination

As instructors, our most important job is to set an alluring stage upon which you can discover the joys of fitness. We can write the original script, but you must interpret it. We can give you stage directions for safety, theatrical cues, tips and guidelines, but *you* are the star. If you try to mimic us or any teacher, you'll miss out on your own show, your own movement dynamic, your inner rhythm. Like an actor or actress reading from cue cards, you'll be uninspired and stiff. Straining to duplicate us can make you nervous and tense, whereas making the movements your own will allow you to flow with ease and grace. Knowing that you've claimed center stage for your own wonderfully unique production of *Fitness* is our greatest reward.

Your imagination can help you create an award-winning show. Champion athletes use it all the time, visualizing their ultimate performance, running it through their heads over and over and over. You can cash in on this nifty neuromuscular programming by envisioning yourself as your favorite dancer or picturing how you ideally want to move. Let that mental image keep flowing through your head as you work out, and it will help your body catch on to what you've got in mind. And besides, the fantasy of it all can be a lot of fun.

Feeling and Emoting

For every feeling, there's a physical response, and for every physical response, there's a feeling. As you open up parts of your body, you may tap into feelings you've locked deep inside. Movement is wonderful therapy in this way. It can help you let go, release tensions that build up steely knots in your muscles, clear away the cobwebs of stored emotions that constrict your body—and get the adrenaline of joy circulating through your whole system.

At the same time, your feelings can enrich the *way* you move. That's why we use plenty of vivid imagery, movement dreaming. It can trigger a physical response much more fully than any technical description. Let yourself emote and move with feeling. Your movements will become fuller—and the fuller your movements, the more muscles you'll tone, the more flexibility and strength you'll gain, and the more conditioning your heart will get.

So, once you've intellectually grasped a movement, let yourself sink into the sensation and passion of it. You'll spark that rich right-brain creativity that takes the work out of your workout.

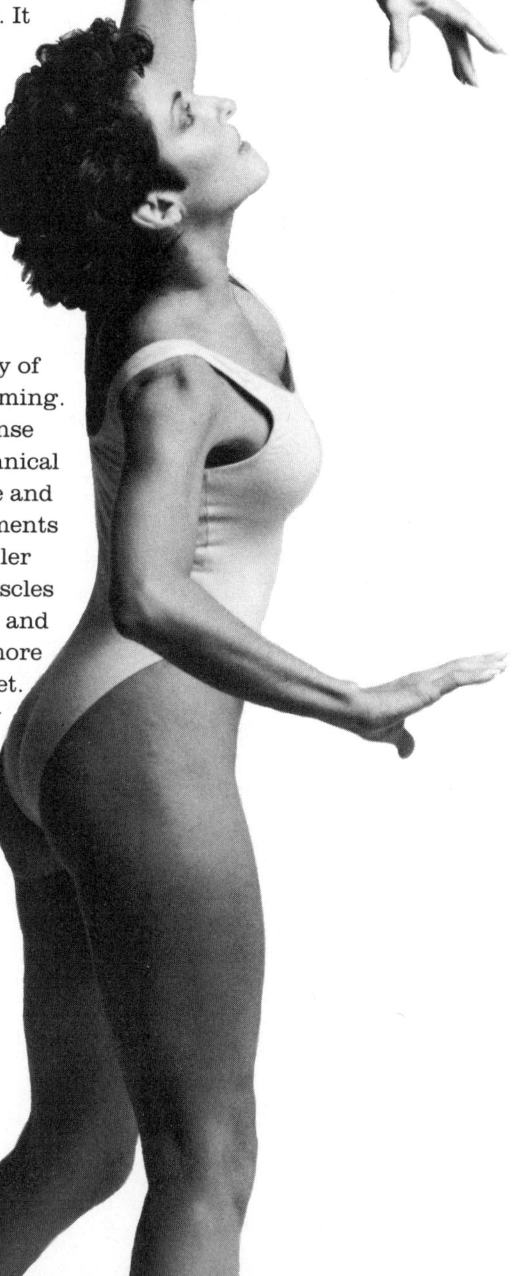

Honoring Your Body

We all start out with different physical parameters that define our range of motion, flexibility, and points of strength; different body types and shapes; different needs; different ways of speaking through our bodies; different movement philosophies. If you honor your parameters, they will fluctuate. If you work with your body type, respecting its limitations and appreciating its possibilities, you will change faster with less risk of hurting yourself. If you respect your own special needs and evocation of movement, they will help to guide you on a safe and sure path to where you ultimately want to be.

Goal Setting

Where is it that you ultimately want to be? Before you begin working out with us, take some time to consider what brings you here. What are your motivations, your goals? Are you trying to lose weight? If so, a little or a lot? Are you trying to get your buttocks and thighs in shape for that tropical vacation that's coming up all too soon? Or gear up for that winter ski vacation so that you're strong and limber enough to take five extra runs down the slopes? Are you working on upper body strength and quick reflex to give your tennis game an added edge? The more you know about why you're exercising, the more efficiently you'll work and the more motivated you'll be to stick with it on days when being prone on a couch looks more appealing than gearing up to work out.

Most of our students start out wanting to lose weight, to change the shape of their bodies, and are delightfully surprised to discover that the NIA Technique gives them so much more than just a particular look. For example, the NIA Technique increases spine flexibility for greater agility, which translates into very practical things like having more fun roughhousing with the kids, gardening, even making love. Every time you move with our technique, you put a little more life back into your body, making it stronger and more supple, fluid, graceful, balanced, lean. You'll have more energy, be able to do more, more comfortably, every single day. The NIA Technique will make you not only look better but feel better, glow from the inside out.

No Pain, More Gain

We want you to feel that glow throughout your whole workout, not just at the end and not just as you move through the day. Exercise is not meant to hurt. Contrary to what has been a fanatical fitness credo, harder is not better; moderation with consistency will get you much further. More and more fitness experts are urging a return to commonsense fitness as research unveils the greater benefits of moderation.

Don't try to be a fitness warrior. Too many people have been intimidated into a ridiculous attitude that if you don't hurt, if your muscles don't "burn," if you don't press up against the "wall," you won't accomplish anything. Well, it's just not true. A burning sensation in your muscles is caused by a buildup of lactic acid—a symptom of the breakdown of the normal chemical balance in your muscle fibers. For example, if you burn through pain in your quadriceps, your muscle tissue can break down and fatigue set in so that your body grabs onto whatever it can to support your movement, compensating with muscles that are meant to act as stabilizers and causing muscle pulls, cramps, and a breakdown in body alignment.

At any point during a workout, if something doesn't feel right, stop. Make an adjustment and keep adjusting until the movement does feel good. That may mean not sinking as deeply toward the floor, not reaching or twisting as far, not circling your arms as wide. We want you to enjoy non-impact aerobics. If you feel good, you'll be back for more, and the more you come back, the more fit you'll get. Motivation is hard to sustain if you're in pain. Enthusiasm is hard to conjure up if you're not having fun.

Working Within Your Comfort Zone

Working within your comfort zone means that you don't hurt, that your shoulders don't creep up around your ears, that you're not gasping for breath, that your muscles aren't screaming at you. A warm, low-level aching in your muscles, especially if you're new to exercise, may be okay if it doesn't last long.

Movement should be alive and loose, not stiff, not full of tension.

Working within your comfort zone, you'll feel steady and well balanced, in relaxed, not tense, control. At the point where you feel comfortable and strong, you work efficiently, effectively, and build up, rather than break down. If you push yourself past that point, you're flirting with injury, the kind that can put a permanent halt to your exercise or show up later as nagging problems. Driving yourself just doesn't pay off. For minimal additional physiological benefits, you run a greatly increased risk of hurting yourself.

The key to monitoring your workout so that you stay within your comfort zone is to be alert to and honor your body every moment of every single workout, to pay attention to what it's telling you. Just because you felt strong and worked hard yesterday doesn't mean that you should feel strong and work hard today. And vice versa. Every time you move, you're in a different body—literally. It even changes within the time frame of a workout as your muscles lengthen, your joints loosen, your blood vessels enlarge from the extra pump of blood that sends oxygen surging all throughout your body.

Little body cues are indicators of things that need adjusting—foot placement, step width, pelvic release, eye-hand contact, knee absorption—to keep you on the rich side of fitness. Are your knees beginning to fill with a low-level ache? Is your back feeling strained? Is your neck getting tighter and tighter? Is your spine rigid? Minor changes in posture and positioning can make all the difference in how you feel and what you achieve.

We'd love to be right there with you to show you the marvel of subtle shifts—how, for example, during sinking movements you can spare yourself knee pain just by keeping your calves perpendicular to the floor with your knees lined up with your second toes or by lifting your toes to rebalance your weight. We've used highlighted tips on the photographs in this book as the next best thing to being there; they alert you to give special attention to the placement and posture of your body at a particular point. Again, once you've grasped the technicalities visually, concentrate on the good feel, and as you grow more accustomed to the good feel, you'll move more instinctively in a safe, efficient, and comfortable way.

Fitness Phases

As you master a new level of fitness, you may feel a settling in, a velvety ease. As you stretch further, stepping off that plateau toward the next level, you may feel very unsettled, as though your stride has been broken. Passing through fitness phases is like climbing through the ranks of any endeavor, whether it be the challenge of becoming a low-ranked *A* tennis player after being a top-ranked *B* player or learning a new musical score after mastering an easier one. Be especially kind to yourself as you broach new levels. If you respect the ongoing change and acclimation within your body, it will, in return, honor your desire and be a steady, trustworthy partner on your fitness journey.

You Know Best

You are your own best guide on that journey, because you alone know what sits well with your particular body. Trust your body, your instincts and intuitions. If you have wide hips or long limbs, widen your stance to create a sound base; if your back is weak, keep your leg lifts low and cushion them by sinking into your supporting leg. If you're new to exercise, make your movements small and close in to your body. If you've just painted your kitchen and your upper body is sore, let your arm work be floppy and loose. If you've spent the day on all fours in your garden, do more pelvic circles to release the tension in your back. In other words, adapt your workout to you, right now. Exercise, like life, should not be static, but flow and ebb as you flow and ebb.

The human machine doesn't take well to unreasonable demands but is wonderfully adaptable if you treat it right. That means taking the time to build strength, endurance, flexibility, balance. A fast-food mentality about fitness is not unlike a starve-and-splurge dieting syndrome that can be more damaging emotionally and physically than doing nothing. Fitness is for the long haul, for a lifetime. Give yourself the immense gratification of developing it with patience, consistency, and joy. Be good to yourself, to that magnificently intricate enterprise called your body.

3/STARTING OUT RIGHT

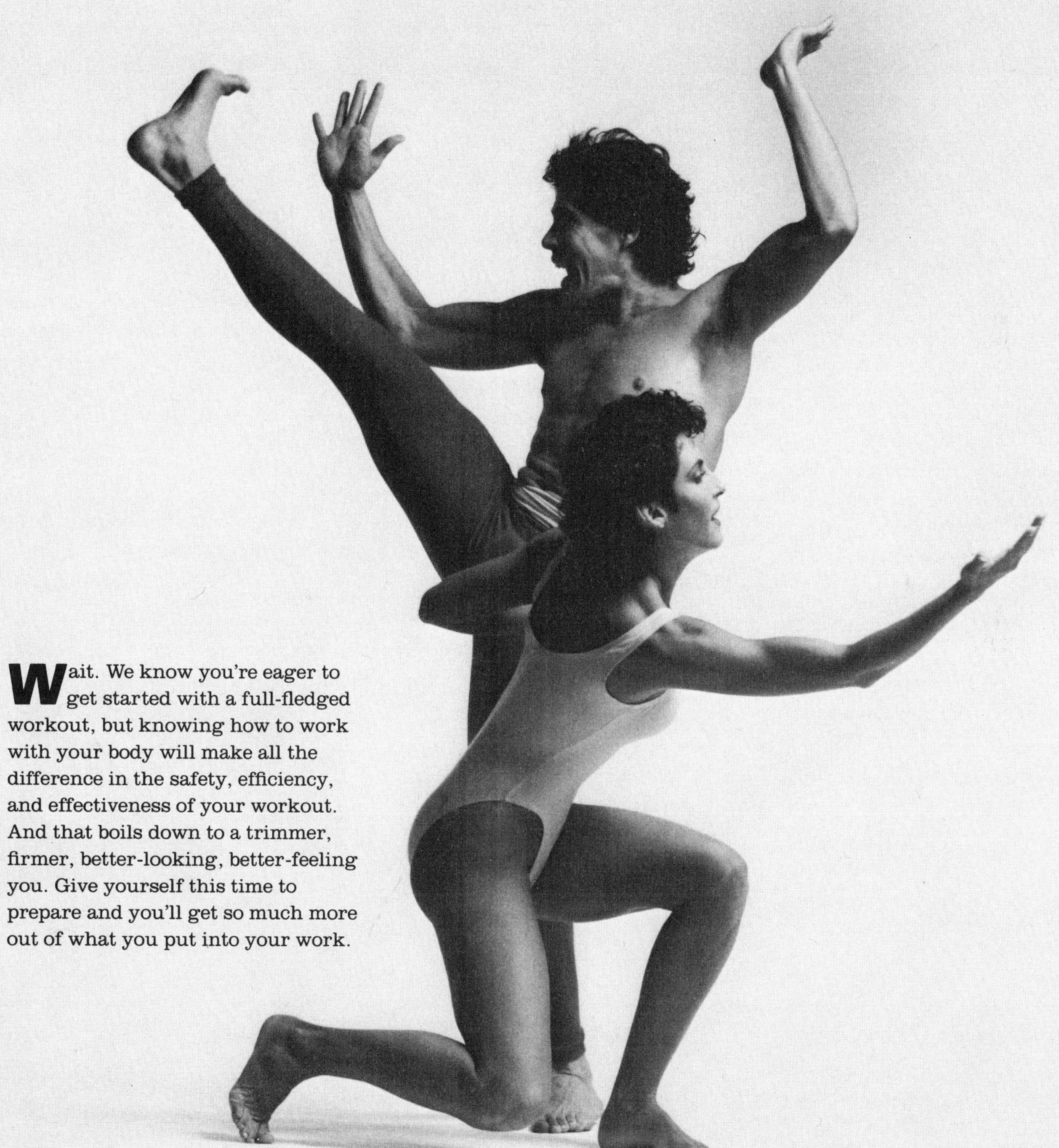

Wait. We know you're eager to get started with a full-fledged workout, but knowing how to work with your body will make all the difference in the safety, efficiency, and effectiveness of your workout. And that boils down to a trimmer, firmer, better-looking, better-feeling you. Give yourself this time to prepare and you'll get so much more out of what you put into your work.

BODY WEIGHTS

The NIA Technique's three main body weights are the head, the chest, and the pelvis. For now, keep them aligned as you work so that your head is well balanced over your chest, your chest is centered over your pelvis, and your pelvis is evenly balanced over your feet. The alignment will prevent strain on your neck, shoulders, and lower back. Check periodically to be sure that your head and chest aren't jutting forward, that your buttocks aren't thrust back. Imagine opposing pulls through your head and pelvis: one drawing you gently upward toward the ceiling through the crown of your head, the other gently drawing your tailbone straight down toward the floor. Keep those pulls gentle so your neck is fully relaxed and your pelvis isn't overly tucked. The pull through your tailbone will stretch and protect your lower back and work wonders for a firmer, sleeker torso.

Imagine a cushion of air at your waist that allows you to lift your chest up off your pelvis and another at your neck that allows you to lift your head up off your shoulders so that your spine can lengthen and breathe. Those cushions act as shock absorbers to keep you beautifully loose and aligned. As you train your body to work in this way, you'll find that you move through the rest of your day with more grace and energy, walking tall and sleek.

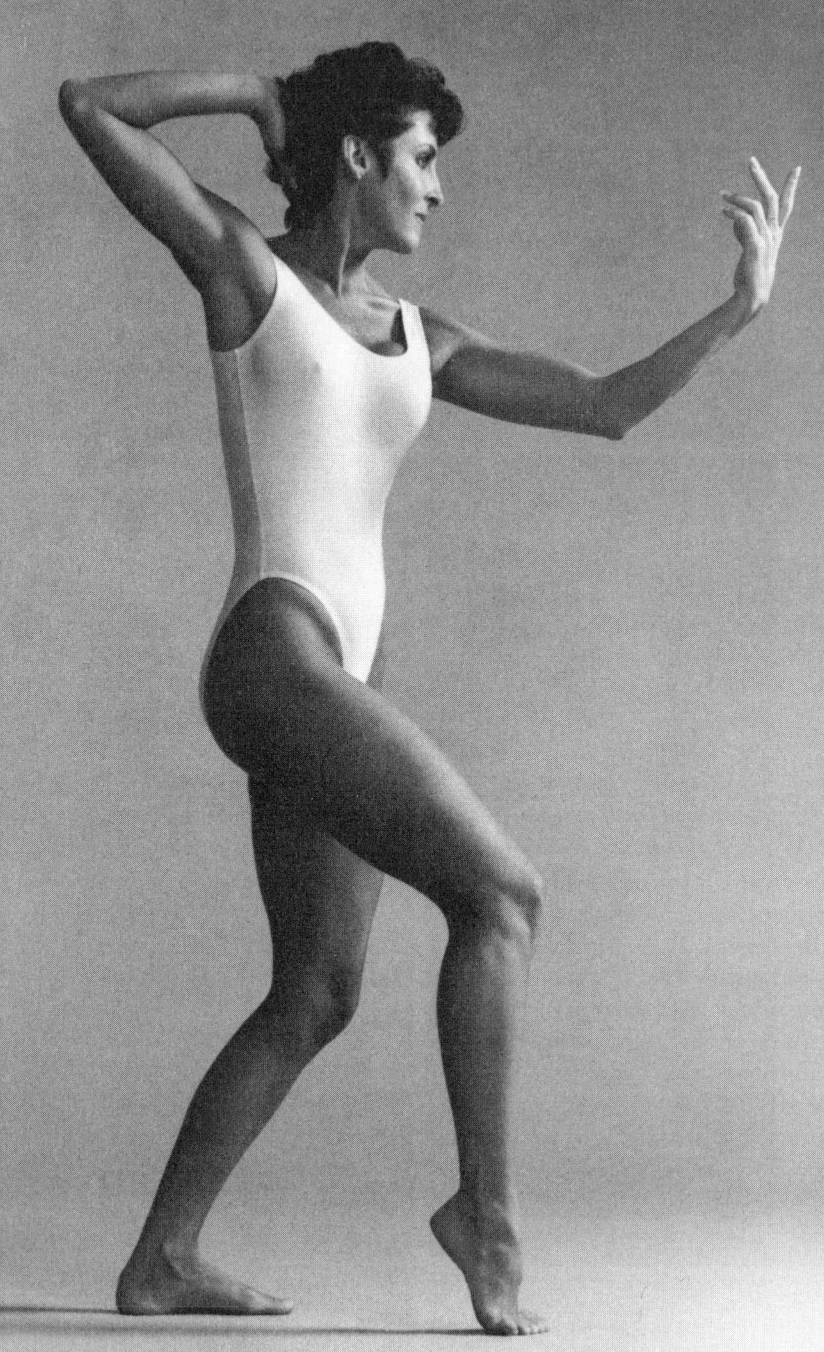

BALANCE

Balance equates with stability, and that equates with safety. Your balance begins with your feet. Feet don't lie. They let you know immediately if something is amiss with your carriage (see Foot Stances, page 40).

Press middle finger down

If you begin to feel wobbly while you're working out, don't worry. You can regain your balance in a number of ways. First, check to see if your head has eased forward, your chest pushed out, your buttocks thrust back—and then readjust. Focus on the floating alignment of your body weights, feeling the pull of your tailbone down toward the floor, your chest directly above your pelvis, the pull upward through the crown of your head.

Opposing motions are wonderful moderators of balance. When you sink, feel a pulling upward through the crown of your head. When you rise, feel a pressing down through your feet. When you rotate, imagine your torso as two overlaying cylinders so that, as the outer cylinder rotates right, the inner cylinder rotates left—as if one cylinder is inside another. Work opposing arms and legs together, letting them sway with the natural rhythm of your body as they do when you walk (right arm and left leg forward for counterbalance). Opposing motions not only help to keep you balanced but work your body systemically for overall toning and conditioning.

Your range of motion makes all the difference in balance and efficiency. If you sweep your arms too wide or step out too far, you'll throw off your balance and end up chasing the motion instead of getting the most out of it. Control the spacing of your movements to fit your pace. When you work slowly, you have time to make your motions wide and broad; when you pick up speed, pull your movements in closer to your body.

BALANCE = STABILITY =
EFFICIENCY = SAFETY

Did you know that you can recover your balance with a finger? By pressing down with your middle finger, you stabilize your upper body and balance your right and left sides.

BREATH

When you work out, you may become so intent on the movements that you forget to breathe. Shallow breathing will all too soon leave you feeling tense and exhausted, and tension and exhaustion put you at risk for injury. Think oxygen. Besides getting gorgeous on the outside, you want to give your insides an invigorating oxygen bath.

Be constantly aware of your breathing, feeling the internal ebb and flow. Keep it steady and natural, following the rhythm of your body in motion, inhaling through your nose and exhaling through your mouth. The slower you move, the deeper you can breathe, and the deeper you breathe, the more you increase your lung capacity and spine flexibility. If you concentrate on a rich, full exhalation, your body will take care of the filling on its own. The only forced breath we use is the karate "Yeet!" which is an explosive, from-the-gut exhalation that protects your lower back from strain and tightens your abs.

Think relaxation. Every now and then, remind yourself to relax so you open up your flow of oxygen to all parts of your body. Check to see that—

- your neck hasn't tensed up
- your shoulders haven't crept up around your ears
- your body weights are soft and aligned
- your joints are loose and fluid
- you're using only the amount of effort necessary for the motions

As you become more efficient and proficient, you'll feel more and more relaxed as you work out.

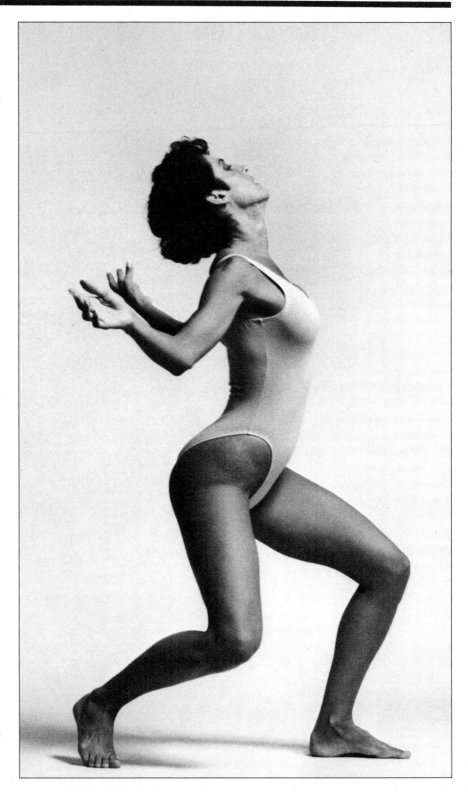

For exercise to be aerobic, it must be performed at your training heart rate. That rate varies with each individual.

HOW TO TAKE YOUR PULSE RATE

1. Place the tips of your first and second fingers on the carotid artery, on the front strip of muscle running vertically down your neck or on the radial artery, on the inside of your wrist just below your wrist bone. You may need to squiggle around a bit until you feel the good steady pulsing of your heart.
2. To find your pulse rate, count the beats of your heart for 10 seconds and then multiply by 6.
3. If you're just beginning exercise, take your pulse rate every 5 or 10 minutes. If it's high, be sure to slow down. If it's low, slightly increase the intensity of your work, using the tailoring tools in Workout I (page 67).

To determine your training heart rate, the American College of Sports Medicine recommends the following formula:

Training Heart Rate

220 minus your age equals your maximum heart rate. Subtract your resting heart rate* from your maximum heart rate and you have your heart rate reserve. Now, multiply your heart rate reserve by 0.7 and that equals 70% of your maximum heart rate. Add your resting heart rate to come up with your training heart rate.

220	
− 30	your age
190	your maximum heart rate
− 60	your resting heart rate
130	your heart rate reserve
× 0.7	
91	(70% of your maximum heart rate)
+ 60	
151	your training heart rate

Carotid Artery

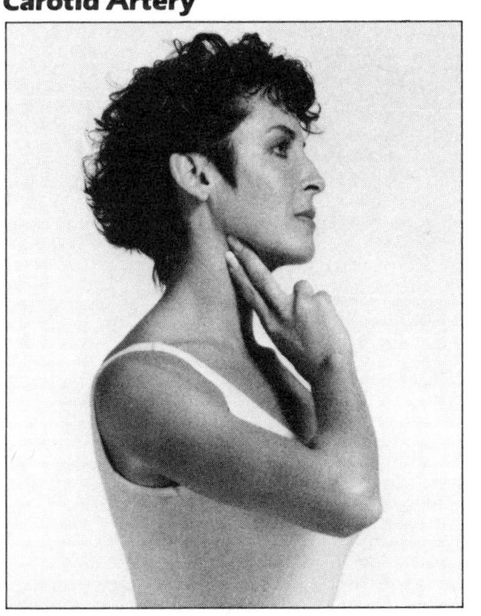

Radial Artery

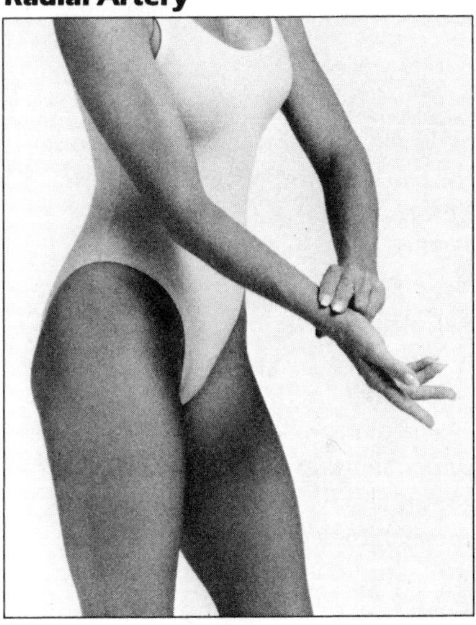

THE FID FACTORS—FREQUENCY, INTENSITY, DURATION

For aerobic exercise to provide good cardiovascular conditioning, the FID factors must be met.

Frequency For maximum effect, you should exercise at least three times a week. Unlike jump aerobics, which should be done only on alternating days to give the body recovery time from ballistic pounding, the NIA Technique can be done every day as long as you don't do consecutive days of "load" workouts. If you do non-impact aerobics every day, we strongly recommend that you vary the intensity of each workout. In this way you'll more accurately and efficiently meet the needs of your body.

Intensity Your exercise should be intense enough to raise your heart rate to within your aerobic target zone.

Duration You should work within your aerobic target zone for at least twelve continuous minutes.

Increasing any of the FID factors means your body must adapt to new demands, so be very gentle and gradual. This is a point of vulnerability, and you must help your body ease into the change. If you make a dramatic change in any of the FID factors, you're setting yourself up for injury.

*To determine your resting heart rate, count your pulse rate for 15 seconds before getting out of bed in the morning and multiply by 4. Ideally, you should do this for a week and average out your daily pulse rates. By determining your resting heart rate every six months, you can monitor your progress.

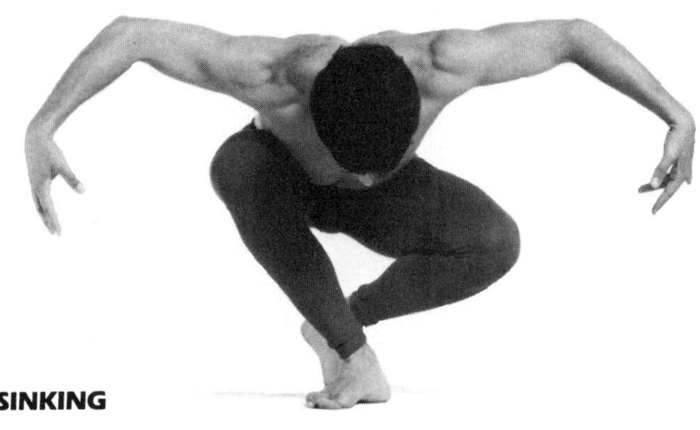

SINKING

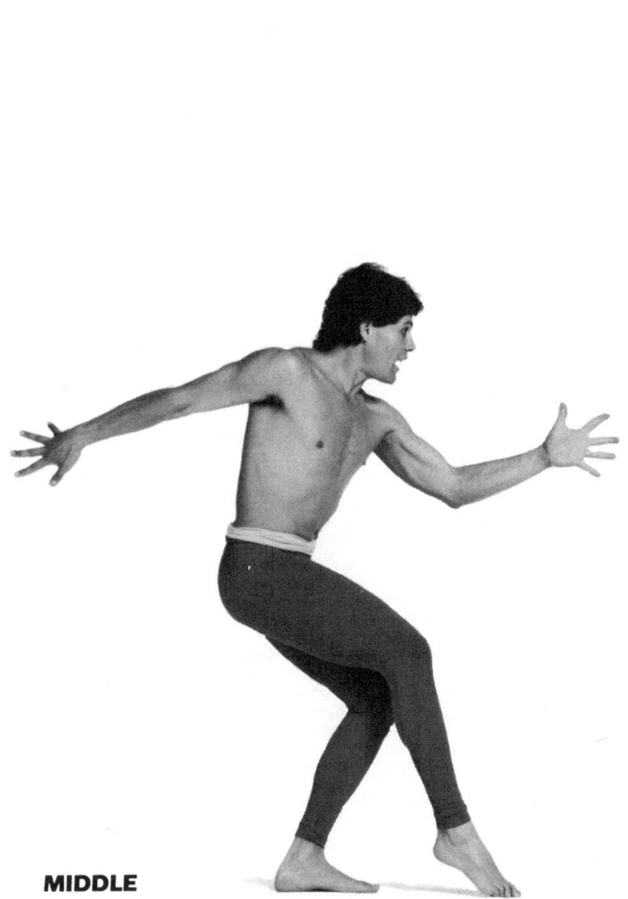

MIDDLE

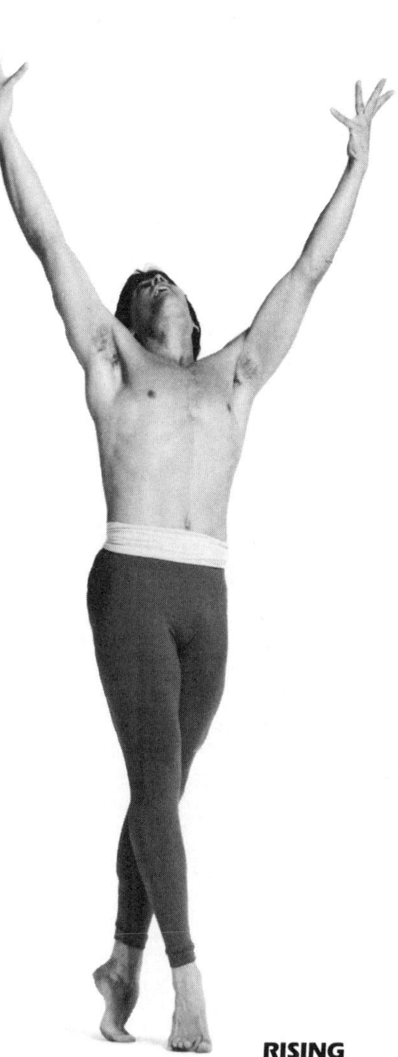

RISING

We work on three different planes of movement for more comprehensive toning, flexibility, and aerobic conditioning. By constantly moving through the three planes of movement, you'll ebb and flow with work/recharge, contraction/release, and avoid building up tension in any single muscle group. Many low-impact aerobics classes overuse the middle plane by holding and working too extensively in a slightly crouched position. Don't do it. Your body needs the recharge of extensions following contractions for the building of healthy, sleek, and comfortable muscles.

The three planes of movement in the NIA Technique are:

- Sinking
- Middle
- Rising

The depth of your plane work depends upon your strength, flexibility, balance, and endurance. The more planes you work on, the more muscles you engage and the harder your heart must pump.

TO LIGHTEN OR LOAD YOUR WORKOUT

- If you're new to exercise, be sure to sink and rise just slightly and give yourself plenty of time to gradually increase your range of motion.
- If you're moderately fit, work on all three planes, but be lenient with your sinking so you don't overextend yourself.
- If you're highly fit, increase the intensity of your workout by lowering deeply and rising high onto the balls of your feet, staying alert to the parameters of your comfort zone. Don't try to be a hero by sinking two inches off the floor. That's incredibly difficult if you're doing it properly with control and precision, and if you're not ready, your body will get back at you in a flash.

The sinking movements ask a lot of your heart, so take it easy. You can readily exceed your aerobic target zone by working too deeply.

Bulk vs. Lean

To avoid building bulky muscles, be sure to give your muscles a full extension for every contraction. For long, lean muscles, you need to use a full range of motion. The NIA Technique is designed to give equal time to opposing muscle groups and to each side of your body, which dramatically increases flexibility and leanness and keeps your body relaxed and ready for the movements that roll one upon the other.

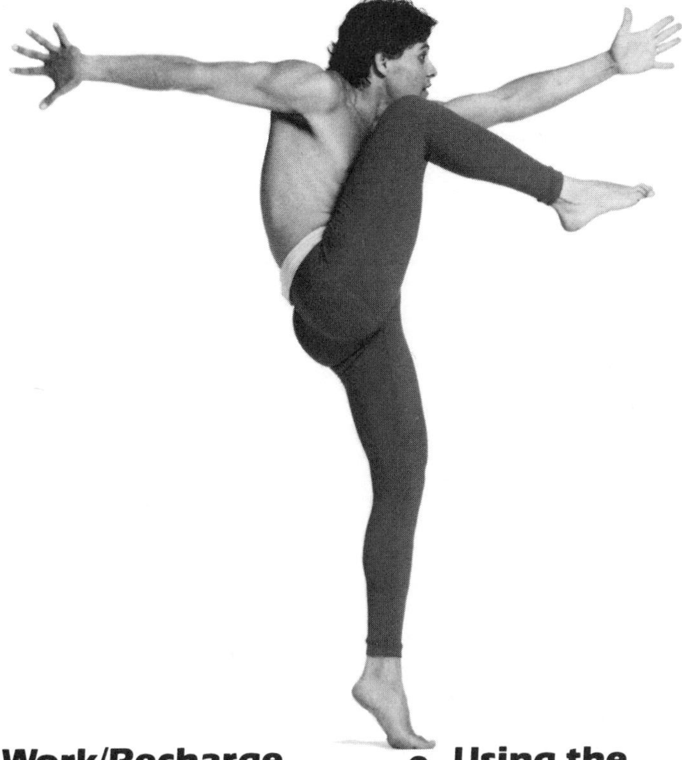

Work/Recharge

Movements of the NIA Technique are designed with work and recharge modes which alleviate tension buildup that can wear you down, leave you aching from overused muscles, or worse, put you at risk for injury. The basis of this work/recharge concept is your breath. Your inhalation is your recharge. Your exhalation is your work. Draw in your energy as you inhale and recharge your motion, filling not only your lungs but your whole body with new energy. If you bypass a full recharge, you'll tire more quickly and miss out on a good symmetrical toning of your body. Then use a whole-body exhalation to put power into your work motion. The more efficiently you utilize the exhalation, the greater paybacks you'll get.

Using the Photographs

Match your body to each movement, starting with your feet and building up piece by piece to your head. Notice that we are your mirror image. Note the direction of your toes, the placement of your feet, the relationship of your knees to your ankles, your hips to your knees, your torso to your hips, your head to your torso. Then work out from your shoulders to your elbows, wrists, hands, and fingers. As you pile the stance up from your base, think in terms of angles and directions. The circles indicate weight distribution as follows:

○ = No body weight
● = Full body weight
◔ = 30% body weight
◕ = 70% body weight

THE CLOCK

The clock is a road map for your feet. Motions in the NIA Technique are directed to numbers on this clock, with you at home base in the center 12:00 directly in front. You rise or sink, tap or step out, pivot on, point, or reach to a specific hour. The simplicity and familiarity of this image will put your mind at ease so that your movements become more spontaneous, fluid, relaxed.

The size of your clock will change as you become stronger and more flexible, able to reach for greater circumferences. Start small and take your time pushing it out little by little.

Take a minute to try out your clock. Imagine yourself standing at home base in the center, 12:00 directly in front of you, 6:00 directly behind you. Then simply touch your right foot to 12:00, 1:00, 2:00, and 3:00. As you continue on to 4:00, 5:00, and 6:00, touch with the ball of your foot. Then touch left to 12:00, 11:00, 10:00, and 9:00 and shift to the ball of your foot as you continue on to 8:00, 7:00, and 6:00.

Your clock movements are done sinking, stepping out, or rising with a variety of tap outs, reach outs, pivots, and points that create rich diversity—all in the name of:

COMPREHENSIVE TONING

ELASTIC FLEXIBILITY

INCREASED STRENGTH AND STAMINA

WELL-MONITORED AEROBIC LOAD

ENHANCED COORDINATION

AN ALERT MIND

FUN

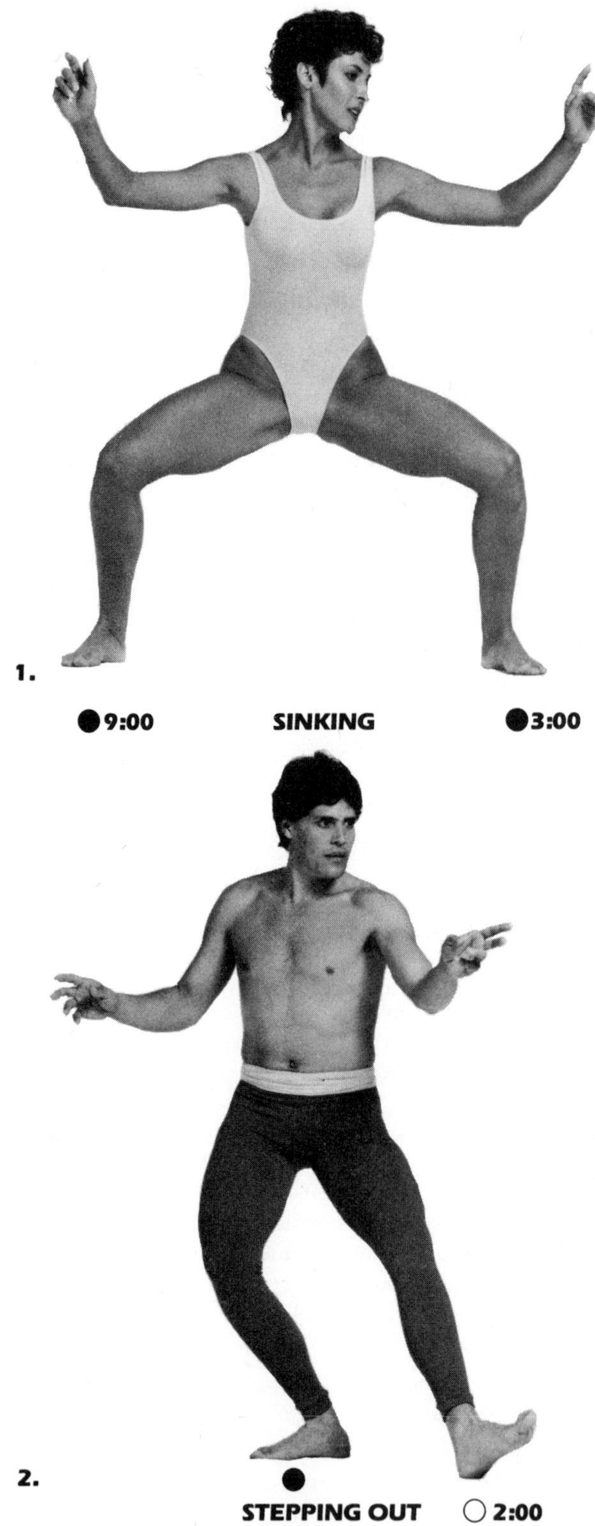

1. ● 9:00 SINKING ● 3:00

2. ● STEPPING OUT ○ 2:00

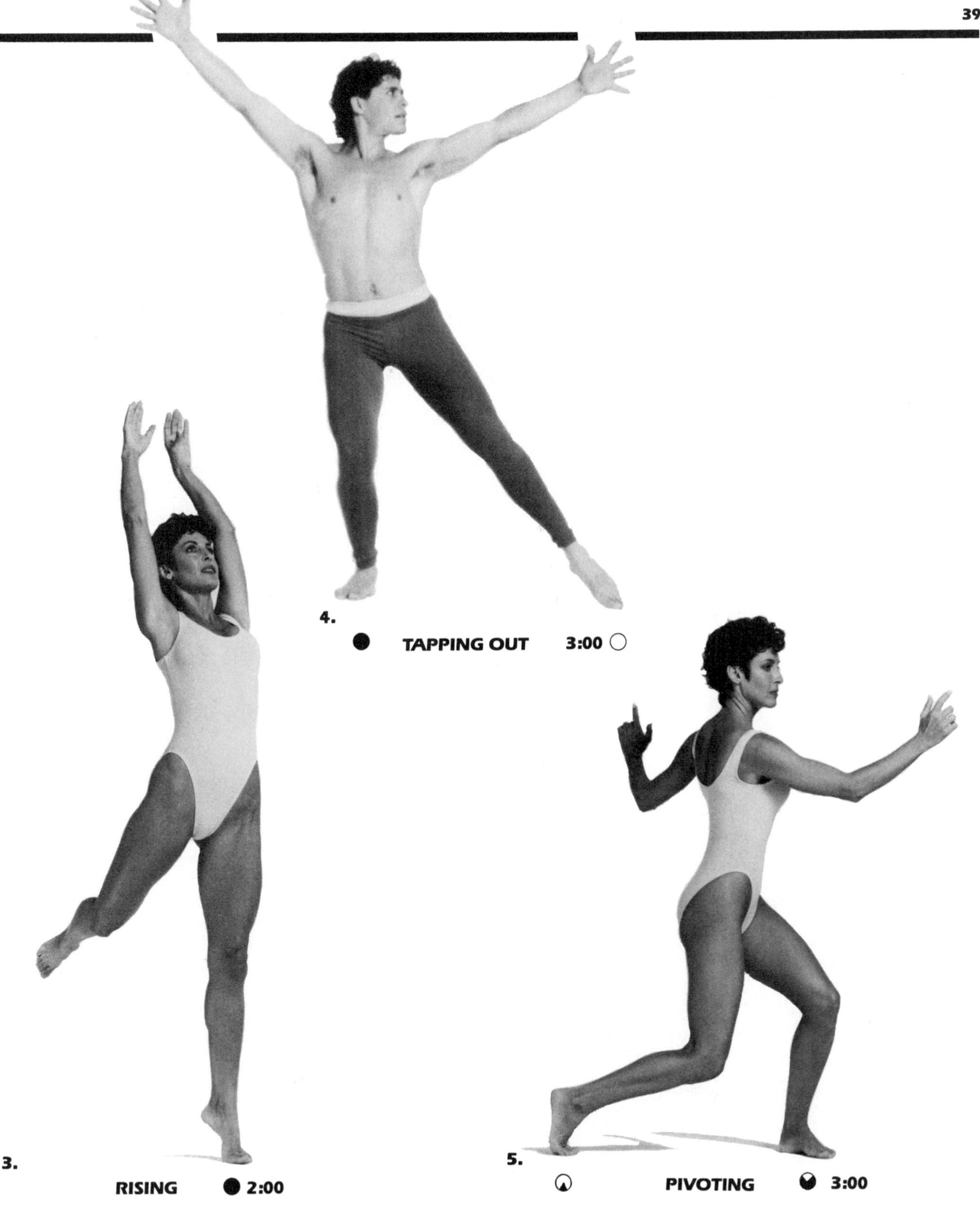

4.
● TAPPING OUT 3:00 ○

3.
RISING ● 2:00

5.
◔ PIVOTING ◕ 3:00

The NIA Technique's Answer to Stability

Feet are often the most neglected, taken-for-granted part of our bodies, in spite of the fact that we rely on them for nearly everything we do.

Think of it:

- How often, if ever, do you work out for your feet, to condition and strengthen them?
- How often do you even think of your feet?
- Do you ever consciously use your feet?
- Do you like your feet?

The better you get to know your feet, the more effective and safe your workout will be. With a solid base beneath you, you can let loose and move more fully.

Without shoes, you'll strengthen your feet and ankles, increase your circulation, flexibility, and dexterity, decrease foot cramping, get rid of callouses, perhaps even heighten your arches. In the beginning, you may develop blisters, but take it as a gentle cue from your body that you may be sliding instead of purposefully placing your feet.

If you're a long-time aerobics student, you may hesitate to take off your shoes. You may have paid fifty hard-earned bucks for them, and besides, anyone who's been around the aerobic block knows that you never, ever, ever work out unprotected. Remember, though, that NIA movements themselves are your protection. Unless you have structural foot problems, your bare feet will be a boon to your workout, sending you signals that help support and balance your movement.

Through non-impact aerobics, we've gained a great respect for the mechanics and functions of the feet and an appreciation of the possibilities they allow. Simply turning them either in or out dramatically changes the toning and stretching of the calf, thigh, buttocks, and hips.

Think of it:

- Your foot is a masterful network of 35 joints and 26 bones held together by 120 ligaments and activated by at least 20 muscles.
- Over 7,000 nerve endings in each foot constantly send messages throughout your body.
- Today you will take some 18,000 steps. By age 70 your feet will have logged 70,000 miles.

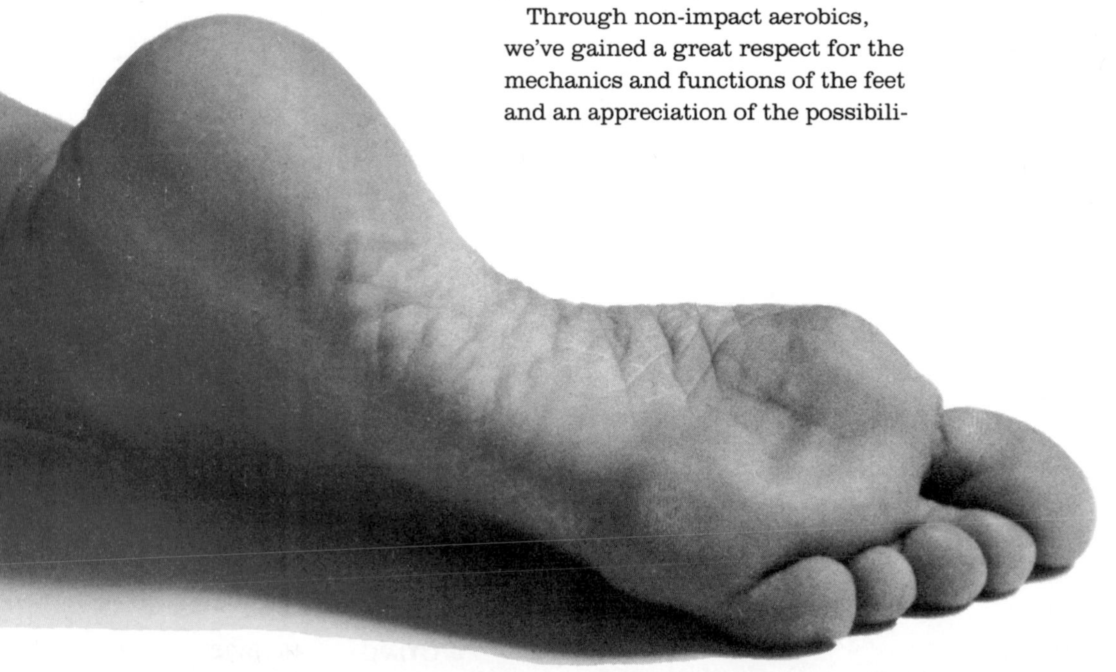

WHY WE DON'T WEAR SHOES

Your feet are platforms upon which to spread the stresses of standing and moving. To be steady and reliable, they must be pliable, strong, resilient. Shoes box them in, constrict their circulation and hinder the mobility of their joints, the full strengthening of their muscles. Working barefooted gives your feet a chance to breathe, to stretch and become more flexible, to flex and become stronger, to touch and be touched. That, in turn, affects everything else you're able to do.

Feet never lie. They're wonderfully forthright and will let you know instantly if something is wrong. The direct contact of flesh with the floor allows your feet to give you a spontaneous, accurate readout on the efficiency and safety of the way you're moving. The moment you feel tension in your feet, you can be sure something is amiss with your carriage. By paying attention to your foot cues given by the proprioceptors, you'll know when to correct your alignment and positioning. Listen particularly to cues that you're pressing too much weight on the inside or outside edges or front of your feet. By keeping your weight evenly spread across the entire surface of your feet, you'll protect your ankles and knees and free up your toes to do their best job of monitoring the safe distribution of your weight.

In a nut, working barefooted will—

- monitor your alignment and positioning
- increase your flexibility and dexterity
- strengthen your feet and ankles
- increase your circulation
- decrease cramping

When you move, think light, feeling a magnetic force drawing you up, all the way from your feet through your legs and torso, lengthening your spine and lifting the crown of your head toward the ceiling. Be light and easy on your feet. A jump-aerobics class can sound like a herd of stampeding elephants. Awareness of the feet is given over to "proper" footwear and stops with the lacing of shoes. But, the jogging and jumping still send three times your body weight crunching down through your shins to your feet and can break down your musculoskeletal system.

We're constantly aware of the feet and how they subtly, elegantly carry our movement. We purposefully place them instead of throwing weight on them. No padding or special sprung floors are necessary because we knead and massage the feet instead of pounding them. No lateral support from shoes is needed because we don't throw weight onto the outside edges of the feet and never rotate on a weight-bearing foot.

If you're wearing shoes, take them off. You're going to become intimate with those wonderfully complex and sensitive carriers. The better you get to know them, the steadier and safer your workout will be.

"The NIA Technique has less impact on the feet and leg joints than ordinary walking because both feet are more in contact with the floor. Because I learned and did most of my teaching on a concrete slab floor, my feet received meticulous training. Instead of height, we stressed and practiced very well-articulated landings using the proper sequence of toes, balls, heels, ankles, and knees to cushion our weight as we came down. Foot coordination and strengthening exercises were done sitting as well as standing. The NIA Technique is physically very sensitive, articulate, and all inclusive and would not be the same without its foundation of meticulously prepared bare feet."

—OEloel Braun
Third-generation dancer and teacher

What Runners Have Learned About Shoes and Pronation

In the December 1984 issue of *Runner's World,* writer David Prokop brings to light a little-known myth about shoes and overpronation, which can strain ligaments, tendons, or the entire leg, causing knee, foot, and ankle injuries, shinsplints, and Achilles tendinitis. "We tend to think of shoes as a supportive, protective aid to runners," writes Prokop, "but did you know that the amount of pronation is always greater when you've got running shoes on than it is when you run barefoot?

" 'It's true: People pronate less when they're running barefoot,' says Tom Clarke, Ph.D., director of research and development for Nike. 'This has been proven by a number of researchers.'

"Clarke explains that when you're running barefoot, the heel is very well shaped to minimize pronation. It's narrow, and has a fat pad that's round, soft and moves over to the inside, adapting as the foot pronates. By comparison, when you're wearing a shoe, the lever arm, as biomechanists would call it, underneath the heel is increased, since the heel of the shoe is invariably wider than the heel of your foot. The longer lever under the heel will tend to snap the foot into a more pronated position. Also, when you're wearing shoes, your heel is in an elevated position, resting atop the cushioning. This softer material—the midsole—offers a lot more room for deflection than the fat pad underneath your heel. In other words, you can sink down much more into the midsole material on the medial (inner) border of the shoe than you can into the fat pad under your heel. The fact that you can deform a shoe midsole much more as your foot rolls inward, while the longer lever under the heel serves to whip your feet into a more pronated position, explains why we pronate more in a shoe no matter how much rear-foot control it provides."

Prokop goes on to quote Barry Bates, Ph.D., head of the University of Oregon's biomechanics laboratory, who conducted a study of rear-foot control and discovered that "a good shock-absorbing shoe" could promote injury among people with rear-foot control problems. Bates explained it this way: "When you're standing on a piece of sponge rubber, obviously it's a much different feeling than standing on a hardwood floor. Your foot can kind of roll around in the spongy rubber, whereas it's much more inclined to stay firmly planted or fixed on the harder material. So by putting the foot on softer material, which is what we do when we put on a well-cushioned shoe, we decrease its stability. When the foot starts to roll or move to the inside in the action of pronation, the soft material allows the inside of the shoe basically to collapse, and it doesn't provide support underneath the inside of the foot. So the foot rolls over farther than it would on a firmer surface."

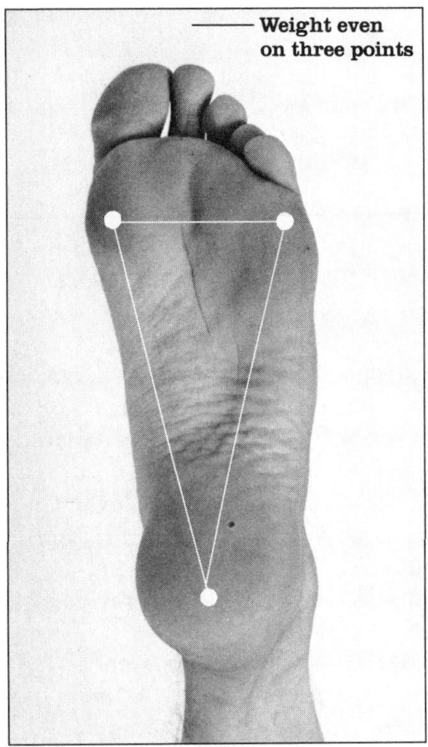

Standing comfortably, lift up your toes and feel for the balance within each foot, your weight equally distributed on three points that form a triangle: your heel and the inside and outside edges of the ball of your foot.

Sole

Your feet provide a secure base of balance if you use them well. Don't play favorites with the inside or outside edges. Distribute your weight equally, evenly across the entire surface of your sole so that your whole foot gets a chance to play.

Tip: Take a look at the soles of your shoes to see what part of your foot you favor. If the edge is worn down on either side, you're pronating (rolling in) or supinating (rolling out). The imbalance can cause strain and risky muscle compensation that can lead to injury. If you tend to roll in, concentrate on pressing through the outside edges of your feet until you feel your whole foot—and vice versa. Pressing down through the weaker side will help to strengthen and correct the muscle imbalance.

During the sinking movements, you might thrust your weight into the front of your foot, pressing your knee past your arch, which puts much too much strain on your knees. To get your weight back where it belongs, lift your toes (not the balls of your feet) and dig your heels into the floor. Throughout, imagine that you have roots growing out of the soles of your feet and reaching deep into the earth.

Heel

When you step forward or laterally, point your foot in the direction you're going and lead with your heel, stretching your calf, strengthening the muscles around your shins, and protecting the thin metatarsal bones in your foot. From the heel, roll through to the flat of your foot, feeling for every cell of every inch of your sole.

Ball

When you step back, always move with soft knees onto the ball of your foot, keeping your heel high. Never step back with locked knees onto the flat of your foot. When you step forward or sideways to rise up onto the ball of your foot, remember to roll first from your heel clear through the whole surface of your sole and then rise up. For now, never step smack on the ball of your foot unless you step back.

Think *balance, equilibrium.* Keep your weight equally distributed. Even when you lead through your heel to roll onto the flat of your foot, even when you rise or sink on the ball of your foot, keep your weight spread across the entire surface of the part that makes contact with the floor. Don't let your feet roll in or out.

Foot Alert

If you have any foot abnormalities, you may need the support of a shoe. To be sure, check with your doctor. Keep in mind, however, that foot pain doesn't necessarily indicate a structural problem, but often is the result of lack of conditioning of the foot and leg muscles. Foot abnormalities often announce themselves through pain felt in the knees, hips, or back.

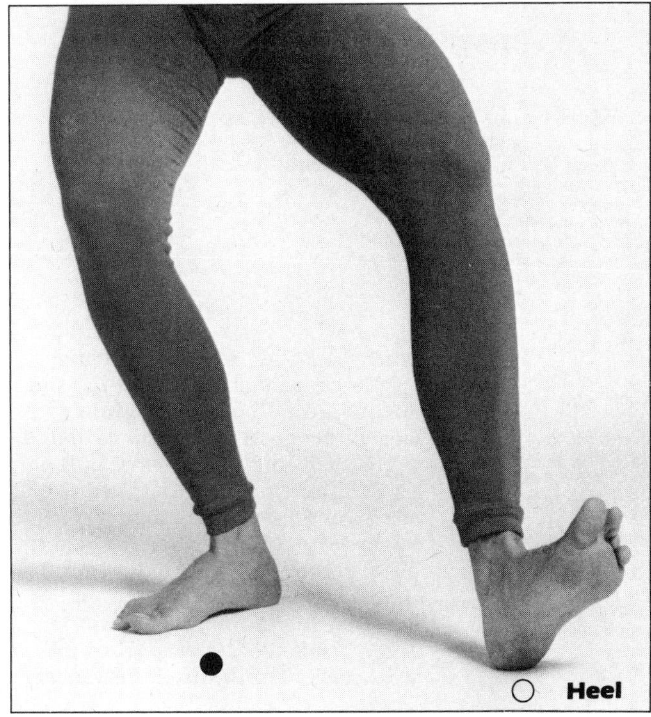

Heel

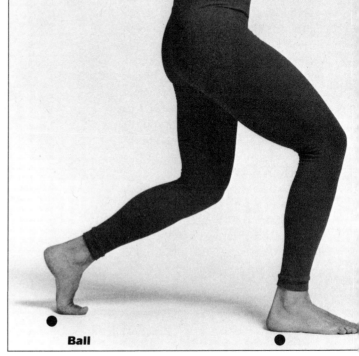

Ball

The NIA Technique's Answer to Beautiful, Strong Legs

Your legs are beautiful pillars of strength that can support a more comfortable and relaxed spine. The following leg stances provide a secure base for sinking, rising, shifting, lifting, and traveling, which take the place of jumping and jogging. The stances give you more toning, trimming, and firming benefits than tedious floor work.

The closed, riding, and one-legged stances require a great deal of strength, flexibility, balance, and stamina and should be used primarily for advanced workouts. The hip and *A* stances are a good place to begin. Always feel for your comfort parameters and allow yourself plenty of time to gradually increase the challenge of your stance, the depth of your sinking, the height of your rising, the extension of your reaches, and the range of rotations.

Since the NIA Technique is based on the full, efficient use of your leg muscles, mobility through your hip socket is very important. If you're constricted in your hips, you'll tend to compensate with your lower back. To avoid undue strain, focus on the spacing of your movements and the alignment of your body weights. Don't worry if you can lower only an inch instead of a foot.

Imagine lighting a fire in your hips and melting the ice around your joints so that you gradually begin to move with greater mobility, fluidity, and ease. Take it easy and you'll feel results soon enough.

Closed Stance

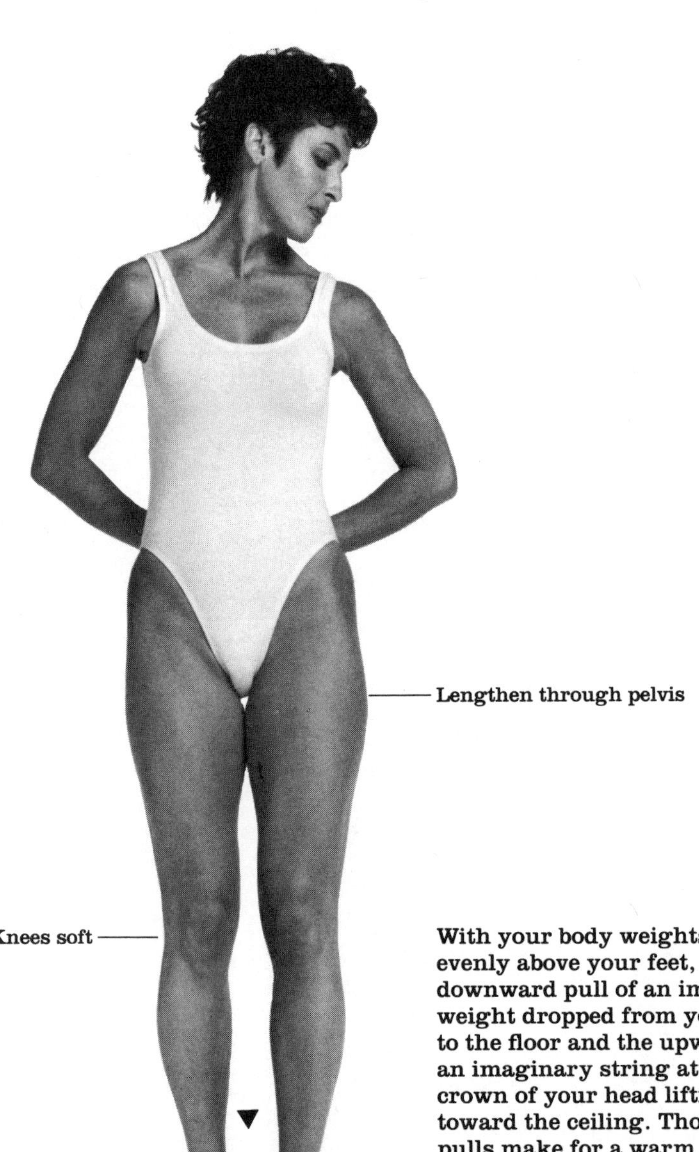

With your body weights floating evenly above your feet, feel the downward pull of an imaginary weight dropped from your tailbone to the floor and the upward pull of an imaginary string attached to the crown of your head lifting you tall toward the ceiling. Those opposing pulls make for a warm stretch through your lower back, a gentle lengthening through your spine, and a relaxed extension through your neck. Think lifted. Feel loose, fluid.

Hip Stance

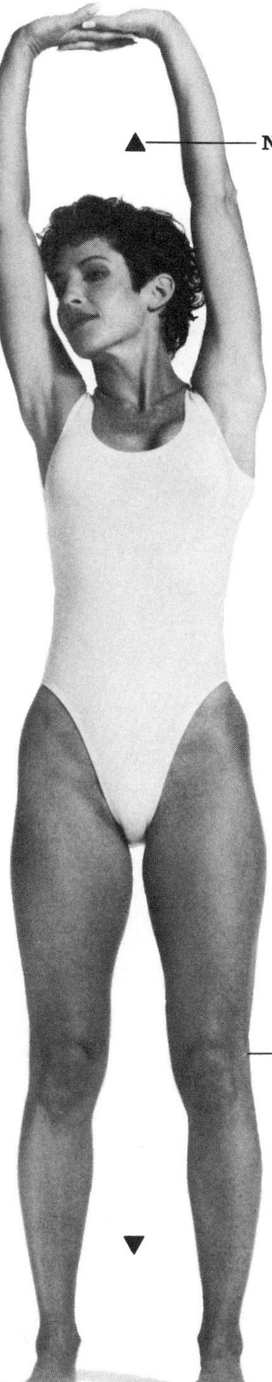

NIAligned

Knees soft

Feet parallel below hips

"A" Stance

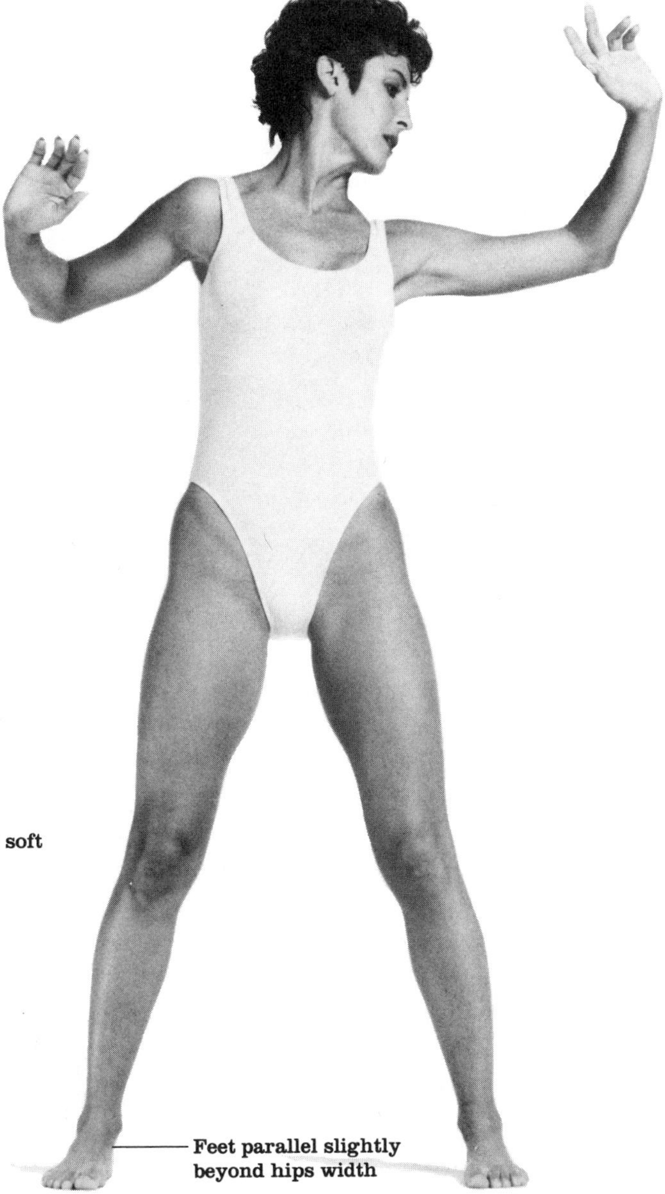

Feet parallel slightly beyond hips width

Riding Stance

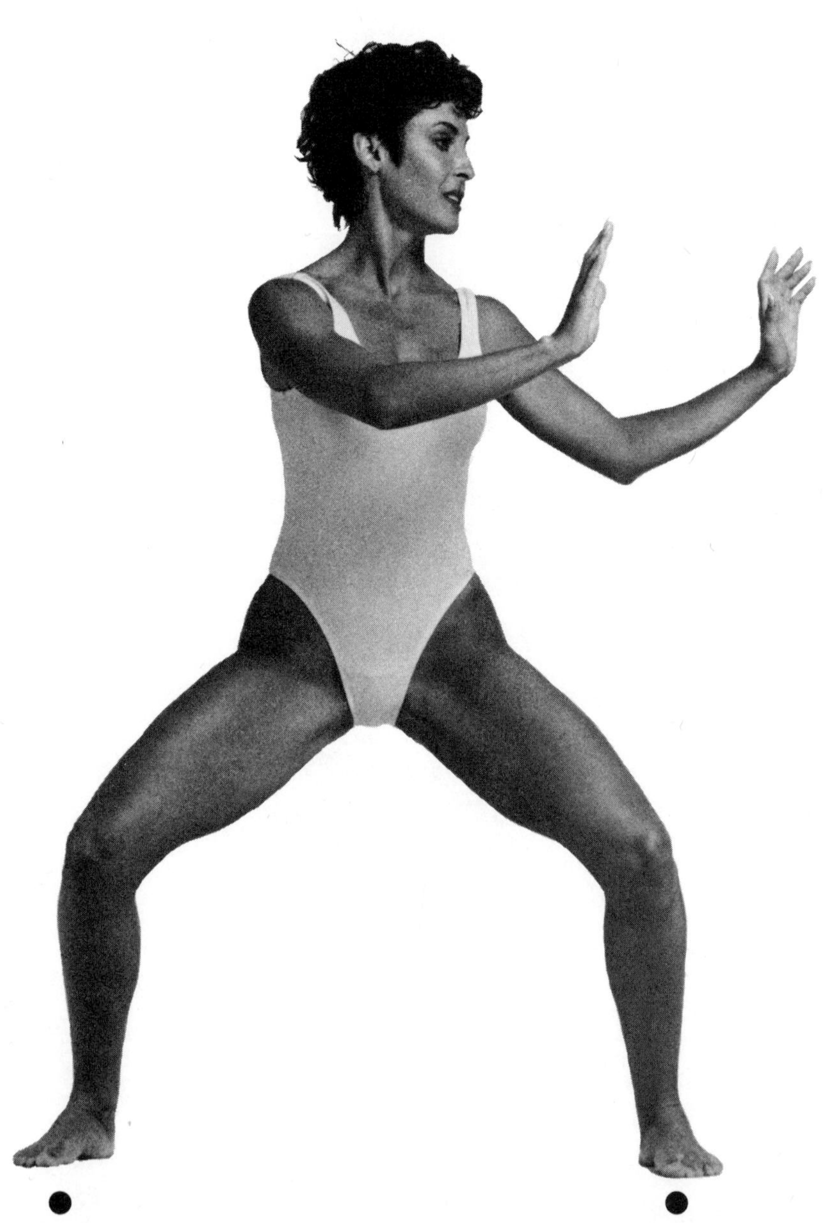

We call this our sumo wrestler pose. How far you extend the pose will depend upon the flexibility in your hips, inner thighs, and lower back. Keep it comfortable, with your buttocks relaxed. Your legs are far apart, as though you're riding a very fat horse; your horse will get fatter the more flexible you become. Your feet are parallel, not turned out. Lift your toes to make sure your weight is evenly distributed.

By moving through center in a riding stance, instead of a hip or *A* stance, you'll increase your aerobic load and push out the circumference of your clock.

ONE-LEGGED STANCES

One-legged stances are both challenging and graceful—challenging because of the balance and upward alignment required, graceful because of the elegant variety of poses. Always be on the whole foot that supports you and lengthen upward from your foot to the crown of your head. Keep your hips balanced over your supporting leg, not collapsed to one side.

To increase your balance when you work on one leg, *breathe* into and focus on the leg that supports you and be sure—

- your weight is evenly distributed in your foot,
- your supporting knee is bent comfortably.

Never swing a straight leg forward. The momentum of the thrust can force your leg past the point of your established flexibility and strain your lower back. Instead, draw your knee up first and then extend out, either pointing your toes or pressing through your heel.

TO LIGHTEN, touch below your knee; **TO LOAD,** touch above your knee.

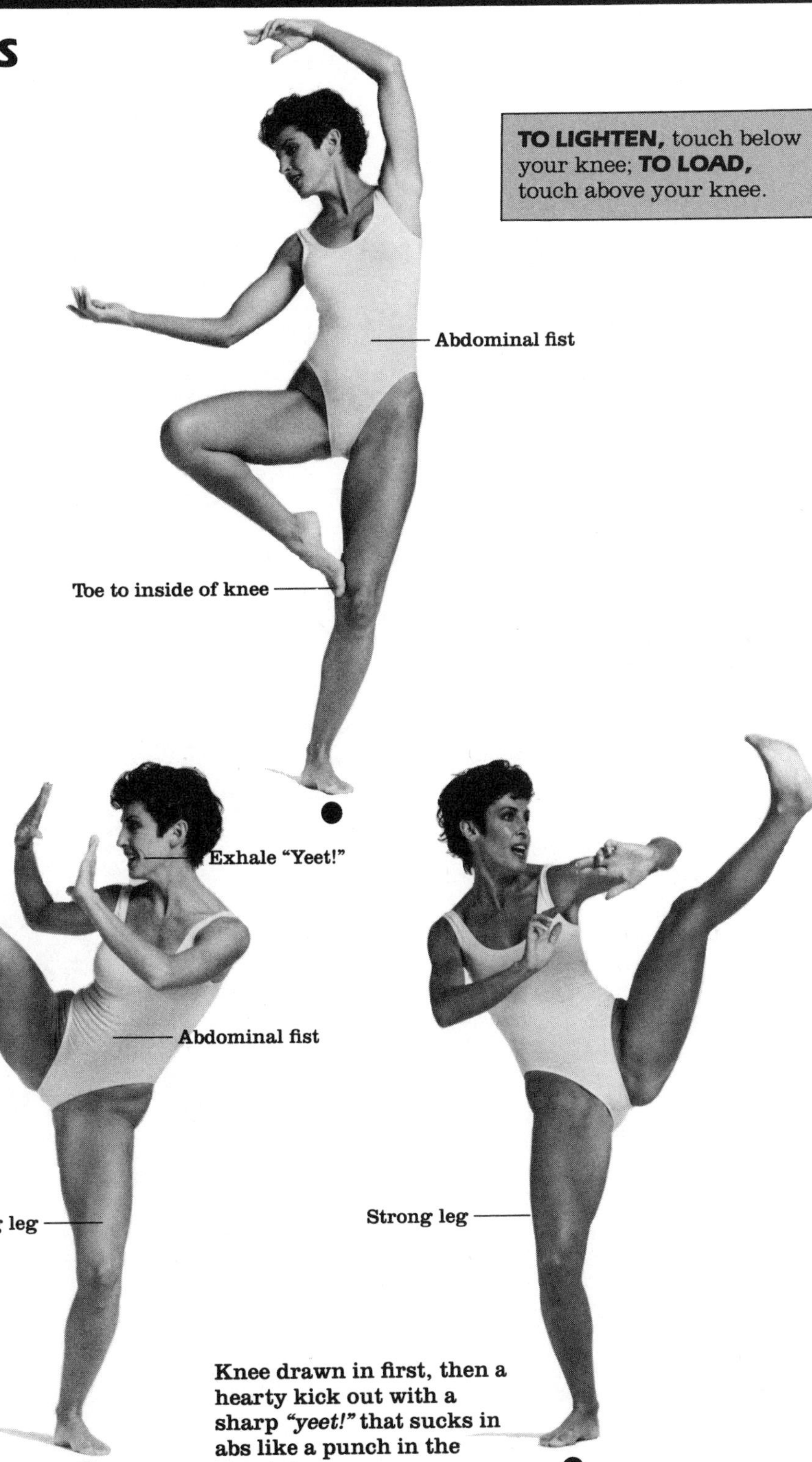
Abdominal fist
Toe to inside of knee
Exhale "Yeet!"
Abdominal fist
Knee into chest.
Strong leg
Strong leg
Knee drawn in first, then a hearty kick out with a sharp "yeet!" that sucks in abs like a punch in the stomach.

HOW TO USE YOUR KNEES

The knee is the largest joint in your body and the most exposed joint below your waist. Unlike the elbow, it must bear the body's weight. Unlike the hip joint, it's not protected by thick thigh muscles and pelvic bones. Unlike your ankle joint, it's not close to the ground with stabilizing support from the foot.

We ask a lot of our knees, marvelous, multi-purpose hinges that they are. Their wonderfully complex mobility and capacity to swivel, turn, twist, and bend are the very things that make them so susceptible to stress and injury. In spite of the fact that the knee is protected by a cap, stabilized by four ligaments, and supported by thirteen muscles, it remains, in fact, quite vulnerable. Where the hip is a ball-and-socket arrangement, the knee is just two huge bones gliding back and forth against each other.

The NIA Technique movements are designed to protect your knees, but *you* have to monitor your alignment and positioning, heeding the messages your bare feet give you. If you feel tension in the front or along the inside and outside edges of your feet, chances are your knees are out of alignment and taking too much strain. Here's how to adjust:

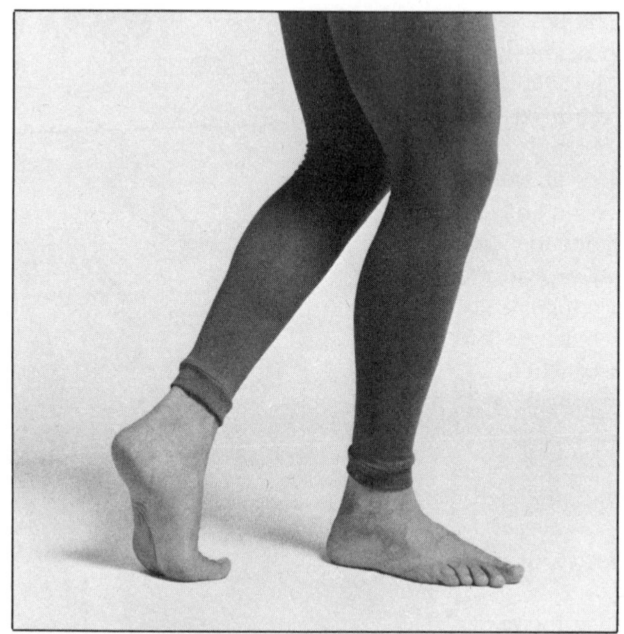

Your knees are always soft, slightly flexed, never locked.

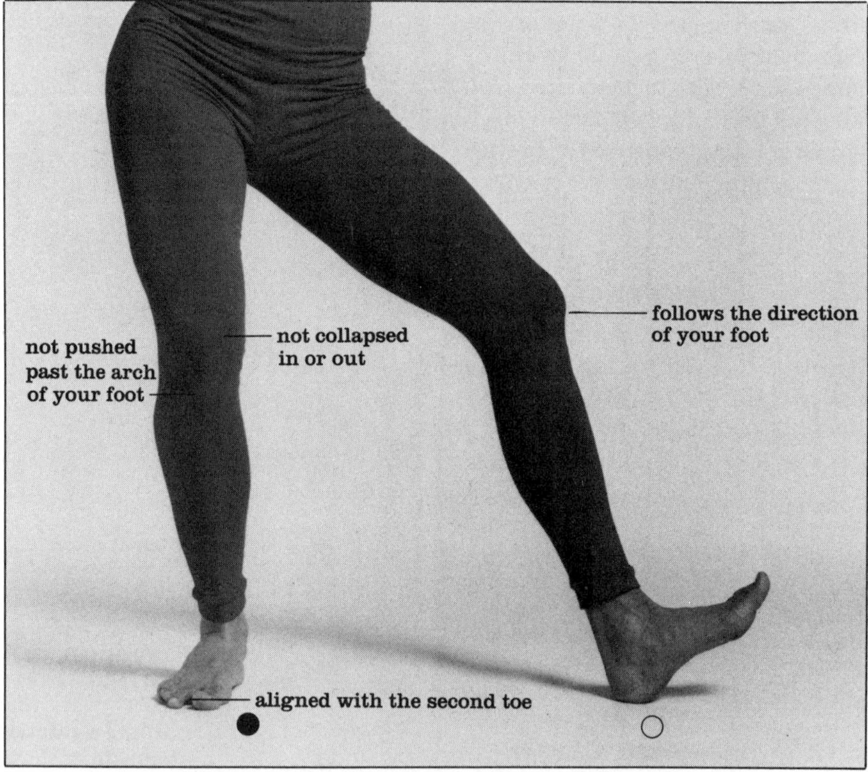

AN OUNCE OF PREVENTION . . .

Overuse, twisting, and poor alignment can wreak havoc on your knees. Here's how to avoid:

Overuse Don't sink too deeply, too soon, especially if you haven't been using and strengthening the muscles around your knees. Keep your lowering motions slight until your knees have a chance to adapt to the strength and flexibility necessary to accommodate your weight safely.

Twisting Don't twist your knee. Turn your hip, knee and foot in the same direction. Put your hands on your hips and, as you rotate your torso, consciously take your hips with you. A sure sign that you're overtwisting your knee is your feet wanting to roll in or out. For the moment, you're safer letting your feet turn in the direction they want to turn in order to release the pressure.

Rotating When you rotate your leg, first empty it of weight, bring your heel up so you're on the ball of your foot, and then rotate your whole leg from within the hip socket. Place your hands on your hips to be sure they remain still and squared front.

Poor alignment The most common misuse of the knee is the forward thrust while lowering. To avoid doing this, lower your buttocks back away from your knees—just as you would if you were lowering into a chair. Notice how your hip flexes instead of your waist, how your knees barely ease forward. The counterbalance of your chest leaning forward is slight. Since you're not hyperflexing by sticking your buttocks way out, your chest likewise doesn't have to hyperextend forward for counterbalance. Lift your toes to check for proper alignment.

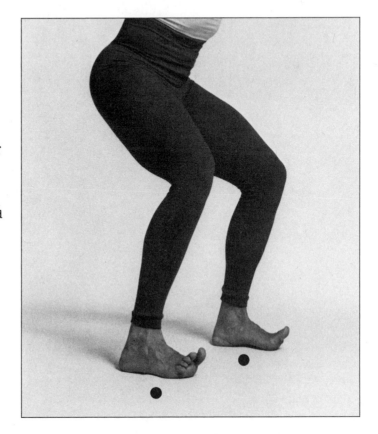

The Loose Connection

Every time you move your pelvis, you tone your stomach and firm your buttocks and legs. Working with a loose pelvis will also elongate your lower back so you don't tense, hold, or overuse those muscles. Freeing your pelvis frees your spine.

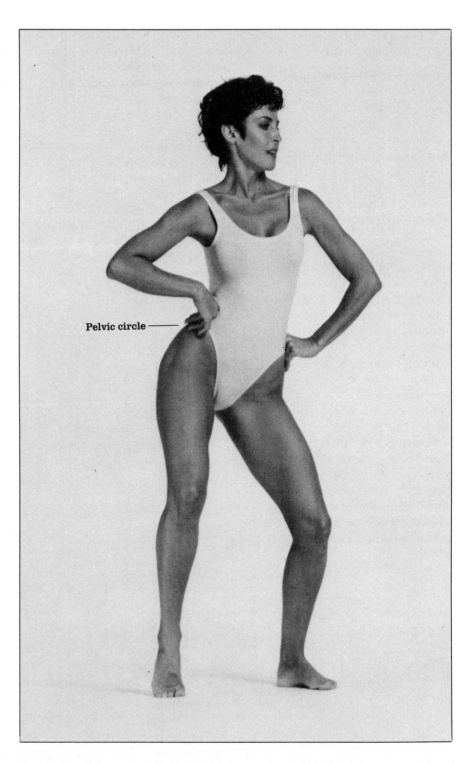

Imagine stirring a pot of soup with your hips.

The NIA Technique's Kinetic Ab and Back Work

Your torso is the core of your body, the weight between your head and pelvis. Most of us tend to tilt forward or backward, so pay special attention to keeping your torso well aligned and mobile for safety and more efficient abdominal toning. Eventually, good alignment will become a habit.

YOUR ABDOMINALS

For sleek, firm abdominals, focus on using them throughout your entire workout. You can tighten those abs without struggling through searing sit-ups, without gritting your teeth and forcing yourself to press through the "burn." Don't punish your abs, just use them.

Breathe Deeply. The simple mechanism of oxygen intake works the muscles between your ribs, stretching and contracting and toning your torso.

Exhale "Yeet!" You won't believe what a difference this makes in the toning of your abdominals. Exhale with gusto, letting go an explosive from-the-gut *"Yeet!"* Don't be shy.

Lengthen. If you purposefully lengthen before you rise or twist, you work your entire torso.

Contract. Besides being the most natural and safe way to round your spine, contracting your abdominal muscles whenever you round over will tighten them up in a flash. Never drop your chest weight to round over. Instead, exhale and draw in those abs as you slowly round down. Always exhale to contract your abdomen. This will protect your lower back and give you sleek abdominals.

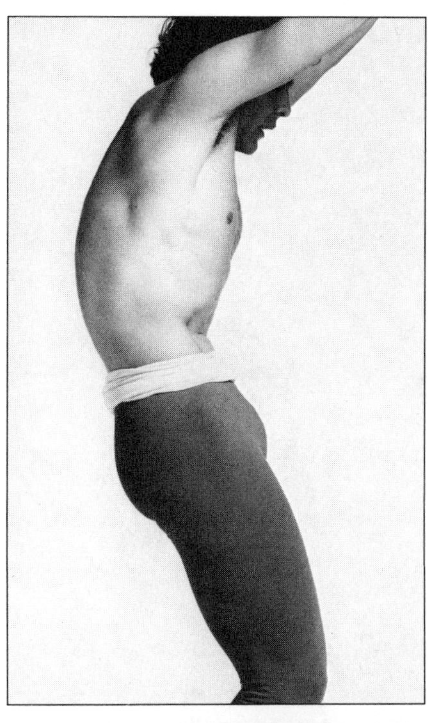

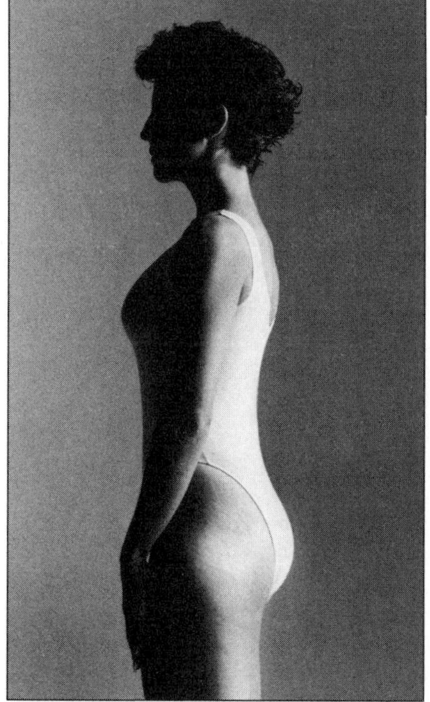

Abdominal Fist. Whenever you exhale, feel your abdominal muscles contract, not your buttocks squeeze. Imagine making an abdominal fist, being careful not to overtuck your pelvis. And keep that imaginary weight, the one dropped down to the floor from your tailbone, working for you. You'll get firm abs fast.

YOUR SPINE

Your spine is an elegant curve of thirty-three vertebrae. By working with that curve as you twist and rotate your upper body, you'll become stronger and more flexible. When your spine is strong and flexible, your hips and shoulders are free to move in a greater range of motion, opening up a whole new store of energy. By exhaling on twists and relaxing with the motions, you'll gradually increase your range of motion.

Focus on rotating your body around your central axis: a flexible, movable spine. Always start by lengthening first, feeling your ribcage draw up away from your pelvis and your head lifting up away from your shoulders. The lengthening is particularly helpful if you're tight or stiff.

Always rotate and twist without force. Keep in mind that twists and rotations may be difficult if your spine is stiff. Take it easy. A little motion is better than none because it helps you gradually loosen up. Work with your body. Twist or rotate only to a point where the tension is equal on both sides of your neck and both sides of your body. Imagine lifting your skull up off your shoulders and neck.

Open

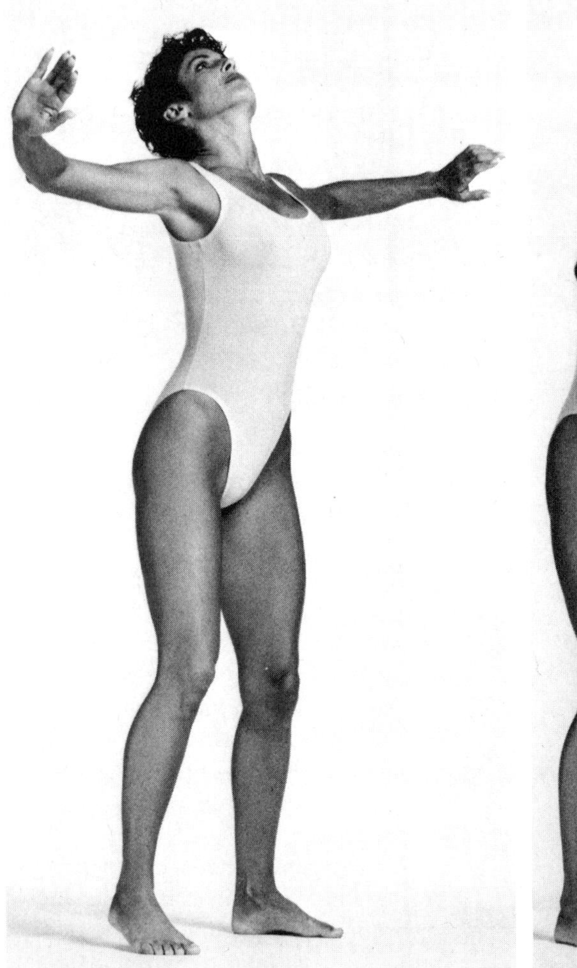

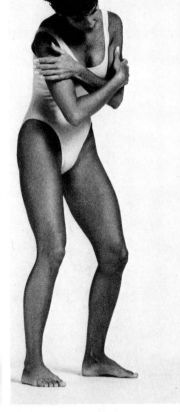

Inhale slowly, fully, and feel the wide stretch along the front of your chest as it expands. Imagine being terrifically proud.

Close

Then *exhale* completely and contract your abs, rounding your spine. Imagine being terribly sad. Initiate the movement from the core of your body, your shoulders and arms following, not leading.

Twists

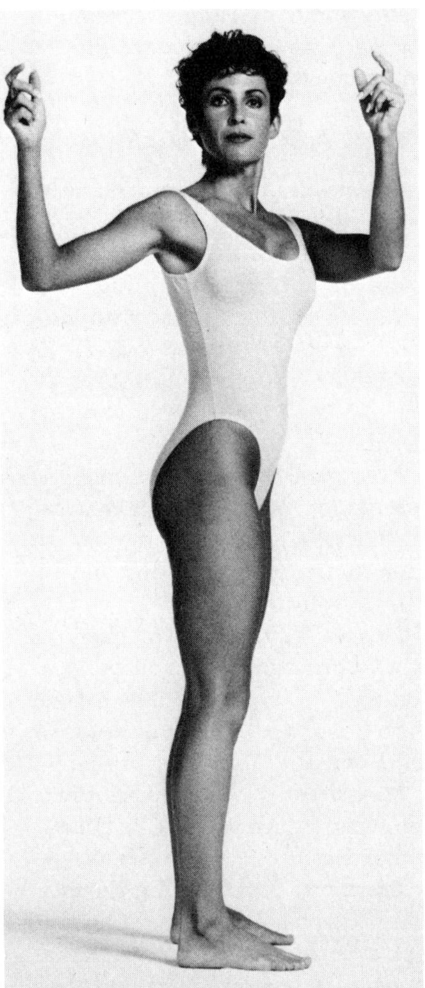

Pretend you're holding a large picture frame out in front of you. Grow tall and twist, leading with the core of your body and following with your head so that you look through the center of the frame. Imagine wringing out your torso like a wet towel.

The Delicate Balance

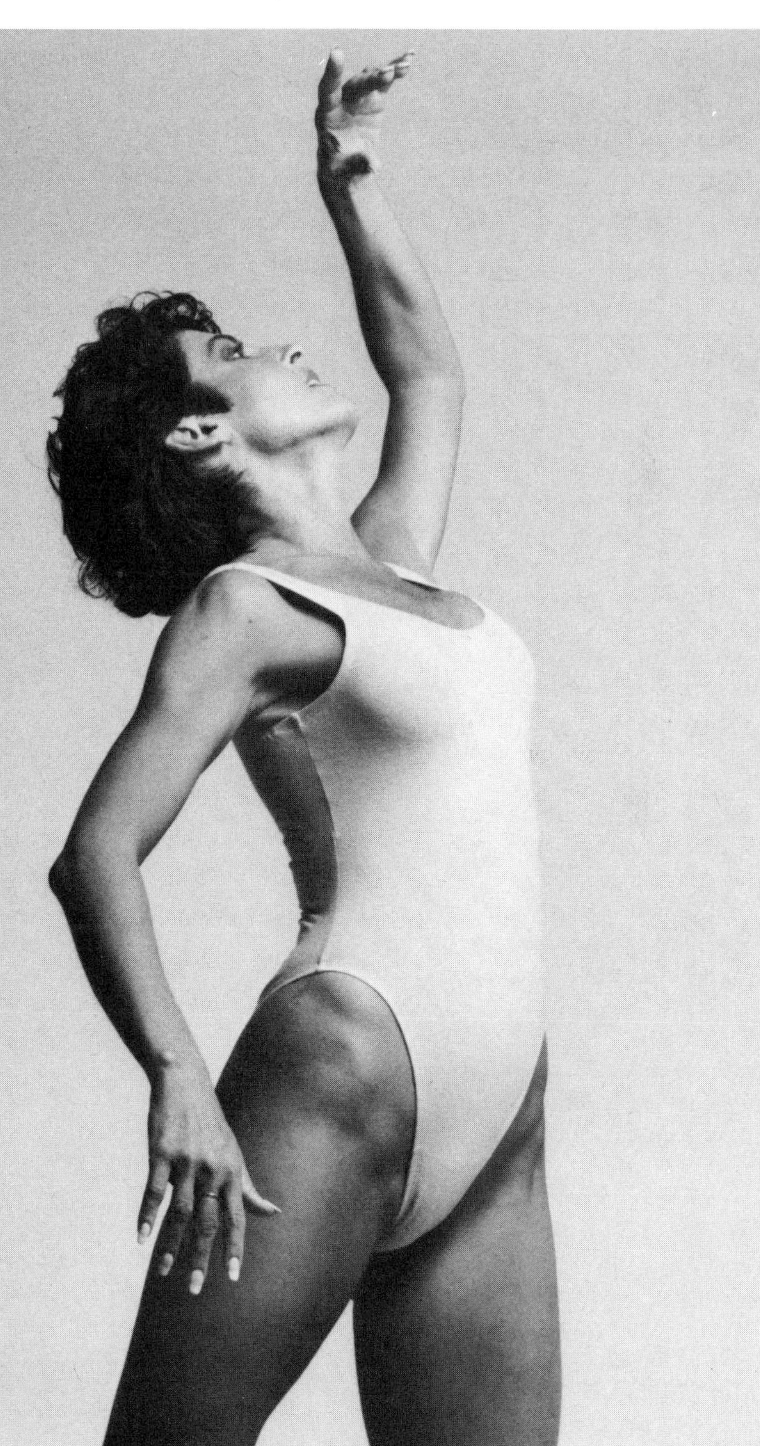

Your head is the heaviest of your body weights and has a tendency to fall off balance, jutting forward or falling backward. If you work with your head dropped forward, you can strain the back of your neck and your lower back. To correct, keep your eyes gazing at horizon level and focus on relaxing your neck. Remember the cushion of air at your neck and lift your head up off your shoulders. Imagine your head sitting on two ball bearings at the base of your skull and being free to roll around on those bearings.

Let your head follow your hands as you work out in order to increase the flexibility and range of motion in your neck. Holding your head rigid builds up tension in your neck. Move it. Let it flow with the rest of your body. Think fluid, loose, lifted. Keep your facial muscles and jaws relaxed. Imagine water running over your face.

The NIA Technique's Answer to Sleek, Lean Arms

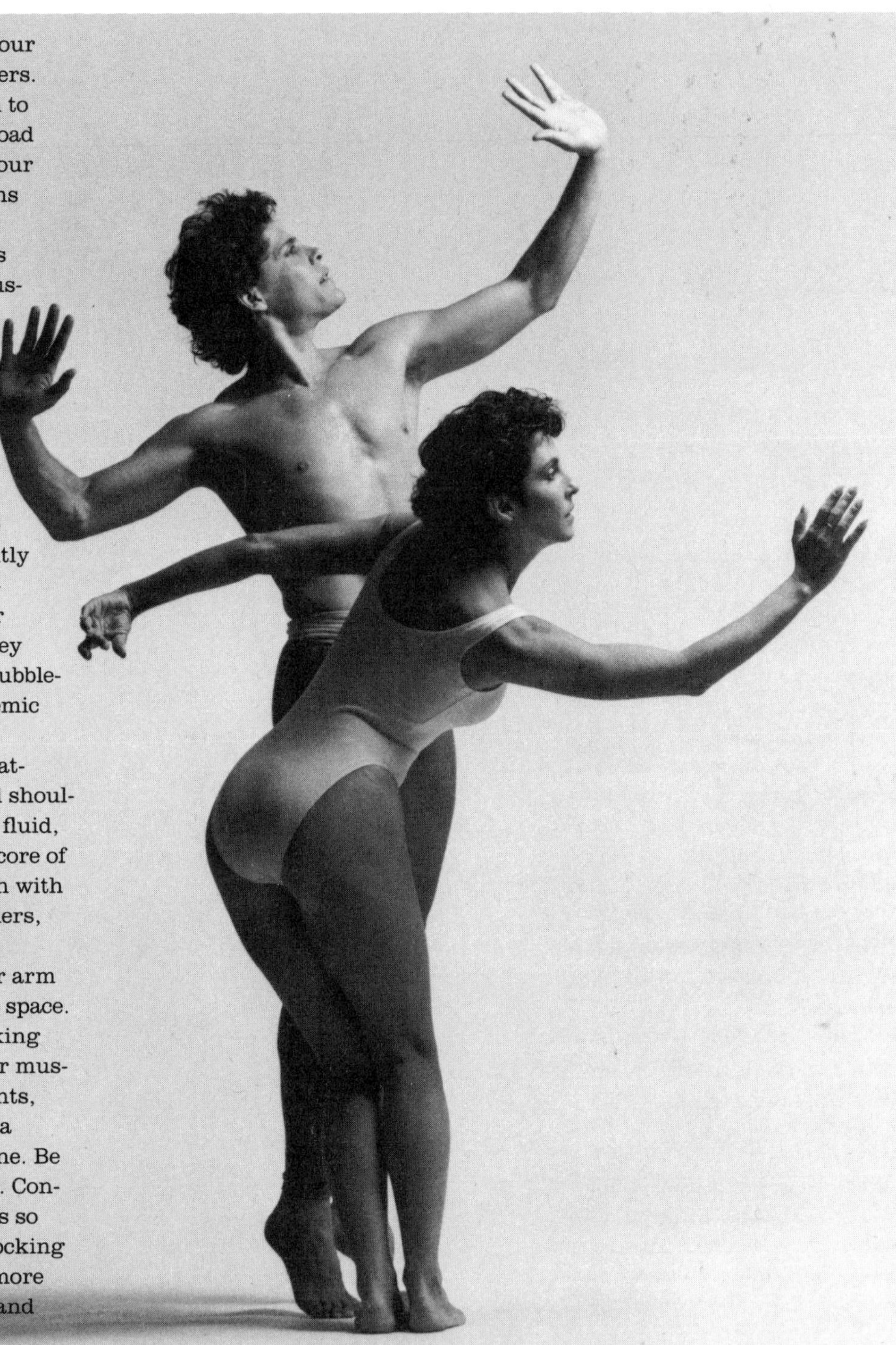

There are six joints from your fingertips to your shoulders. Take advantage of all of them to work your entire arm in a broad range of motion. Sweeping your arms in wide, circular motions and getting your shoulders, elbows, wrists, and fingertips involved engages all your muscles and gives you nice, even definition with increased flexibility. For example, instead of the linear bicep curl (pumping your fists toward your shoulders with your arms extended to either side), imagine pulling bubble gum off your shoulders, tightly squeezing your fingertips together and leading with your wrists as you stretch the gooey stuff out to either side. The bubble-gum pull gives you full systemic toning and stretching.

Remember, your arms are attached to your shoulders and shoulder blades. To be relaxed and fluid, initiate movements with the core of your body, following through with your shoulder blades, shoulders, and then arms.

Visualize and think of your arm movements as calligraphy in space. Keep all your joints soft; locking your joints doesn't work your muscles. By working all your joints, you'll tone more muscles for a sleeker, more symmetrical line. Be sure not to snap your elbows. Controlling your arm movements so that you extend just shy of locking will protect your joints and more efficiently work your biceps and triceps.

TO LIGHTEN

- use fewer body weights, dropping first the fingers, then the wrists, then the elbows, until you're using just your shoulders
- keep your arm movements close in to your body
- do fewer repetitions

TO LOAD

- add weights, starting with the torso, then the shoulders, elbows, wrists, and finally the fingers
- make your movements fuller, broader, more controlled
- do more repetitions without a "burn"
- be more passionate

REACHING OUT AND OPENING UP

Whenever you reach and open, feel an extension running out and beyond your fingertips and lengthening upward through the crown of your head so that you tone all the way from your tailbone up, strengthening your abdomen and back at the same time that you lengthen and strengthen your arms. Be careful not to overextend or throw your arms. If you're tight through your upper body, be especially gentle with your opening up and reaches. Stay comfortable, loose, and fluid.

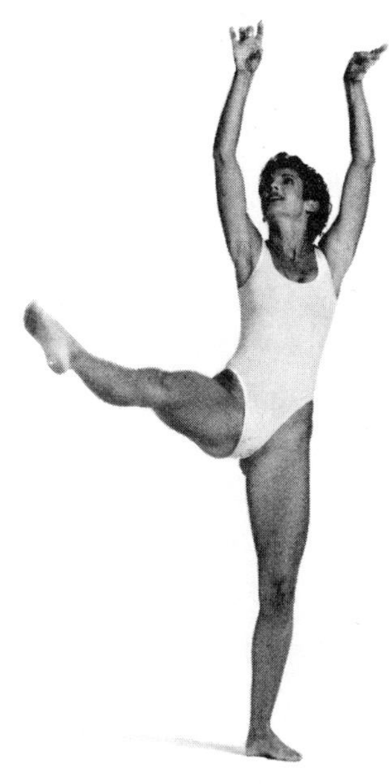

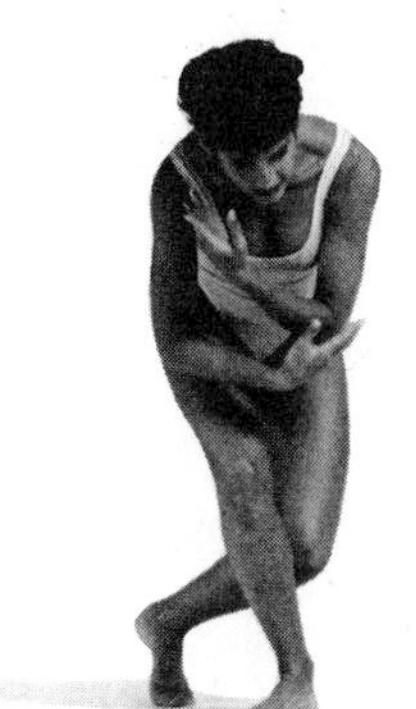

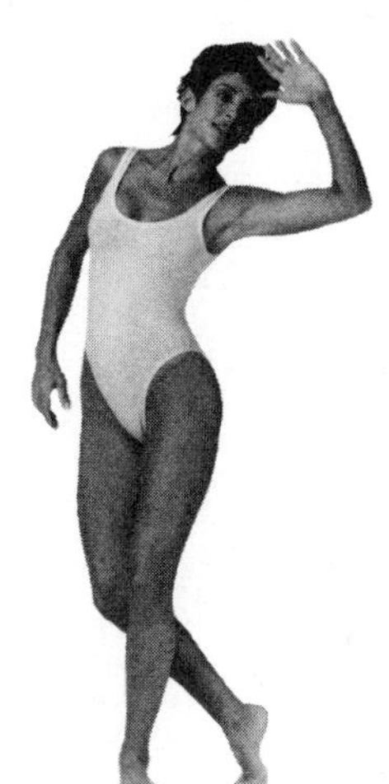

RECHARGING BY DRAWING IN AND CLOSING

For greater staying power and muscle balance, be sure to draw your arms back in to the center of your body after reaching out. The drawing inward recharges your motion while keeping you relaxed so you don't overuse or build up tension in your arms or shoulders.

RELEASING AND BUILDING UP INSTEAD OF BREAKING DOWN

If you feel particularly tight through your shoulders, lead with your elbows as you circle your arms, working your shoulder girdle with your arms for a nice massage. If your whole upper body feels like pressed steel, start your arm movements by simply rolling your shoulders and then gradually add arm weights (your body parts), by first moving the elbow, then tying in the wrist, and finally the fingers. The closer in to the core of your body you move your arms, the less stress your shoulders have to deal with and the better chance you have of building strength. Remember, getting fit means stressing your body just enough so that it can adapt and adjust to the new demand and not break down. Don't overwhelm it. Go slowly.

BUILD STRENGTH, NOT STRESS

Expressive Signatures

BREASTSTROKE

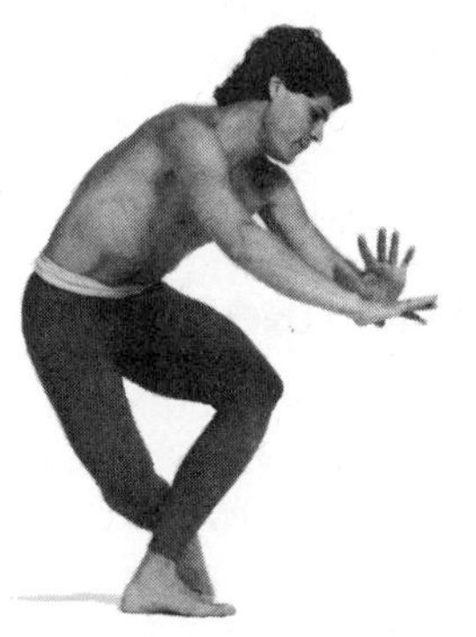

Feel the stretch across your back as you push the water away.

TOUCHDOWN

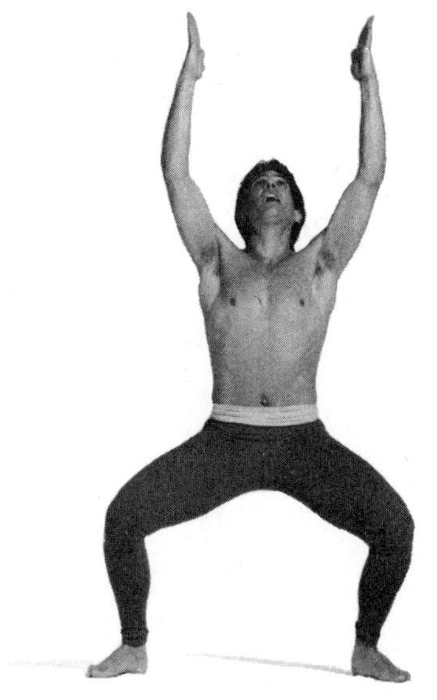

Feel the stretch along the sides of your body.

WELCOME THE WORLD

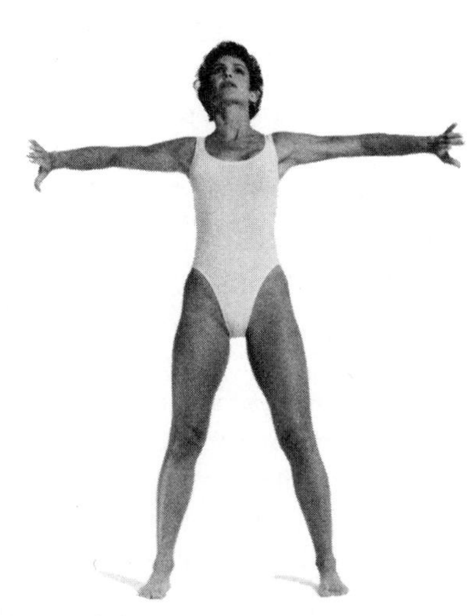

Feel the stretch through your chest.

HAND SHAKE

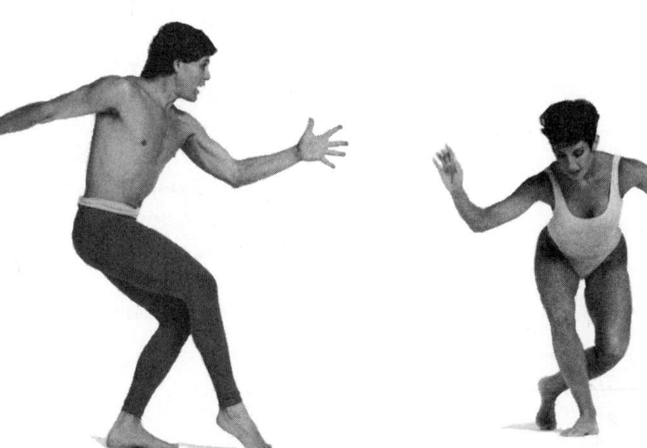

Feel the contraction through your chest as you reach out to shake

WINGS

Feel the stretch across the top of your shoulders as your wings draw down.

WIPE FOREHEAD

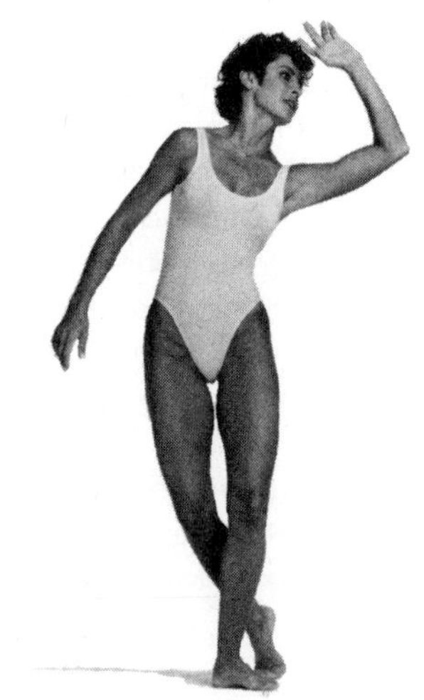

Feel your torso twist and trim as you wipe your forehead.

GRAB THE SUNLIGHT

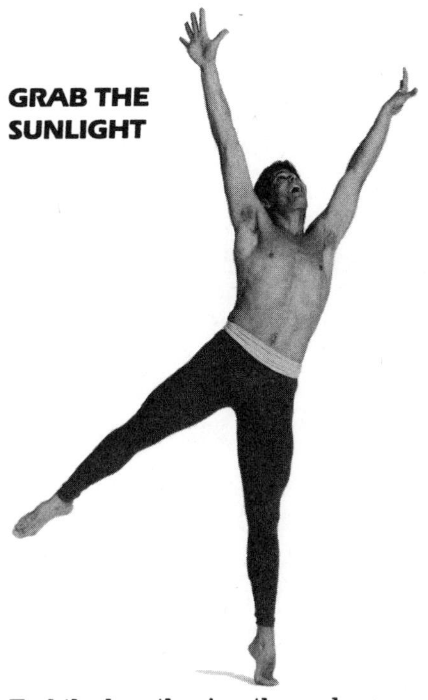

Feel the lengthening through your arms.

TABLE WIPE

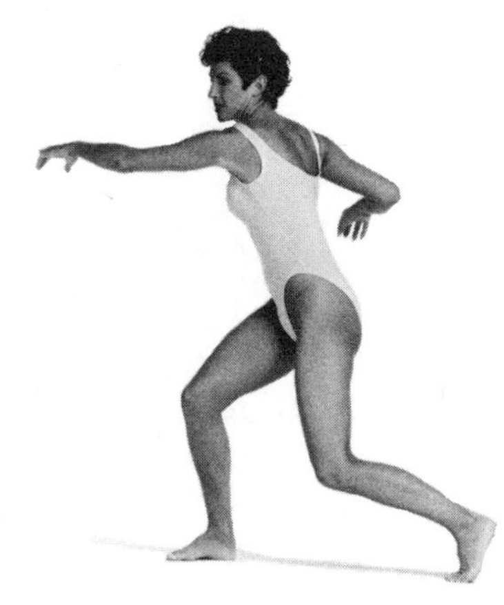

Feel the rounding of your spine, the contraction of your abdomen.

PUNCHING BAG ARMS

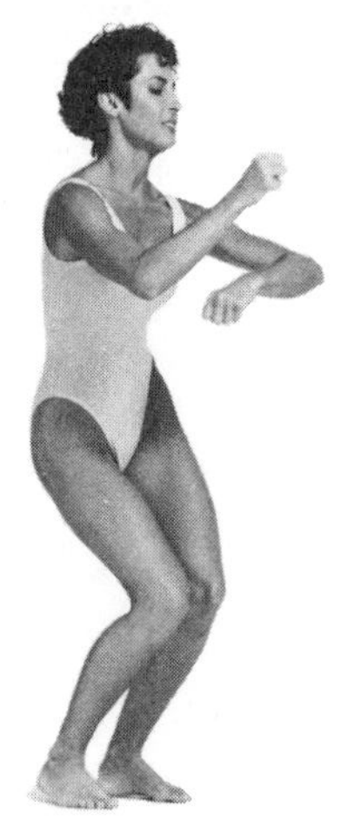

Feel a contraction through your chest as you roll and punch.

DRAW RAINBOWS

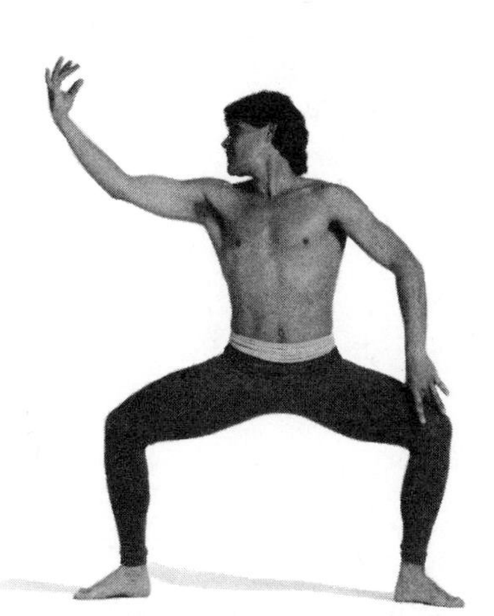

Feel the side of your torso contract as you draw your rainbow.

HULA HOOP WIPE

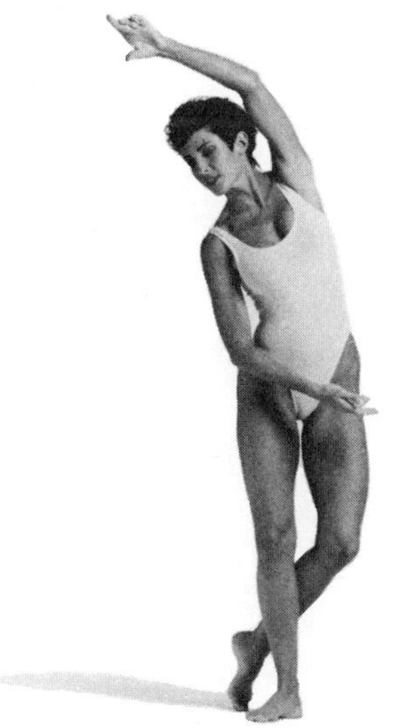

Feel the opposing stretch and contraction along the sides of your body.

A Word About Using Your Whole Arm

To avoid tension buildup in your upper body when using full arms, focus on moving your forearms, wrists, and fingertips fluidly and lyrically like a conductor. Your upper arms and shoulders will follow and stay relaxed.

The Little Guys Make a Big Difference

You can raise your heart rate with your fingers. The following finger movements will markedly increase the intensity of your workout and strengthen and define your hands and forearms.

CREEPY CRAWLER

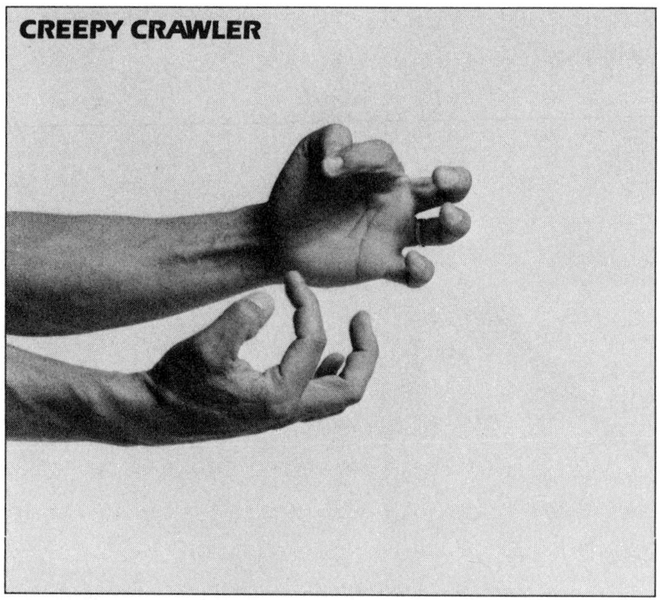

Wiggling all your fingers and both thumbs, feel a heat building up through your hands to your forearms. Use Creepy Crawlers to increase dexterity.

LIGHTNING RODS

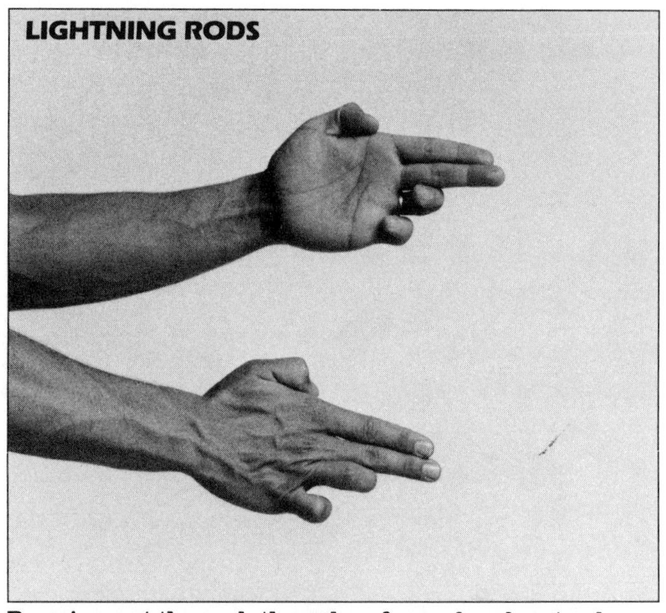

Pressing out through the palm of your hand, extend your first and second fingers, cock your thumb, and fold your fourth and fifth fingers down. Use Lightning Rods to intensify arm work.

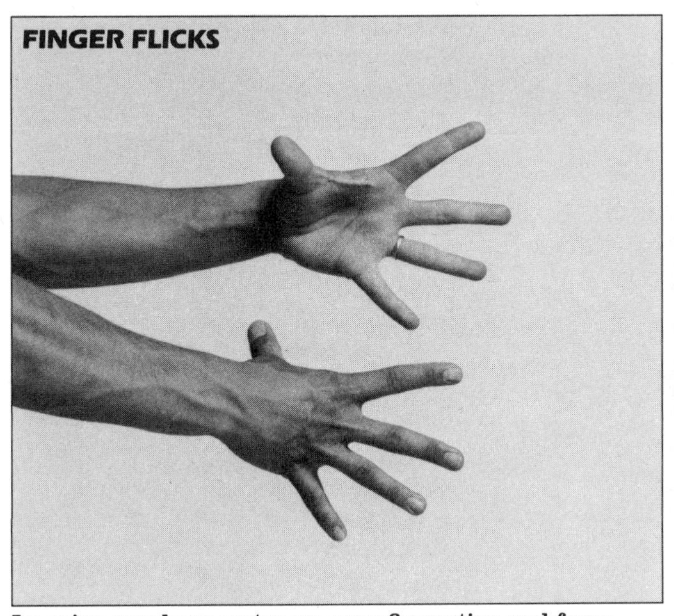

Imagine you have water on your fingertips and forcefully flick it off, starting from a closed fist and extending fully. Use Finger Flicks to avoid "tennis elbow."

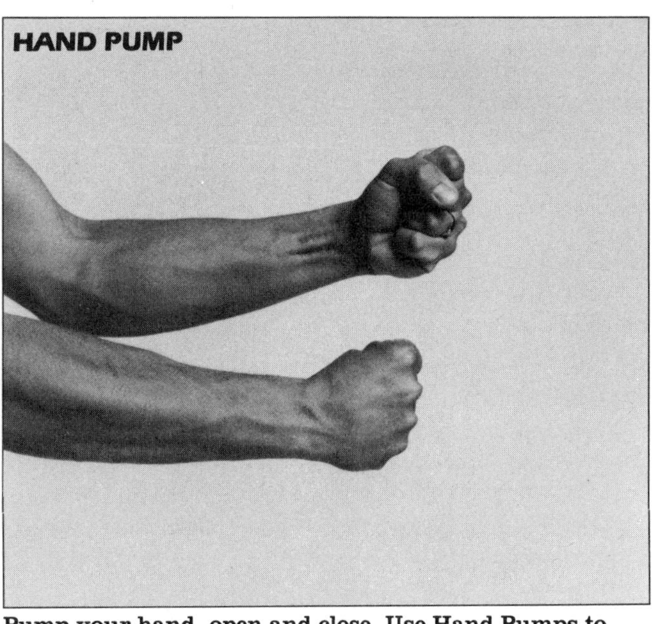

Pump your hand, open and close. Use Hand Pumps to increase wrist strength for racket sports.

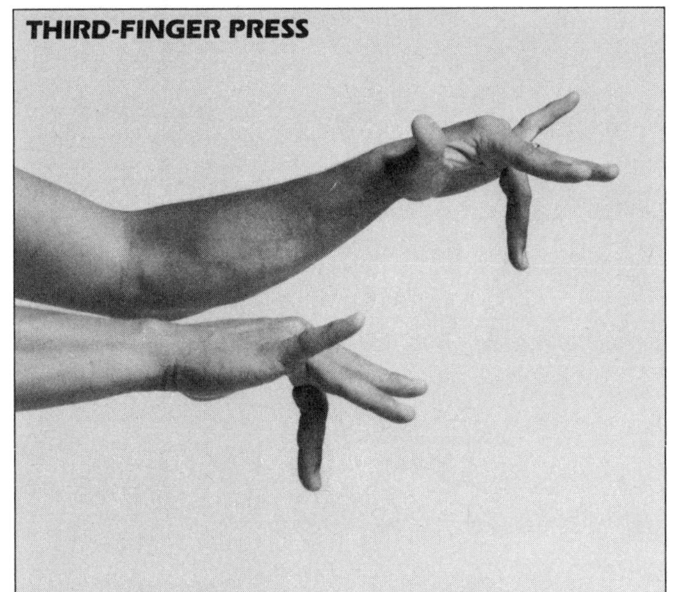

If your balance falters, use the Third-Finger Press to steady yourself. With your hand extended, press your third finger down.

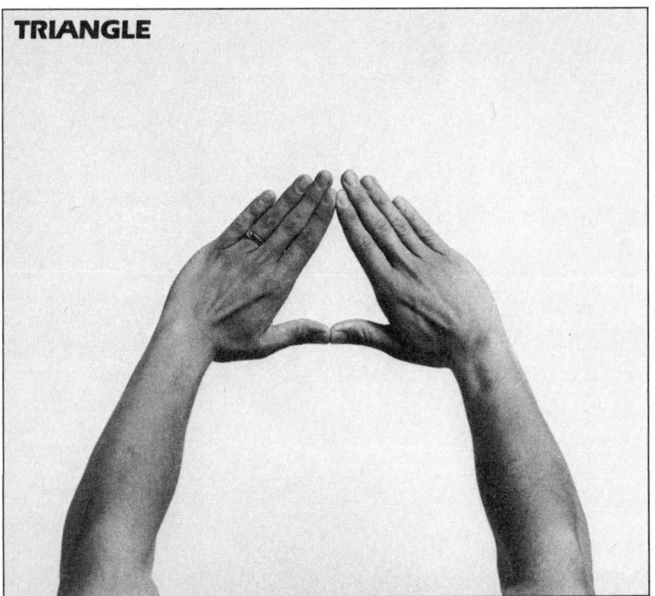

For focusing and centering, use the Triangle. Thumbs and forefingers together, palms away.

Stress Signals and What to Do About Them

Pay very special attention to these body cues and take action if you experience one. Over and over we hear from medical experts that the aerobic injuries they treat have persisted for months unattended. Don't be so unkind to yourself.

Because we're not right there to help monitor your work, we're counting on you to listen to your body and take very good care of it.

SIGNAL	ACTION
Abnormal heart action • irregular pulse • fluttering, jumping, or palpitations in the chest or throat • sudden burst of rapid heartbeats • sudden drop in pulse rate	Stop! Walk slowly until your heart rate returns to normal. Don't exercise again until you've seen your doctor.
Pain or pressure in the center of your chest, in your arm or throat	Stop! Walk slowly until your heart rate returns to normal. Don't exercise again until you've seen your doctor.
Dizziness Lightheadedness Sudden incoordination Confusion Cold sweat Glassy stare Pallor Blueness or fainting	Stop! Lie down and elevate your feet or put your head down between your legs until the symptom passes. Don't exercise again until you've seen your doctor.
Continued high heart rate 5 to 10 minutes after you've stopped exercising	Slow down the next time you work out and monitor your heart rate to keep it at the lower end of your target zone. If you still have an excessively high recovery heart rate, see your doctor.
Nausea	Lighten the intensity of your work and be sure you're giving yourself plenty of time with a full Heat-Up and Ease-Out.
Gasping for air after working out	Lower the intensity of your work and continue lowering until you can hum a tune to yourself while you work.
Prolonged fatigue even 24 hours after working out Insomnia	Lower the intensity of your work and give yourself more time with the building up again.
Side stitch (diaphragm spasm)	Slow down and purposefully breathe deeply into the spasm until it relaxes.
Joint or muscle pain	Stop and adjust your alignment.

CONGRATULATIONS! YOU NOW HAVE A FIRM FOUNDATION FOR A SAFE,
EFFECTIVE, EFFICIENT WORKOUT. SO LET'S GO!

4/GET READY

Workout I is for everyone, exercise neophytes as well as advanced jump aerobicisers, athletes, and dancers. The lighten and load tailoring tools allow you to gear up or down depending upon what feels right for you. You want to become familiar with these tools before moving on to Workout II. You also want to become—

- very familiar with the movements
- comfortable with your pace, range of motion, and intensity of work
- in sync with your own rhythm
- adept at sinking and rising, shifting your weight, and aligning your body properly

In the beginning, start easy so you get a feeling for the way the movements are strung together. Don't rush. Starting with Workout I leaves you plenty of room to gradually gear up as you become stronger, more flexible and balanced, and more adept at moving the NIA Technique way. If you skip this workout and try to do Workout II right away, you might well end up frustrated and discouraged, your body aching, exhausted, and potentially injured. So be smart, slow, and steady. You're learning a brand-new way of moving, even if you're an athlete, dancer, or jump-aerobics student, and you want to set it correctly in your muscle memory right from the start. Your patience and thoroughness will make all the difference in the efficiency, effectiveness, and enjoyment of your work—and that means a better-looking, better-feeling you.

Unless you're on a thick gymnastics or wrestling mat, don't worry about flooring; the way you move is your protection. Likewise shoes. You can take them off. Really. The flesh-to-floor contact will help you monitor your balance and alignment. Remember, the movements themselves are designed to protect your feet. Without shoes, you can better increase your circulation and dexterity, flexibility and strength. If you just can't abide baring your feet, get a pair of wrestling, gymnastics, or t'ai chi shoes. The more accustomed you get to not being constricted by an athletic shoe, the more enticed you'll be to remove the last layer between you and the floor.

Making It Easy

To give yourself an edge on learning Workout I, take a minute simply to page through it. Notice that we are your mirror image and the slugs give you tips for getting the most out of your work. The circles indicate weight distribution, a solid circle ●, meaning full weight, a clear circle ○, meaning no weight. The boldface titles are your leg movements, the lightface titles are your arm expressions. Look for body angles and lines in the photographs to determine proper alignment, and get a mental image of yourself doing the movements, creating those lines and angles, stepping out with your heel, sinking and shifting, inhaling and exhaling, stepping back onto the ball of your foot, drawing your knee into your chest as you scoop in your abdomen, moving with ease, comfort, and control. Remember, many top athletes use visualization as an integral part of their training, imagining themselves in perfect motion. They attest to the fact that the mental image can prompt the body to duplicate the mind. Take advantage of this neuromuscular programming. Fill your mind with possibilities.

Next, slowly move through Workout I without music, simply getting a feel for each movement until your body relates to it in a smooth and comfortable way. Don't try to get a workout, but aim simply to grasp the motions, first one by one and then as a fluid, continuous whole. Be patient. Workout I will come of its own accord if you let it. If you force it, you'll end up tense, frustrated, aching, and exhausted. Remind yourself to relax—often—and use the imagery to enhance your movement, to create full, systemic conditioning. Drawing rainbows or pulling bubble gum off your shoulders will move you more efficiently, effectively, safely. Invent your own imagery, tickle your right brain, and your work will feel like play, your movements become natural.

When you're ready, put on a nice, easy piece of music with a clear, steady beat and away you go. The easy pace will allow you to focus on balance and muscle work. In the beginning, concentrate on your lower body, from your navel down, doing just the leg movements while your arms sway naturally for balance.

When you have a good command of the leg movements, add your arms, keeping your movements small and close to your body.

When Workout I feels good and friendly, you can work at a faster, but never frenetic, tempo. As you become more adept at moving the NIA Technique way, gradually extend your range of motion by sinking deeper, rising higher, and reaching farther. In this way, you'll increase your aerobic load, work and stretch more muscles for better definition and greater flexibility, and enhance your balance.

The way to learn the NIA Technique:

1. Page through: mental image
2. Rehearsal: no music, develop imagery
3. Opening night: easy music, legs only
4. Second show: easy music, legs and light arms
5. Ongoing: varied tempo, broader range of motion

Music

Let your choice of music match your mood, but don't forget to let your body vote. If you feel snappy in spirit but your body's working through a lag stage, opt for your body's pick of music.

When choosing music, remember that the tempo should be comfortable. If you're chasing the beat, your work will be shallow, exhausting, and not very rewarding. Try something slower that will give you enough time to work deeply and thoroughly.

Don't hem yourself in. Experiment with music. Play. Vary your pace from one day to the next. You'll work differently, feel differently. Open yourself to change; lure yourself with diversity. Even allow yourself to move off beat if your inner rhythm begins to pulse differently.

Repetitions

Far more important than the number of repetitions you do is the quality of your movements and how you feel doing them. You can snap through an entire workout, doing just the right number of repetitions, but if you do the movements wrong, if you don't feel them, you can end up bored and still cool as a cucumber at the end. That would be a waste of your time, no fun, and zero payback for your investment. Focus instead on—

- doing the movements right by feeling for balance and control
- becoming familiar and comfortable with each movement
- getting the very most out of each movement
- generating a comfortable heat out of each motion

That way, you'll have nary a dull moment, will be dripping with the sweat of a great aerobic workout, and glowing with the immense gratification of garnering high interest on your investment.

In the beginning, instead of varying the number of your repetitions, use the tailoring tools below to increase or decrease intensity. Then, when you've mastered the workout sequence, add or subtract repetitions depending on how you feel on any given day. Remember, nobody's watching; nobody's judging your performance. Make it just right for you. Go for feeling good.

Tailoring Workout I

We can't stress this enough.

THE NIA TECHNIQUE
IS MEANT TO BE CHANGED.
BY YOU. FOR YOU.

As you tailor your workout by lightening or loading, feel for—

- being in your comfort zone
- dancing the NIA Technique instead of exercising it

Build the intensity of your workout gradually, respecting the adaptation and acclimation within your body. Don't make a dramatic leap in the intensity of your workout, but use the load options to build sensibly one step at a time. As you become stronger, more flexible, balanced, and adept at moving the NIA Technique way, pick one or two new load options to add to your workout. The easy gradation of your work will keep you on the safe, efficient side of fitness.

In the same way, gear down with lighten options to accommodate your body's fluctuating needs. Remember, it's okay to ease up. If you allow yourself to ebb and flow, heeding your body's cues, you'll get a lot further, faster.

Work/Recharge

Recharge segments are indicated in Workout I; all others are work segments. You can modify intensity by adding or staying longer in a recharge segment if you're feeling tired, or extending a work segment if you're feeling strong. Adapt each workout to fit the way you feel at the moment. Remember, just because you worked hard yesterday doesn't mean you have to work harder today. It's better to vary your daily workouts—hard one day, easy-does-it the next. Honor your own internal ebb and flow.

Heat-Up, Aerobic, Ease-Out

You may be accustomed to conventional stretching as the way to warm up for and begin an aerobic workout and therefore can't fathom where the warm-up is in this workout. We do things differently. Instead of static stretching, we begin to move the whole body right away, using complete motions in a small range to lubricate the joints and knead the muscles, creating pliability and generating heat. We call this heating up. As the core of the body heats up, we expand the movements like the concentric circles that undulate from the point where a pebble hits upon the surface of a still pool. In our former jump-aerobics days, when we were doing conventional, static warm-up stretches, we would suffer periodic muscle pulls, but since using whole-body movement to create elastic flexibility, we haven't pulled a muscle in four years.

As you'll see, the NIA Technique aerobics is one continuous flow, a gradual build. After generating heat from within, gently increasing the heart rate, stretching muscles and lubricating joints, we sensibly begin to engage more muscles, increase the range of motion, the flow of movement, to kindly work the heart at an efficient aerobic rate. A brief pause to check the pulse is followed by an ease-out, a smooth ebbing, taking advantage of the warmth in the muscles to stretch and lengthen, taking the time to relax, to cool off, to step out into a new day. The finale is sweet, a meditative return to a new body.

Start Out Inside Your Body

Where else could you be, right? For starters, mulling over an important project at work. Replaying a conversation with your boss. Making mental notes about something you must tell a friend, your spouse. Compiling a grocery list. Planning a party, a trip. Ad infinitum. The mind is a tenacious traveler unless you tether it to a task at hand. If it's touring while you're exercising, you'll miss out on efficiency, effectiveness, and the rich synergy of mind-body-soul movement, to say nothing of those all-important body cues like "ease up" or "reposition" that can keep you on the safe side of movement.

You'd be surprised at how much your thoughts can affect the way you move. We often preface our non-impact aerobics workouts with this simple exercise below.

When you clear your mind of extraneous thoughts and focus cleanly on the movement of your body, you can stretch a little farther, bend a little deeper, last a little longer, and work a little safer. And that means a trimmer, slimmer, better-looking, better-feeling, healthier you.

Move your arm up and down, reaching for an imaginary shelf that you can barely touch. At the same time, start compiling a grocery list, review all your appointments for the week (keep moving your arm), replay a conversation with a friend (reach up and down), list all the errands you have to run (keep moving), the letters you keep meaning to write. Without letting up an iota on your thoughts, reach up to edge an imaginary can on top of your shelf.

Now close your eyes and feel the beating of your heart, the soft undulating of your breath. Then reach up and down, imagining that you're holding your most treasured piece of fine china. Concentrating solely on the controlled movement of your arm, reach purposefully up to set the china on the shelf. You should be able to reach higher this time.

TO LIGHTEN

Plane Work: Shallow

Decrease your plane work by sinking just slightly and by working on the flat of your feet instead of rising up onto the balls of your feet.

Work/Recharge: Work less, recharge more

Increase the length of the recharge segment and decrease the length of the work segment. Whenever you tire, ad lib and add a recharge motion—Jazz Walk, Cross Behind, or Sink 'n' Rise—or simply walk in place.

Range of Motion: Close to body

Lessen your range of motion by keeping your motions in closer to your body, rounding over less, and rotating just slightly.

Muscle Groups: Core of body, plus light arms or light legs

You can monitor your aerobic load by the number of muscle groups you use. Think of the core of your body as your starting point and every other part of your body as additional weights that load your workout. The more body parts you use, the more you intensify your work.

Trim your workout by dropping one weight at a time, letting up on your fingers, wrists, elbows, until just your shoulders are undulating with the rhythm, your arms hanging loose and floppy at your sides, while the core of your body and your legs carry the rhythm. If you don't want to give up the full upper body toning, keep your arms and torso moving and ease up on your leg work. The key is to be picky about what you want to accomplish and what feels right.

Holds: None

The longer you hold a motion, the harder it becomes. In the beginning, simply move to the beat of the music without holding any of the motions.

Travel: Forward and backward, small steps

If you have room, travel the movements forward and backward for four steps each way, keeping your steps small.

TO LOAD

Plane Work: Deeper

Increase your plane work by sinking deeper and rising higher onto the balls of your feet, focusing on a nice even pace up and down and being especially alert to your comfort zone, to the alignment of your knees, and to not exceeding your aerobic target. Deeper sinking requires more balance, strength, flexibility, and stamina, and demands more of your heart.

Work/Recharge: Work more, recharge less

Increase the length of your work segment and decrease the length of your recharge segment. Do not, however, skip over a recharge segment or you might build up too much tension. The ebbing and flowing is crucial for a healthy workout.

Range of Motion: Broad

Lowering your body's center of gravity, which is two inches below your navel, allows you to extend your range of motion through your ankle, knee, and hip joints. As you sink more deeply, your range of motion below your waist increases. You can also extend your range of motion by reaching and rotating farther and sweeping your arms more broadly. As you do so, you'll increase your aerobic load for greater endurance, and tone and stretch more muscles for greater strength, definition, and flexibility.

Muscle Groups: Core of body, plus all extremities down to fingertips and toes

If you need an extra boost to kick into your aerobic zone, really let loose with the movement of your chest and pelvis, contracting and releasing your abdominal, chest, and back muscles; use all parts of your arms, generating the motion from the core of your body, extending out through your shoulders, sweeping with your elbows, rolling your wrists, wiggling your fingers, and move out with your legs, fully using your toes, ankles, and knees.

HOLDS: Two to four beats

Hold the sinking motions for a count of two to four musical beats. Holding a posture demands greater strength and aerobic stamina, so take it easy. Your body must rally to generate the force from within, whereas continuous movement begins to build momentum that helps propel you.

TRAVEL: Vary patterns, broad

If you have room, use a variety of travel patterns (see illustrations) and move broadly, four steps in one direction and four steps in the opposite direction.

Body Alerts

- Always work in a comfortable range of motion.
- Never let your knees press beyond the arch of your foot.
- Keep your knees aligned with your second toes.
- Lower only to the point where you feel the work in the belly of your muscles, not your joints, never in your knees.
- Lead with your buttocks as you lower.
- Rise and lower slowly and at an even pace without jerking.
- Inhale fully to recharge your motion.
- When you step behind, stay on the ball of your foot so you make lots of light under your back heel.
- Always step back onto a soft, not locked, knee.
- Use only the amount of effort necessary for a motion.
- Never force your range of motion.
- Think fluid, lyrical as you move, reaching for both the relaxation and the work in each motion.
- Your arms evoke and convey feeling; let them speak eloquently for you.
- Relax: Tension depletes your energy and constricts your breathing.

NO PAIN, MORE GAIN

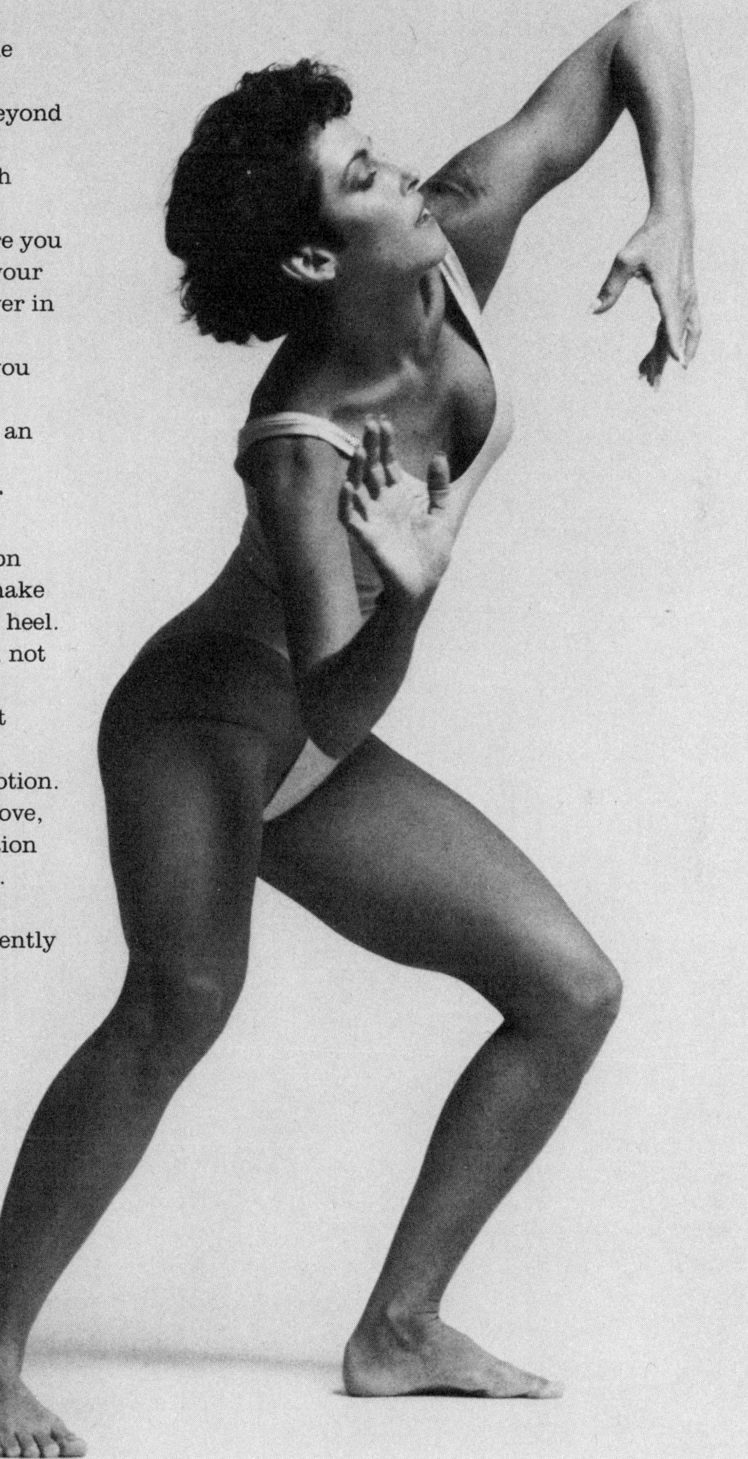

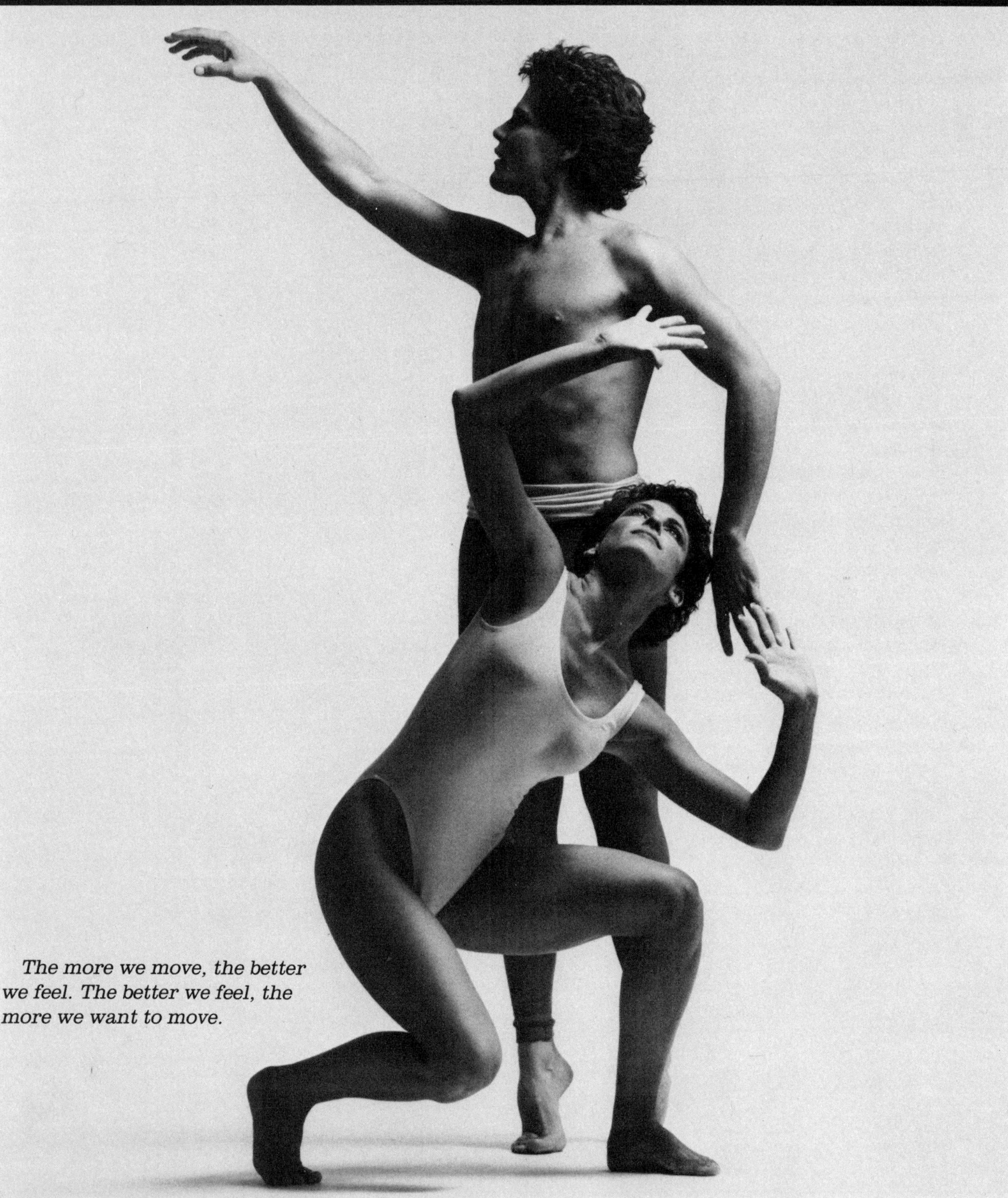

The more we move, the better we feel. The better we feel, the more we want to move.

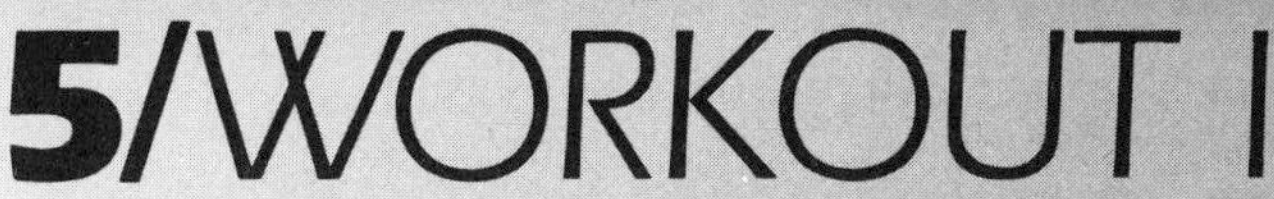

5/WORKOUT I

Put on your music, check your heart rate so you can mark the rise as you move through the workout, and let's begin. Lightly walk in place, your whole body loose and fluid as you find the rhythm of your music. Your count in the workout is always 1-2-3-4 and each 4-count equals one repetition. If you can't readily find a 1-2-3-4 beat, pick another piece of music in which the beat is clear and easy to follow.

When we ask you to do eight repetitions, count—
1-2-3-one
1-2-3-two
1-2-3-three
1-2-3-four
and so on. To catch your beat, walk to the count of 3 and clap on 4; keep going until you've done eight repetitions.

Eventually you'll develop a feel for the duration of the counts and you'll know when you've done the right number of repetitions, even though you haven't been counting the entire time. If you use the same music time and again, you'll know when to change by listening for familiar musical cues.

The count of 1-and-2 is always an inhalation and 3-and-4 is always an exhalation, except for the Spine Roll, Jazz Walk, Charleston, and karate kicks. Try out your breathing with another eight repetitions of the walk-in-place. This is a guide only; if it doesn't feel comfortable, follow your own natural breathing rhythm.

Be sure to read the benefits; they indicate where the changes are taking place in your body and where you should feel the movements.

The Mind Tamer

BENEFITS: To get ready and quiet your mind, to tune in to your body's mood and bring it into unison with your mind, to become balanced, at ease, in sync with the rhythm of your breath, which is the beginning of all movement, to focus on your workout goal.

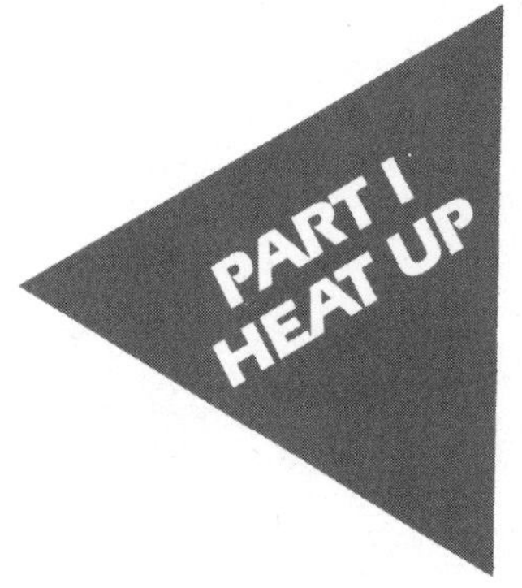

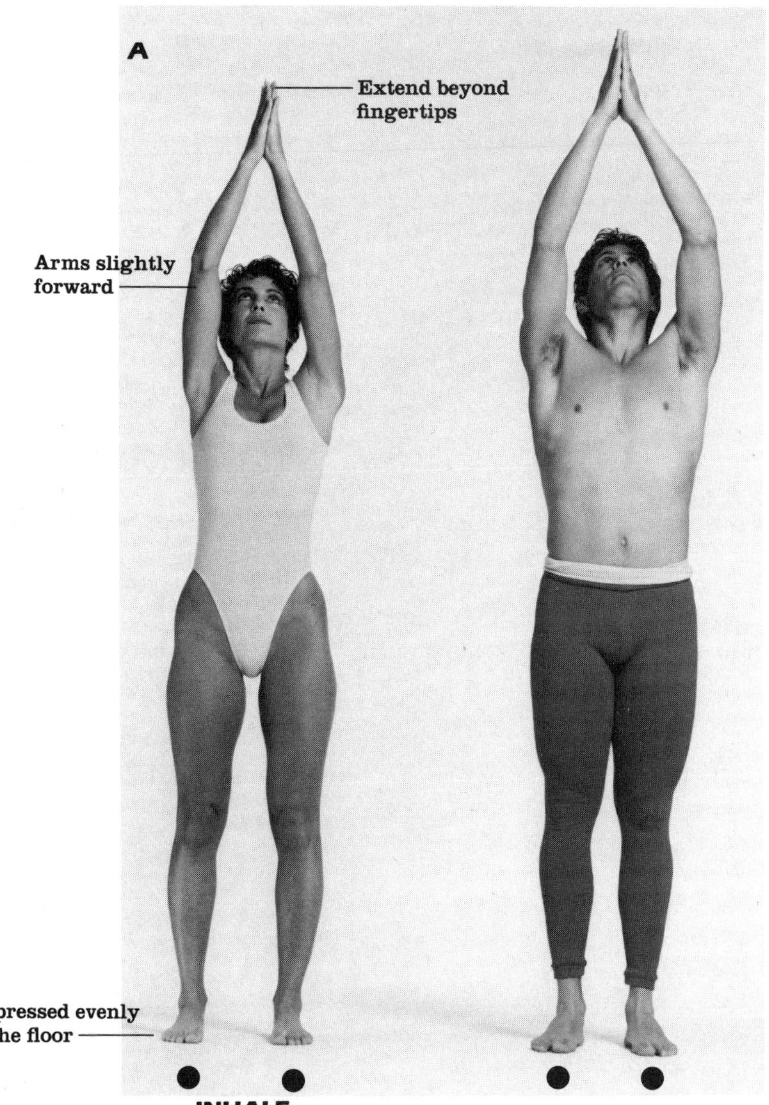

Take two purposeful steps forward into the center of your clock. Do so with feeling, bringing all of your good intentions and energy into this one place. Pause. Feel your body relaxed and centered. Breathe. Inhale deeply as you draw your arms slowly out from the sides of your body, ending up high above your head with a clap of your hands.

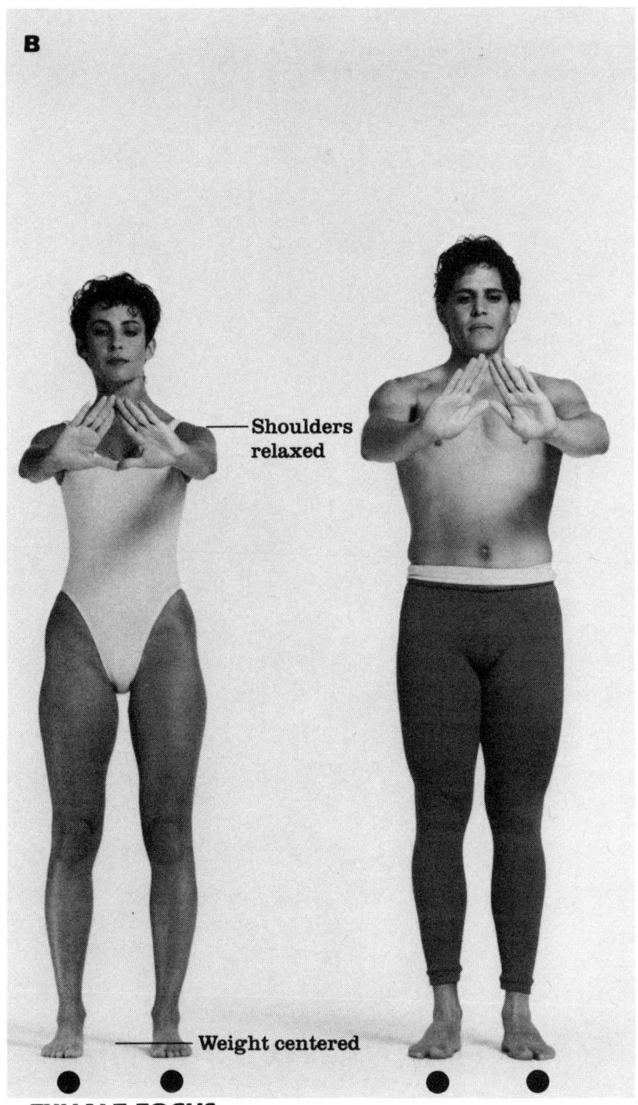

EXHALE-FOCUS

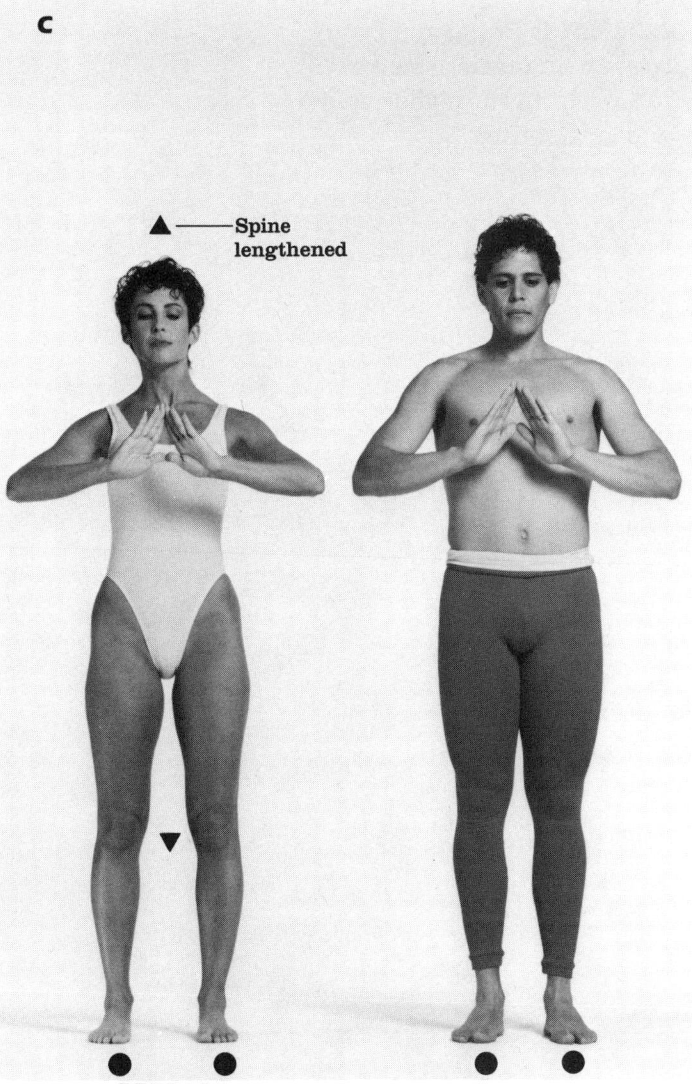

PREPARE

Exhale as you slowly lower your arms, your fingers forming the Triangle. Looking through your Triangle, take a minute to check in with yourself. How are you feeling, mentally, emotionally, physically? Be honest with yourself—and understanding so that you can gear your work toward a rich synergy of mind, body, and spirit. With every workout, take the time to visualize a goal in your Triangle and let it change as you do. Make it as vivid, as colorful, as you can and hold that image as your point of focus throughout the entire workout.

Slowly draw your hands back toward your chest and let them relax to the sides of your body, feeling mentally prepared to move.

STRETCH 'N' SHAKE

Muscle Relaxant

BENEFITS: To warm up your body in an unexerciselike way, to loosen through your spine and extremities.

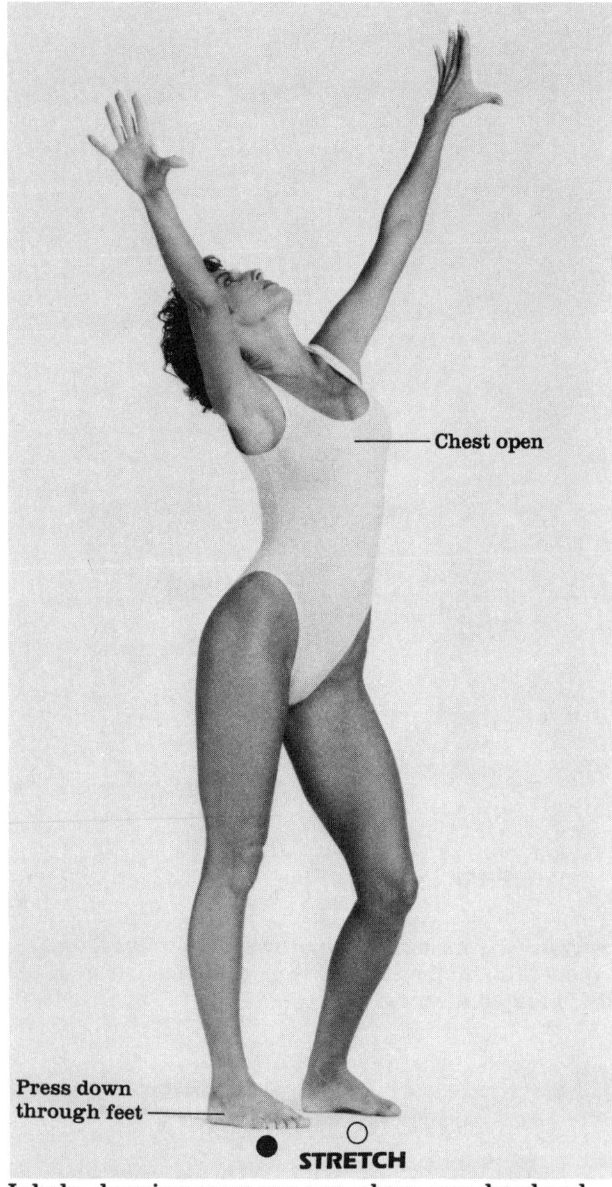

Inhale, drawing your arms up above your head and stretch toward the ceiling like you're just waking up.

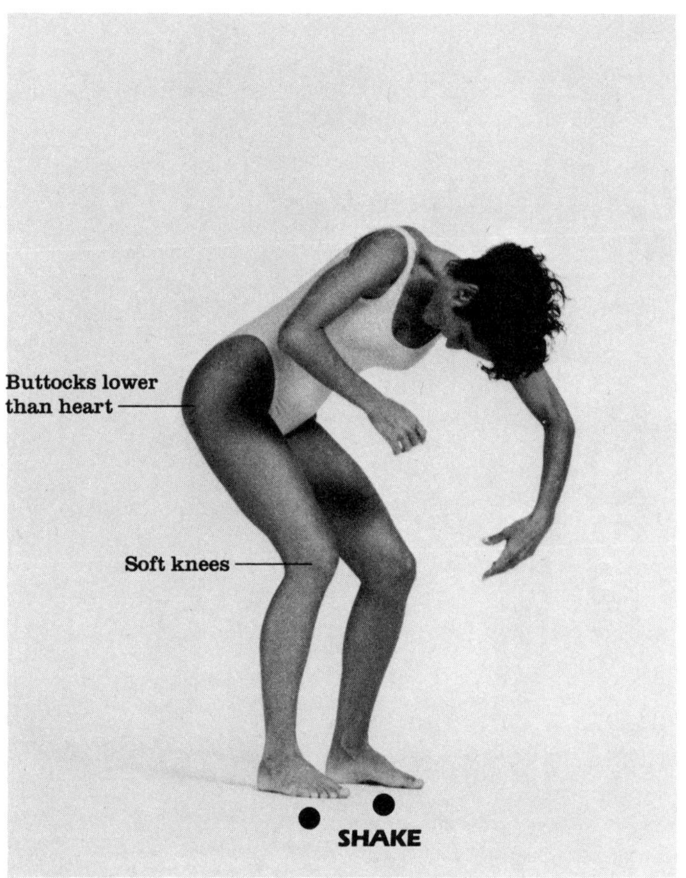

Exhale, letting go as you shimmy and shake—nothing wild, just little jiggles—lightly loosening every joint in your body. As you shake, let your head and chest droop over a little so the weight of your upper body gently stretches the full length of your spine. Still lightly shaking, press your feet into the floor as you round back up, stacking one vertebra at a time, and reaching high to stretch again. Repeat 8 times with feeling. Droop over a little farther each time, waking up more of your body. If you can comfortably and gradually bend all the way down to touch the floor, great. Otherwise, go just as far as you can without forcing the stretch.

Playful Improvisation

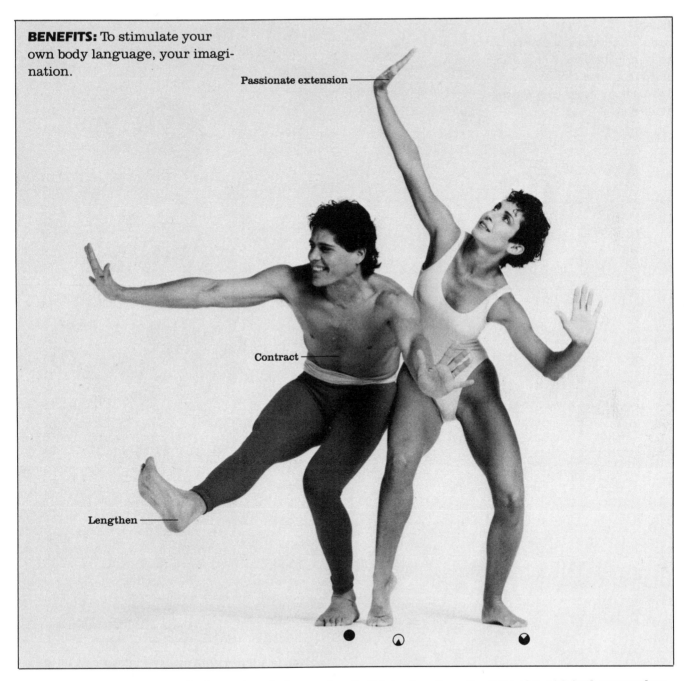

Imagine that you're standing in the center of a large, clear bubble and push on the sides of it with both your palms and fists, stretching up, down, left, right. Work against the light resistance of the filmy, shimmery surface, now sinking slightly to press it with your back, buttocks, knees, shoulders, hips. Inhale when your chest and arms open; exhale when your chest and arms close. Explore, play until you feel ready to go on, at least for a count of 60.

SPINE ROLL

Whole Body Warm-Up

BENEFITS: To increase your spine, hip, and knee flexibility, to strengthen your legs and buttocks, to warm up your whole body in an undulating fashion.

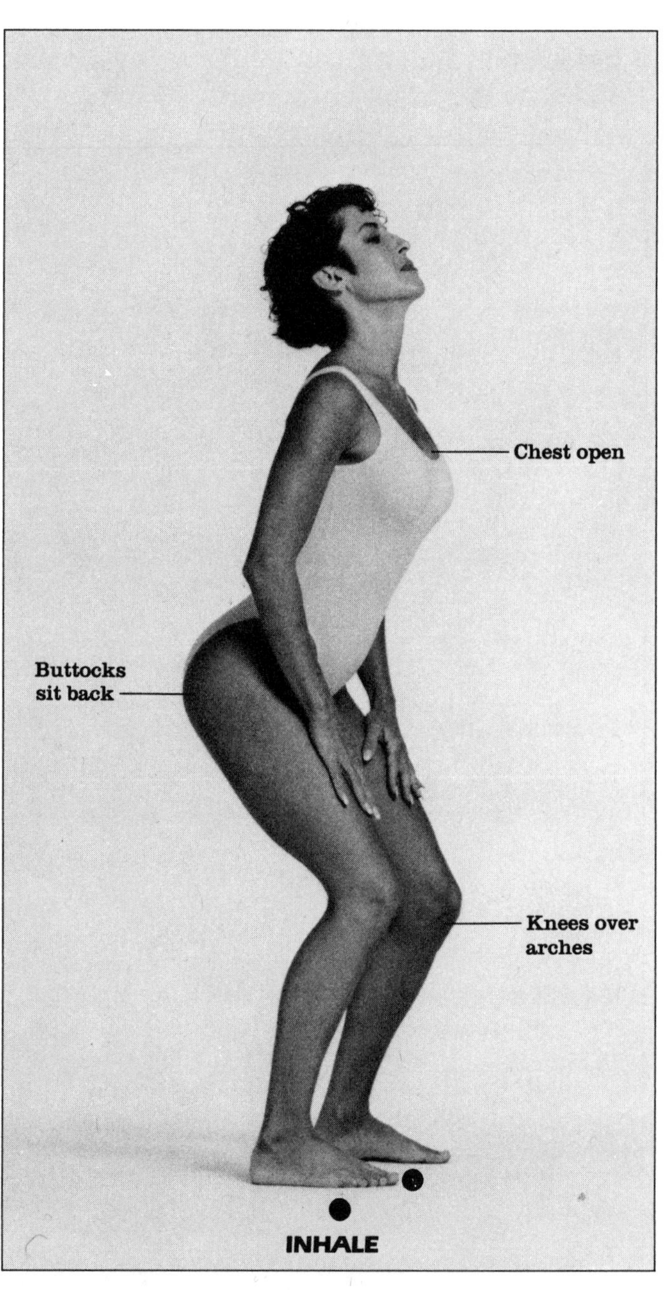

Standing in a hip or an *A* stance, sink onto an imaginary chair, gently sliding your hands down your thighs toward your knees, inhaling deeply and opening your chest. Stop your hands at your knees and lift your toes to check your alignment and balance. Continue inhaling, lowering your buttocks a little more.

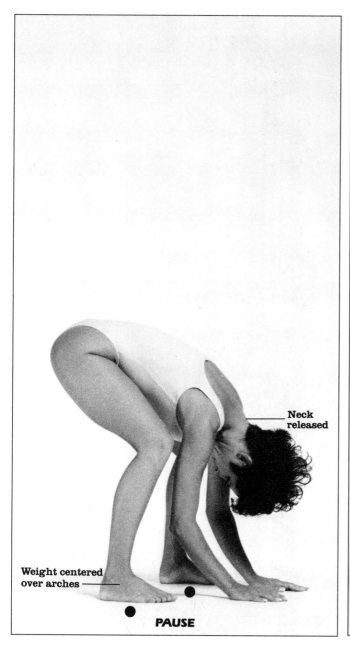

PAUSE

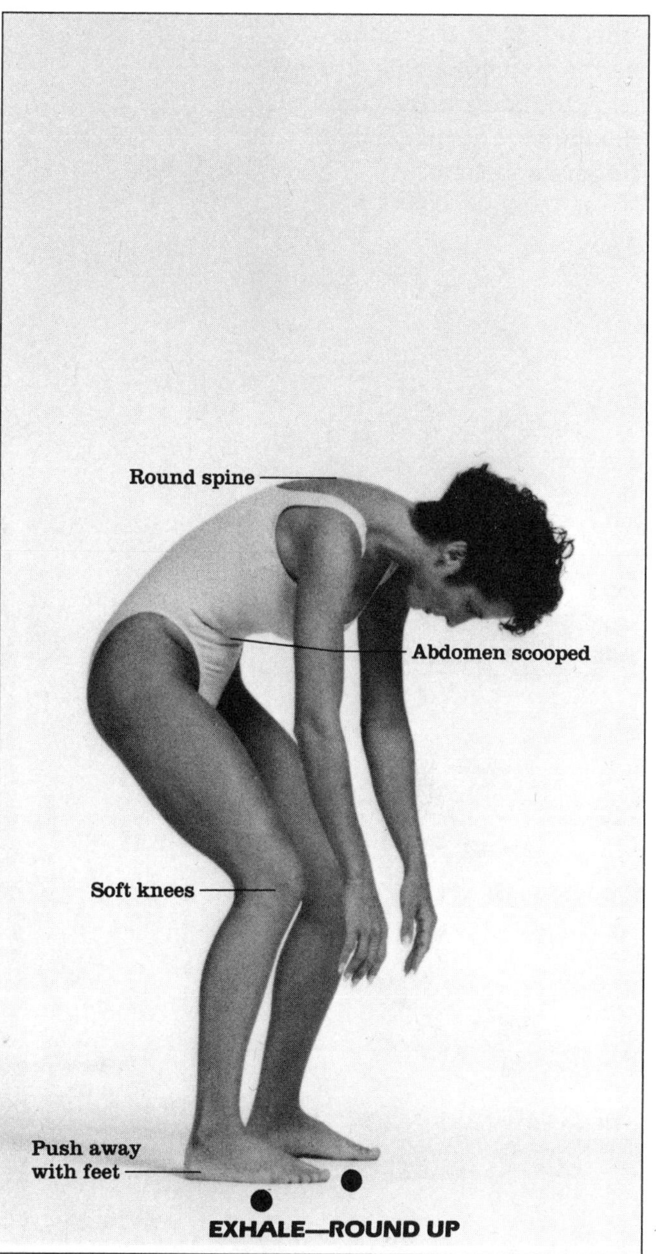

EXHALE—ROUND UP

Finally round over so that your neck releases, your head droops, and you feel a nice stretch along your neck and back. Feel for the lengthening of your spine. Don't overdo. Respect your flexibility so you can coax it a little farther each time.

Using the strength of your legs to push away from the floor, exhale and round slowly back up, stacking each vertebra one at a time, until your head finally tops them all. Roll down and round up 8 times.

Extremity Wake-Up

BENEFITS: To strengthen and define your forearms and lower legs, to increase the circulation, flexibility, and dexterity of your fingers and feet.

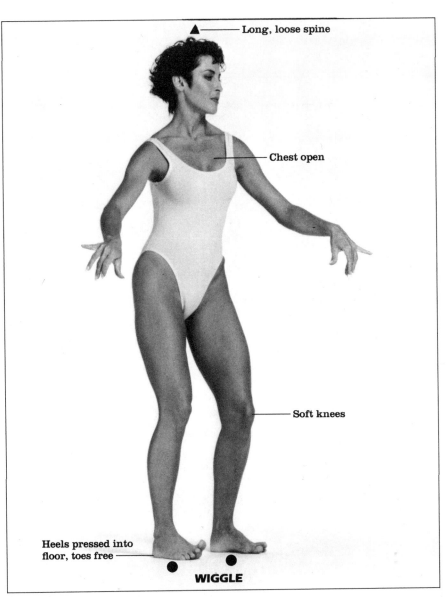

Long, loose spine

Chest open

Soft knees

Heels pressed into floor, toes free

WIGGLE

CREEPY CRAWLER FINGERS

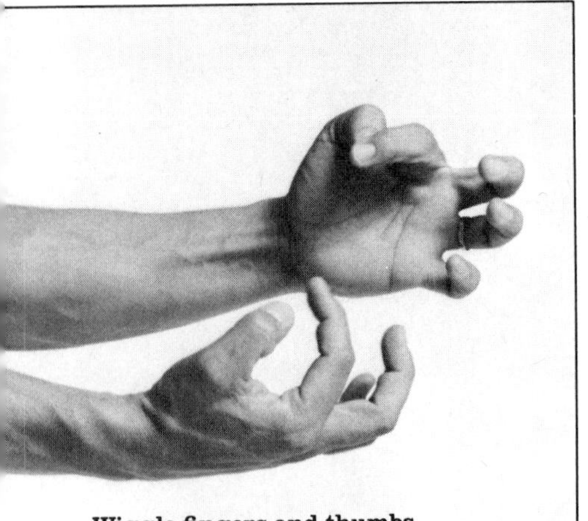

Wiggle fingers and thumbs

Standing in your hip stance, wiggle your fingers and toes, working all the joints, until you feel a nice warmth building up through your arms and rising from your feet into your calves. Imagine being at the beach and squiggling the sand between your toes. If you can't coordinate wiggling your feet and hands at the same time, do one at a time, first wiggling your feet and then your hands. Repeat for a count of 60.

Shin Strengthener

BENEFITS: To strengthen the muscles along your shins, helping to protect against shin-splints, to stretch your calf muscles and Achilles tendon, to tone and increase flexibility of your shoulders, arms, and hands.

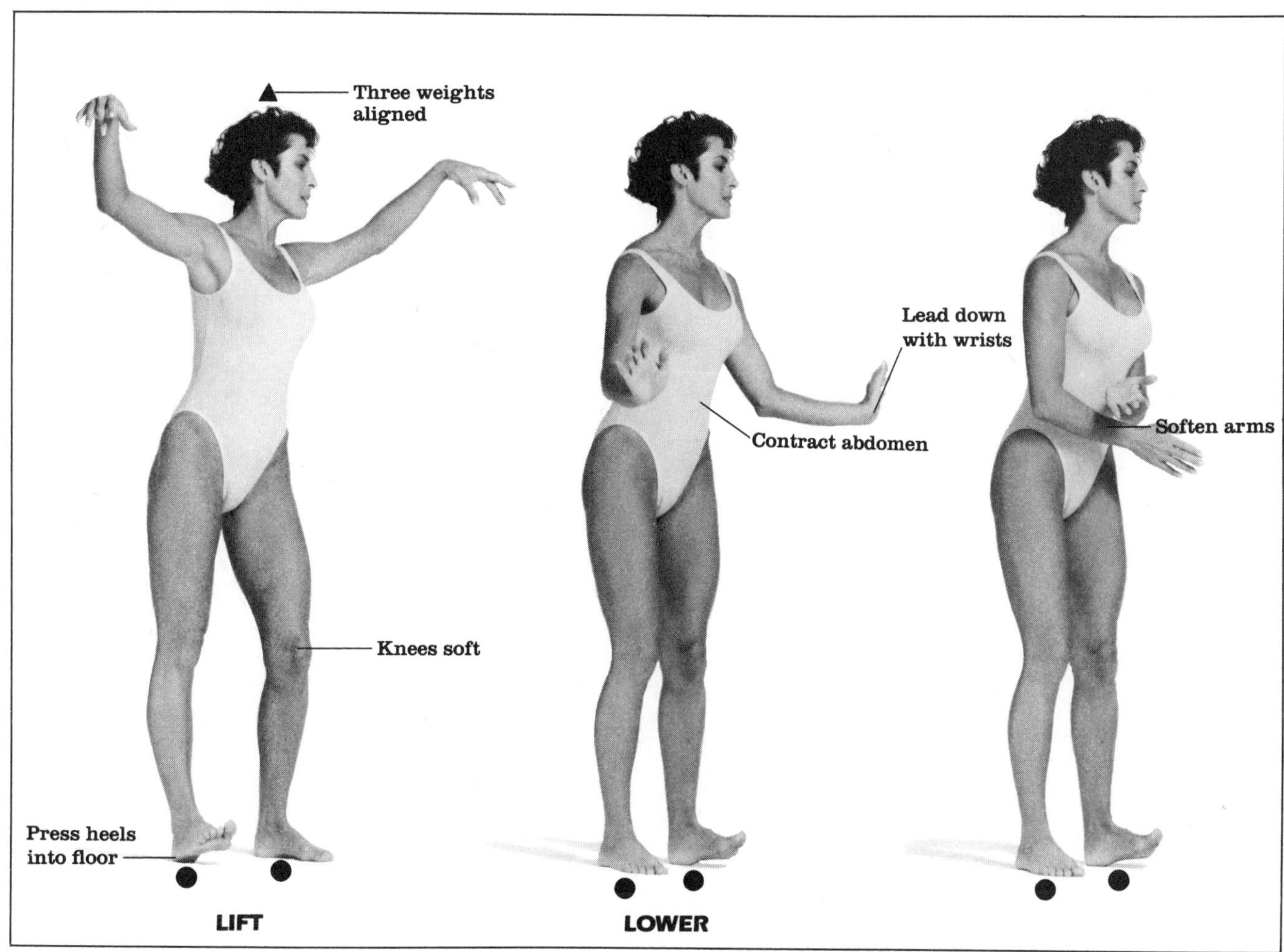

Alternately lift the front of your feet off the floor as high as possible. Don't let your knees snap back or your buttocks thrust behind, but stay soft and feel for the movement through your feet and ankles. Now fly south, drawing your arms up and down like wings, your elbows and wrists loose and fluid. Wiggling your fingers and leading with your elbows, inhale your arms up on a 2-count with your feet; exhale your arms down on another 2-count with your feet. Repeat for a total of 12, counting 1-2-3-one, 1-2-3-two, and so on.

To lighten the movement, roll your shoulders, letting your arms simply hang loosely at your sides, and wiggle your fingers in a disorderly fashion until you feel a nice heat rising up from your hands, through your forearms, and into your shoulders. Simple wiggles help guard against tendinitis by strengthening the muscles around the elbow.

Circular Balance

BENEFITS: To stabilize your ankles, to lubricate the joints in your toes, ankles, knees, and hips, to strengthen your legs and upper body, to increase your upper body flexibility, to enhance your balance, to get a feeling for circular motion involving your whole body.

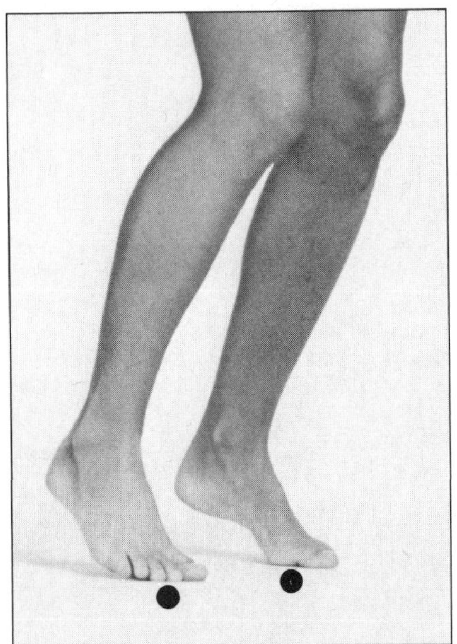

Rock forward onto the balls of your feet and backward onto your heels, moving through the entire length of your feet as you rock back and forth several times. Then rock side to side, feeling the inside and outside edges and the warm massage across the balls of your feet. Finally, tie the movements together, making broad, full circles, your feet pressing into the floor all around the edges. Circle slowly in one direction several times and then reverse, letting your whole body sway with the motion. Feel the warm massage through your lower back, the heat building in your hips to loosen the ligaments, to melt away any constriction. As your hips sweep front, inhale; as they sweep back, exhale. Imagine your hips are sweeping around the inside rim of a hula hoop. Let your arms hang loosely at your sides, using them for balance.

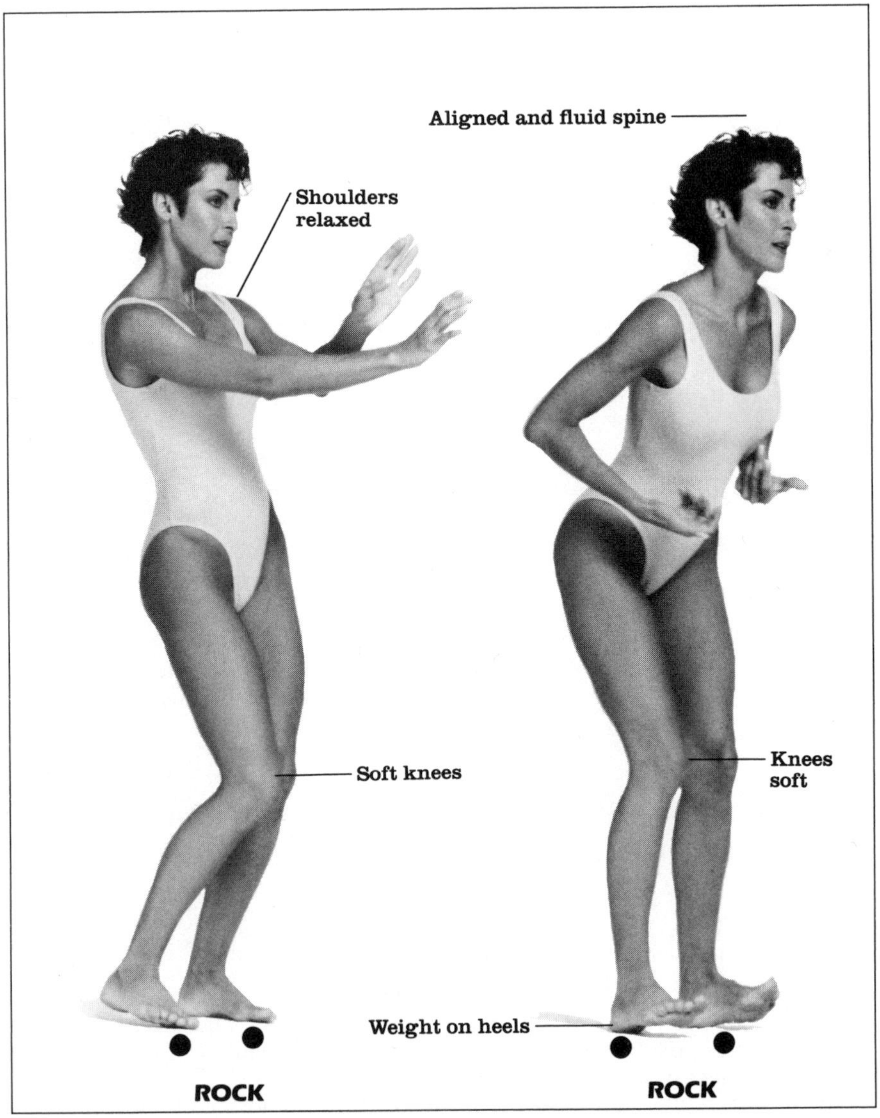

Aligned and fluid spine

Shoulders relaxed

Soft knees

Knees soft

Weight on heels

ROCK

ROCK

Add a breaststroke slightly below shoulder level, inhaling when your arms are wide open to either side and exhaling as they cross in front of your body. Circle your hips slowly in one direction 8 times and then reverse for another 8, letting your whole body become involved in the motion as you breaststroke.

The Whole-Body Press

BENEFITS: To strengthen your feet and calves, to create flexibility in your ankles, chest, and upper back, to give new definition to your calves and shoulders, to enhance your balance.

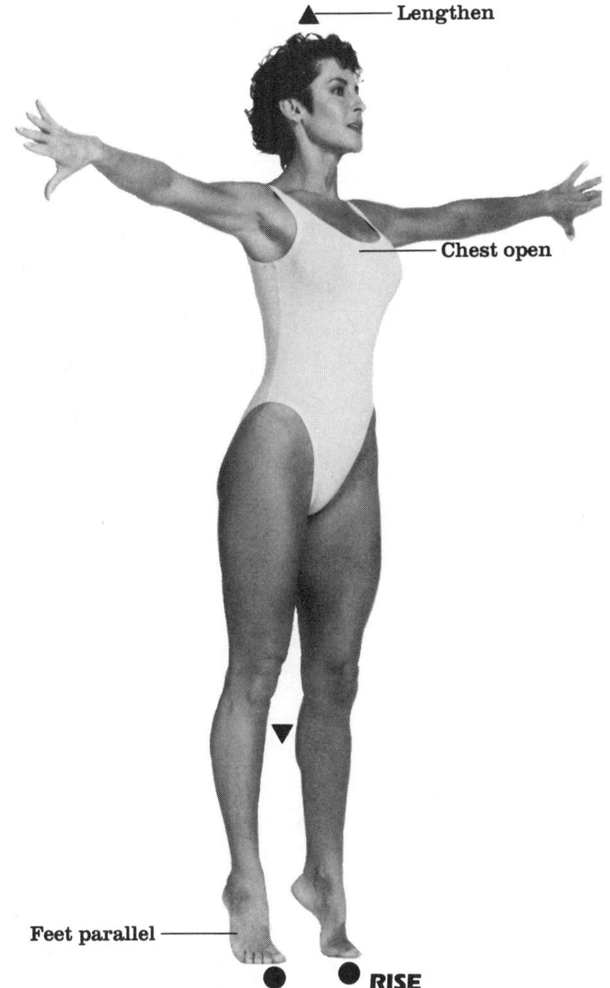

Inhale and slowly rise up onto the balls of your feet as though you're peeking over a fence. Feel the lengthening of your whole spine run up through your neck, the even strength of your legs surging down through your feet. As you rise, spread your arms wide to the side, leading with your wrists, and pull imaginary taffy off your chest, stretching it out to either side and flicking it off your fingers.

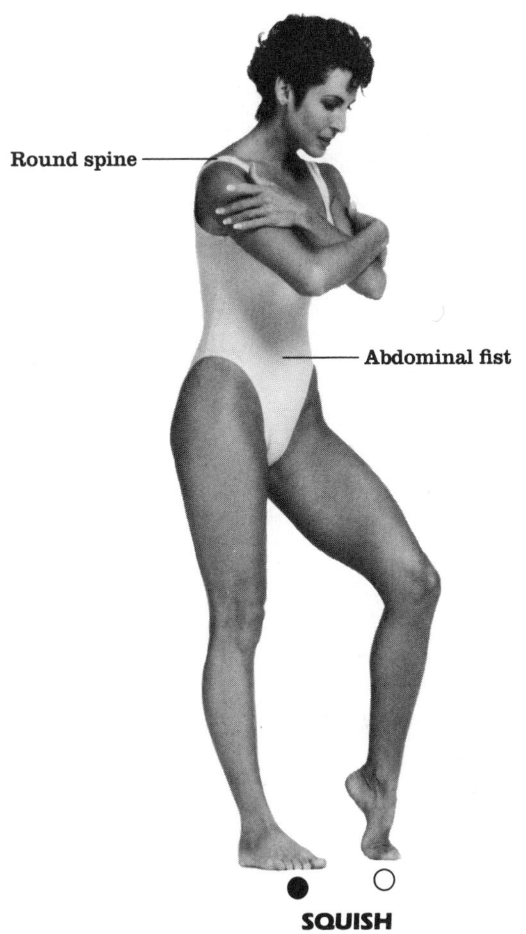

Exhale and soften your right knee to the front as your left heel squishes into the floor and wrap your arms snugly around your body. Rise and lower fluidly, evenly, alternating the heel squish. If you pop off the floor and crunch back down, you won't evenly tone your legs and can create muscle imbalance. Instead, rise up with control, pressing down into the floor with the balls of your feet, using the strength of your thighs, calves, ankles, and feet to purposefully generate the motion, and feeling your calf muscles contract to help maintain your equilibrium. When you lower, squish back down as though you're pushing against a spring. Working against real or imagined tension engages more muscles, which means better definition and greater strength. Repeat a minimum of 16 times, alternating left and right, up 2 beats and down 2 beats, until you feel heat rising up through your entire legs.

The Total-Body Boost

BENEFITS: To trim your inner and outer thighs, to tone your calves and hamstrings, to lift your buttocks, to increase your foot flexibility, to tone and define your upper body, to enhance your balance.

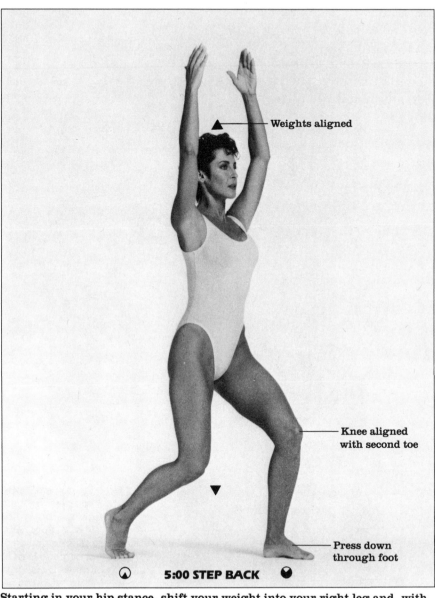

Starting in your hip stance, shift your weight into your right leg and, with control, step back onto the ball of your left foot at 7:00, inhaling as you raise your arms high above your head like a football referee signaling a touchdown. Pause for a moment and feel your balance and strength. If either foot is rocking to the side, adjust by pressing smack through the center of your sole in front or the ball of your foot in back. For stability in the beginning only, turn your front foot in a bit if you tend to roll onto the outer edge; turn out a bit if you tend to roll onto the inner edge. Now, keeping most of your weight on your front leg, slowly sink your back knee comfortably closer toward the floor. Go only as far as is comfortable.

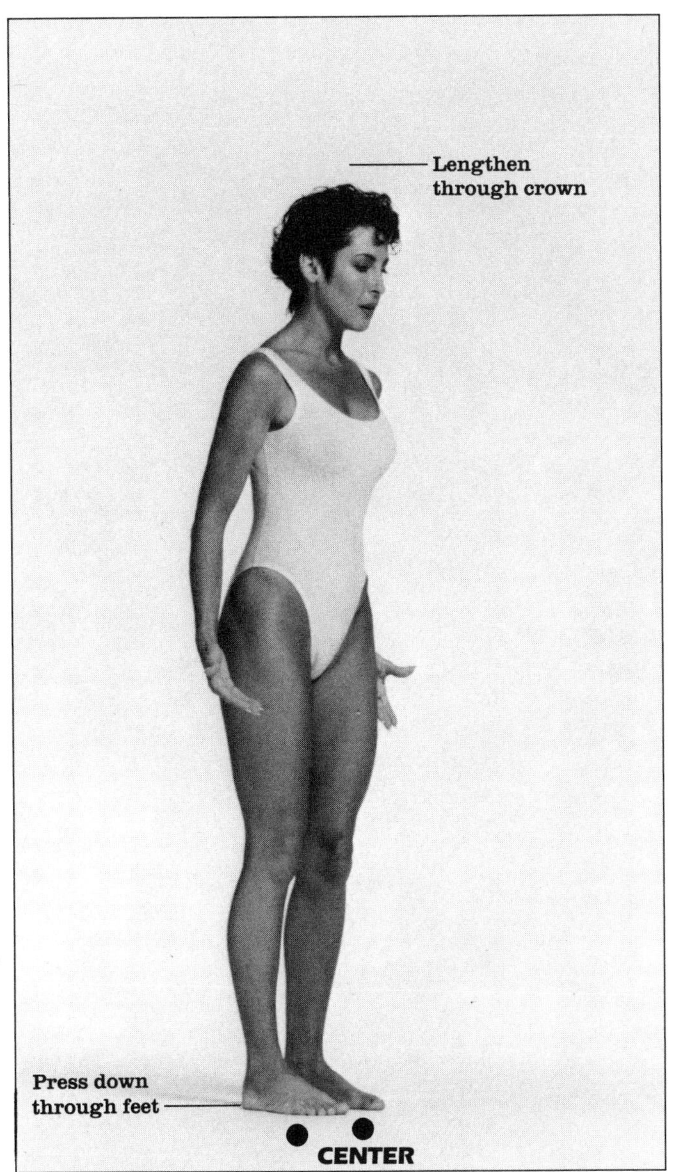

Exhale as you rise slowly, evenly, and sweep your arms down in front of you, returning fully to center. Even though the arm movements appear to be linear in the photographs, trace a full semicircle as you lower.

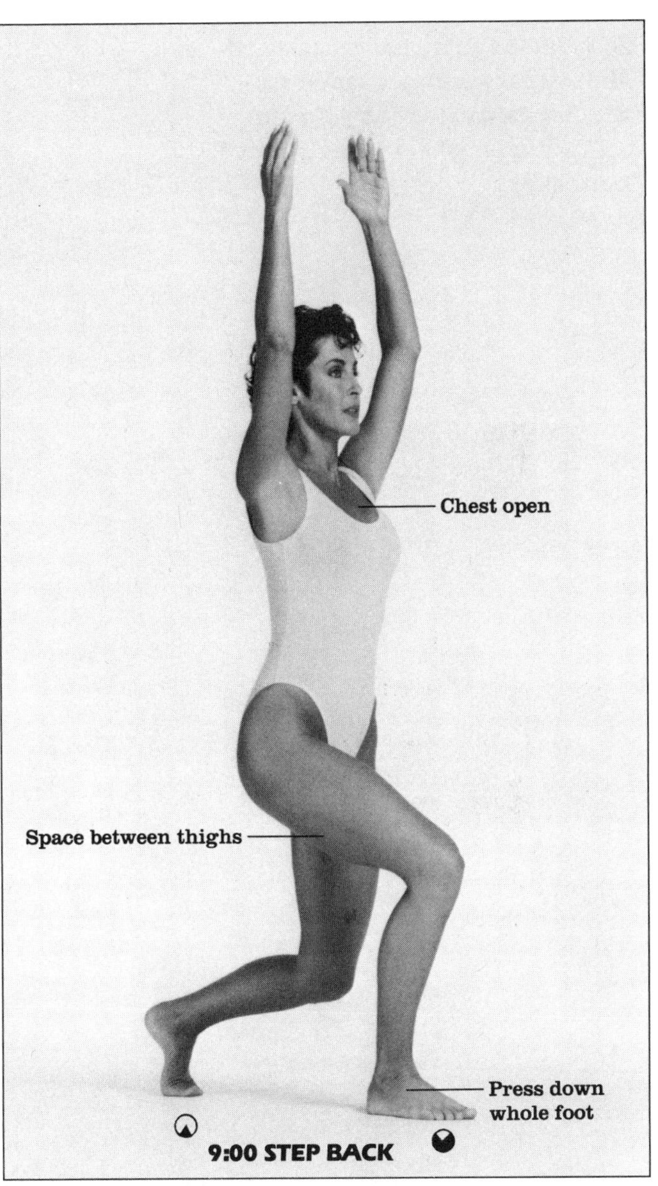

Repeat on the other side, stepping back onto the ball of your right foot at 5:00. Alternate left and right, lowering and rising at the same steady pace. Repeat 16 times altogether, stepping back 2 beats and coming center 2 beats.

YOUR BODY SHOULD FEEL A GENTLE WARMING, YOUR HEART RATE BEGINNING TO RISE.

The Whole-Body Stretch

BENEFITS: To increase back and abdominal strength, spine and hip flexibility, to tone your inner and outer thighs, to trim your buttocks.

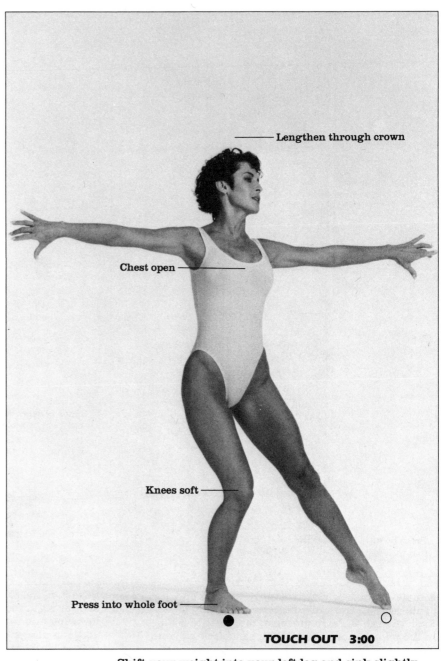

Shift your weight into your left leg and sink slightly as you inhale and, imagining sun on your chest, spread your arms wide to either side, reaching out with your right leg to touch your toes to 3:00. Feel the strength of your supporting leg.

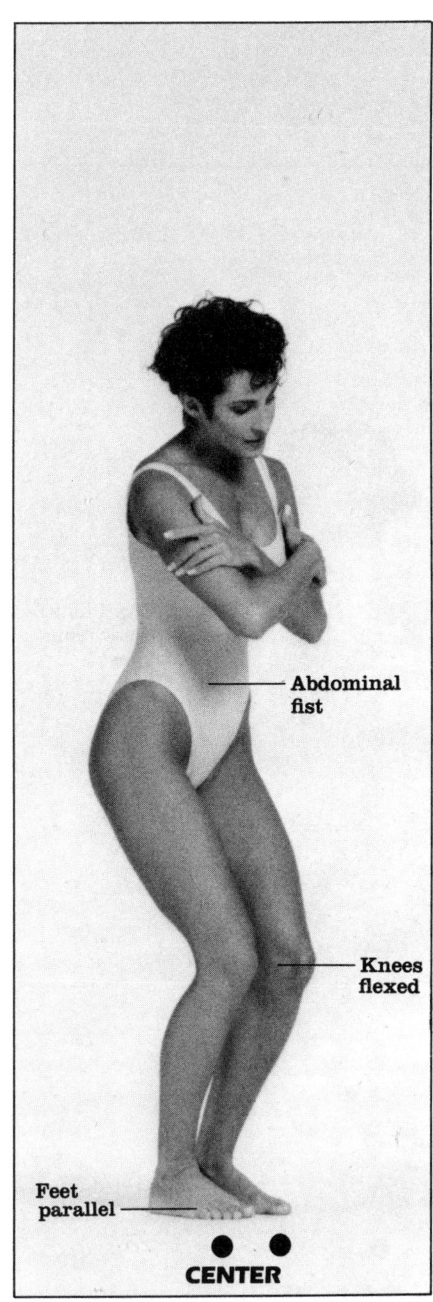

Imagining sun on your back, exhale as you bring your right leg back to center, contract, and hug yourself.

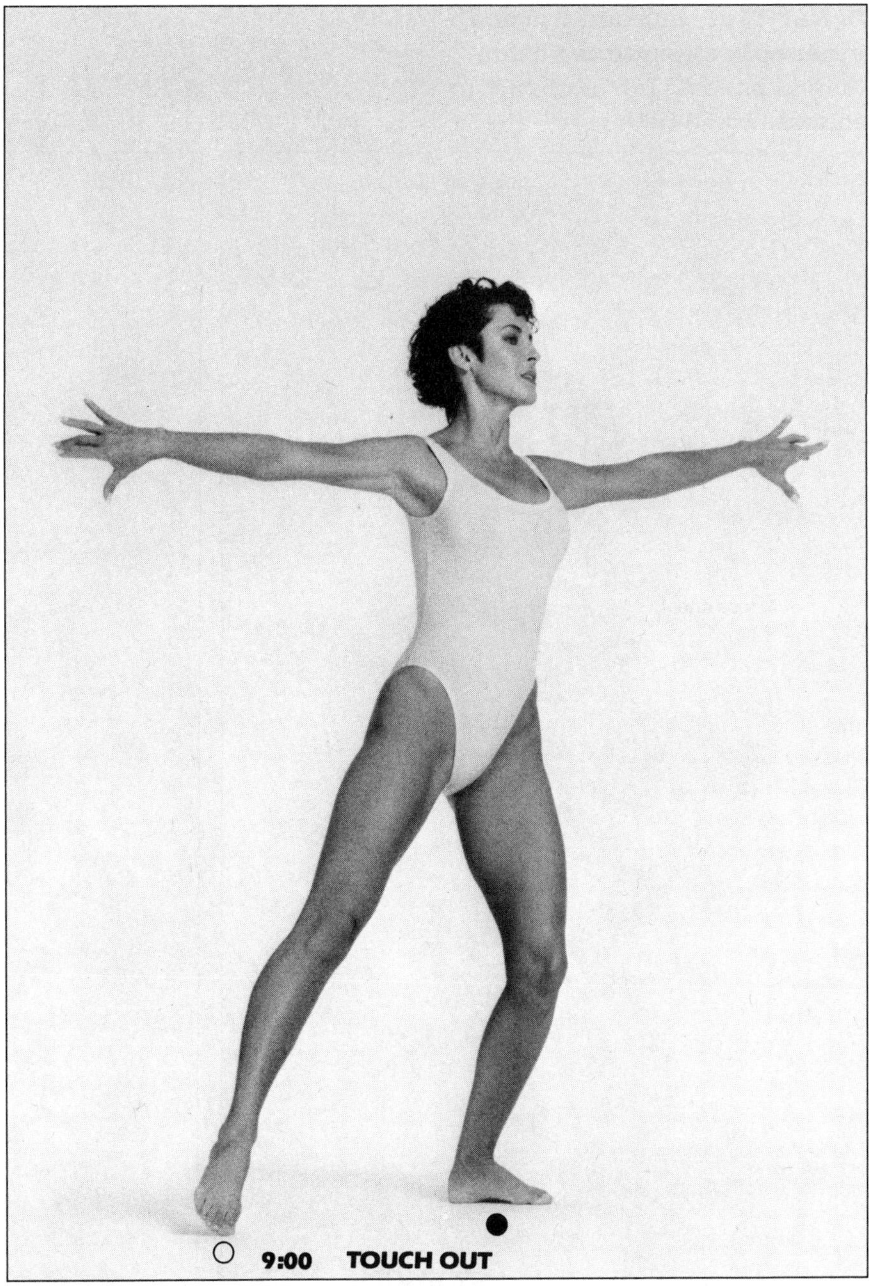

9:00 TOUCH OUT

Then inhale and touch left at 9:00. Alternate left and right, repeating 8 times on each side.

The Speed Walk

BENEFITS: To increase arm and upper body strength and definition, to promote hip flexibility, to enhance coordination.

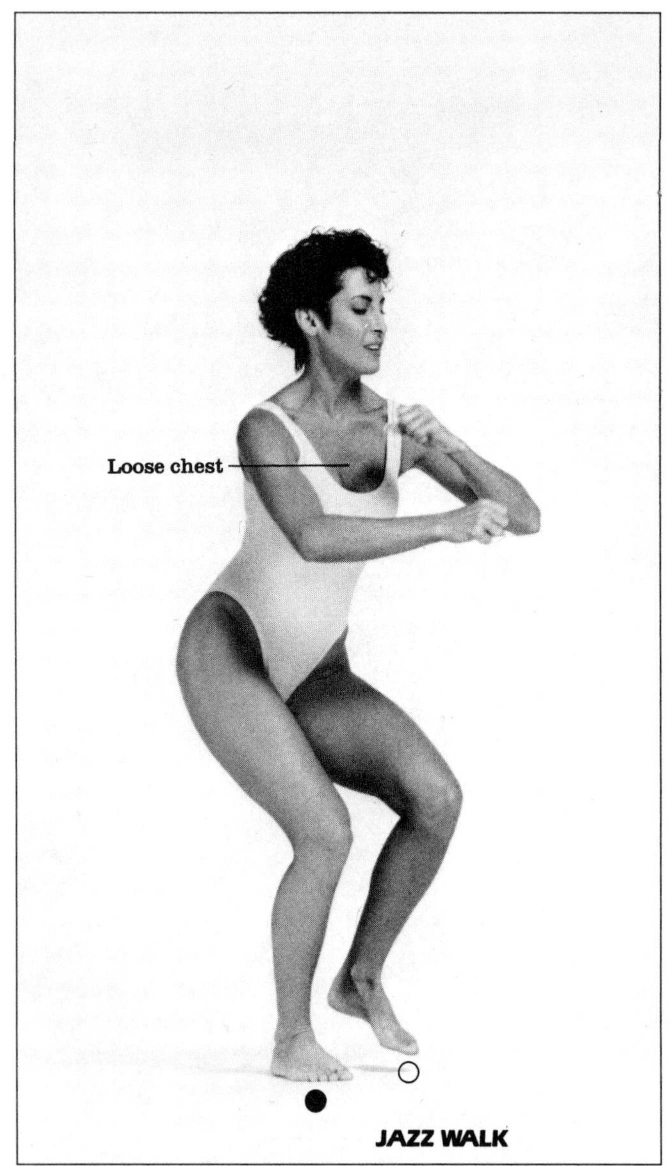

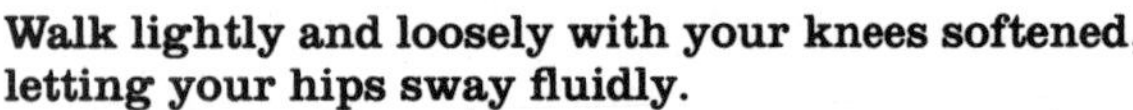
Walk lightly and loosely with your knees softened, letting your hips sway fluidly.

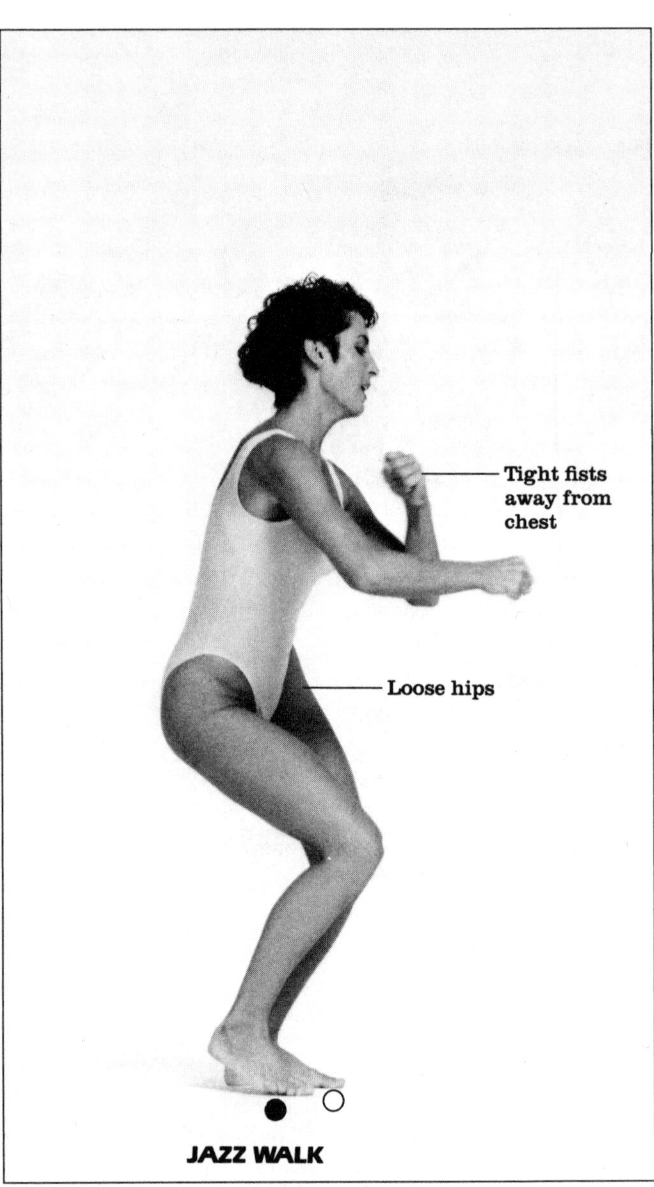

With your arms at shoulder level, rapidly circle your forearms, punching an imaginary bag. Counting with your right foot only, repeat 24 times. Inhale and exhale.

SINK 'N' PIVOT/TABLE WIPE

Torso Trimmer

BENEFITS: To extend your range of motion through your hips, to increase your spine and torso flexibility, to tone your buttocks, inner, and outer thighs, to create chest definition.

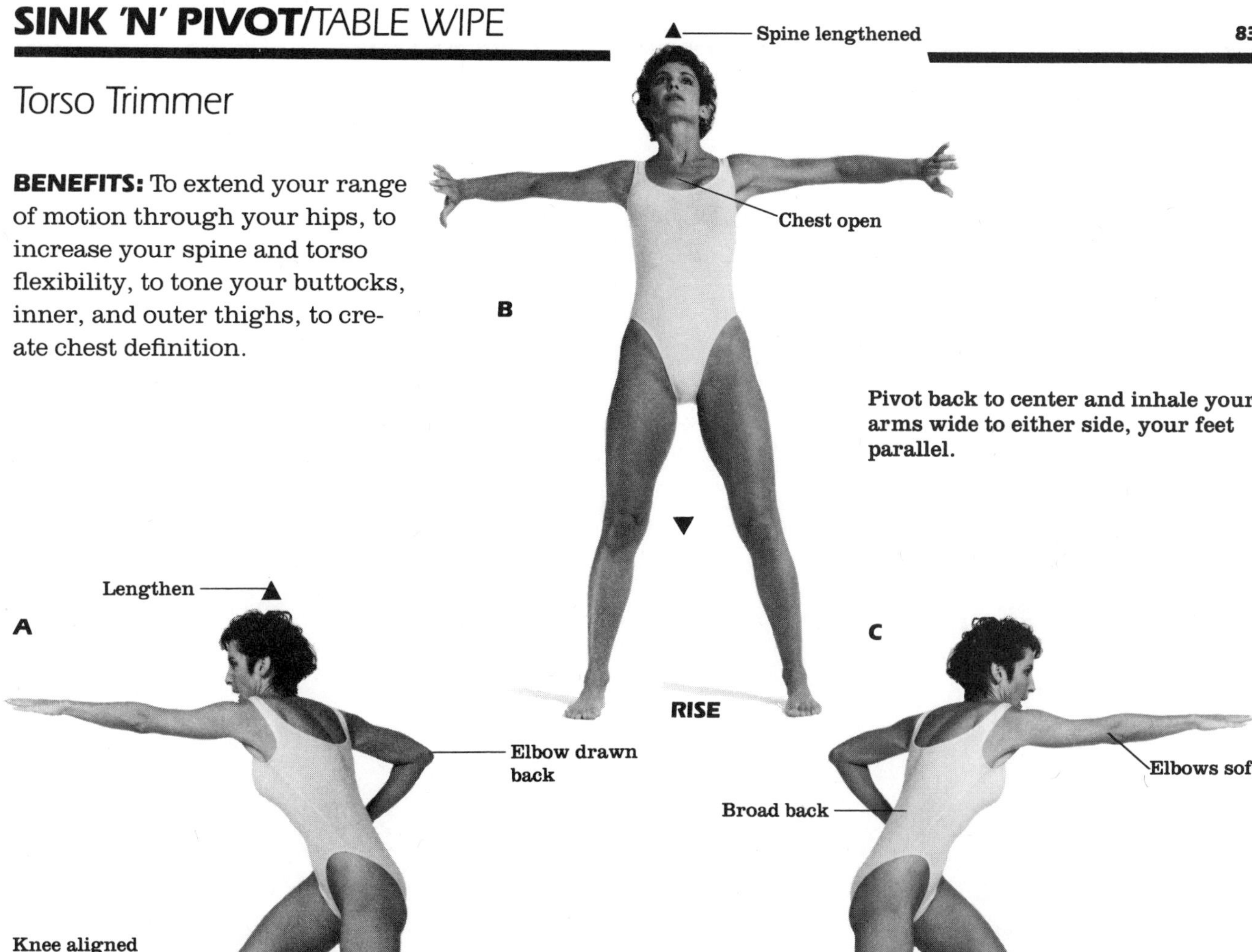

Pivot back to center and inhale your arms wide to either side, your feet parallel.

9:00 SINK-PIVOT

In your *A* stance, sink your weight into your left leg and pivot the ball of your right foot at 3:00. At the same time, exhale as you reach out wide with your right arm and wipe off an imaginary table at chest level, sweeping from right to left, your arm following the rotation of your torso. Pause.

SINK-PIVOT 3:00

Repeat on the other side, pivoting at 9:00. As you pivot, be careful not to *thrust* your hips into your supporting leg or you might strain your knees. If you feel pressure in the knee of your supporting leg, let your foot turn out, decrease the pivot of your free leg, be sure to finish your pivot with both feet turned slightly out, and turn more with your torso, less with your hips. Never turn a leg that has weight on it. Empty first by shifting your weight off the leg and then rotate. Continue alternating left and right, 8 times on each side.

Tummy Tightener

BENEFITS: To tighten your abdominals, to tone your frontal thighs, to increase the strength and flexibility of your upper body, to trim your torso, to whittle your waist.

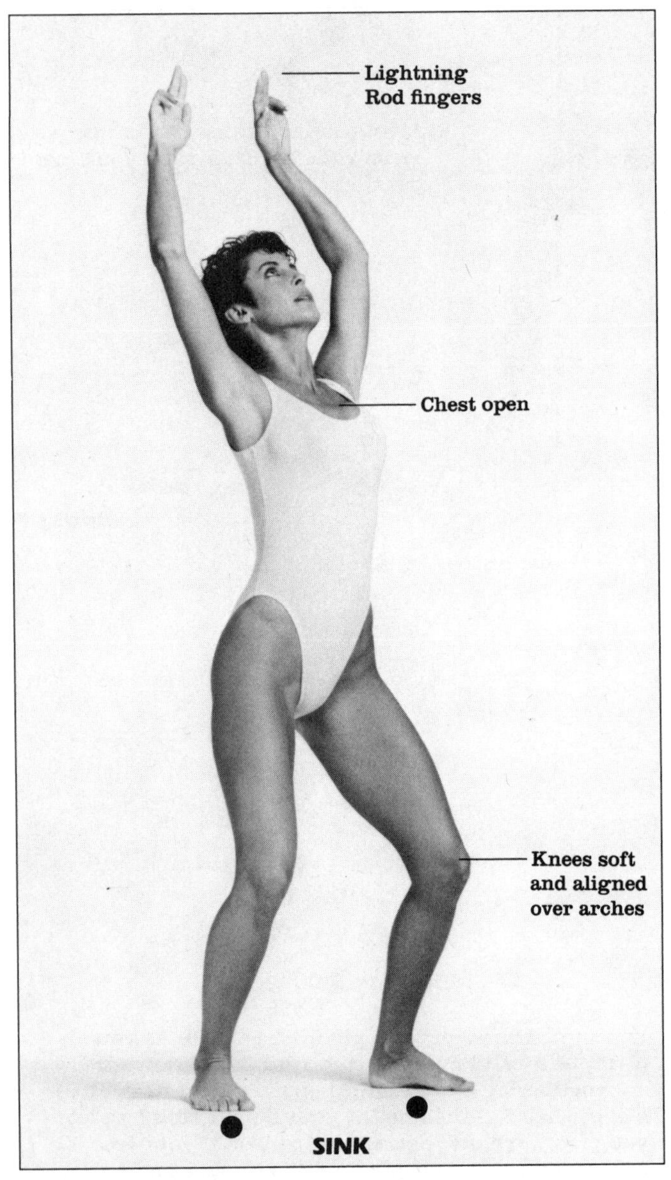

SINK

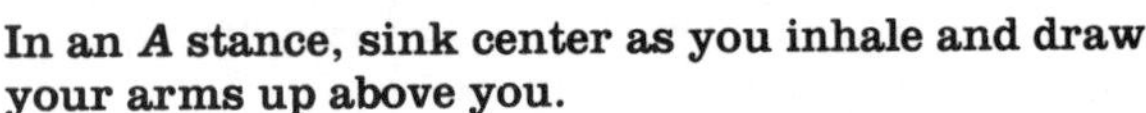
In an *A* stance, sink center as you inhale and draw your arms up above you.

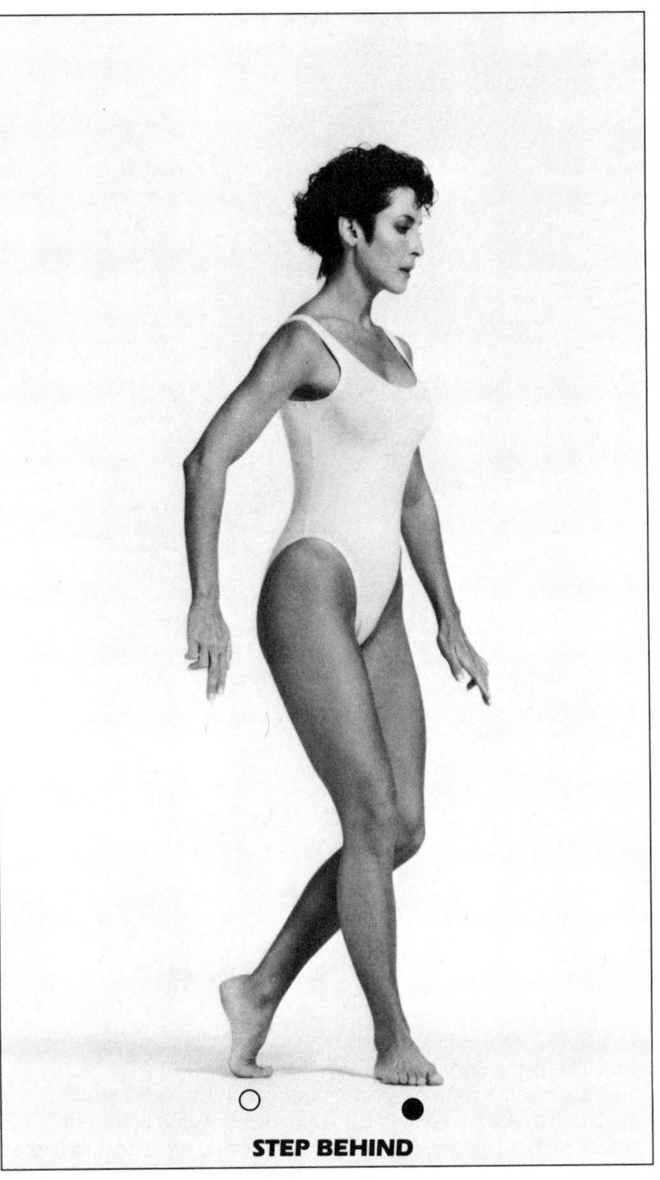

STEP BEHIND

Shift into your left leg and cross your right foot behind, your arms beginning to float back down.

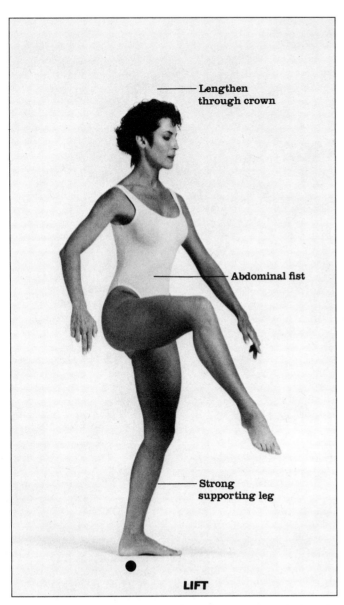

LIFT

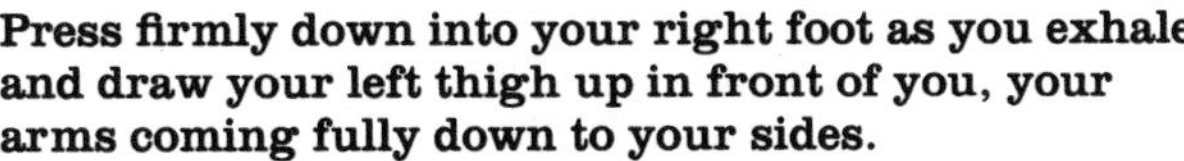

Press firmly down into your right foot as you exhale and draw your left thigh up in front of you, your arms coming fully down to your sides.

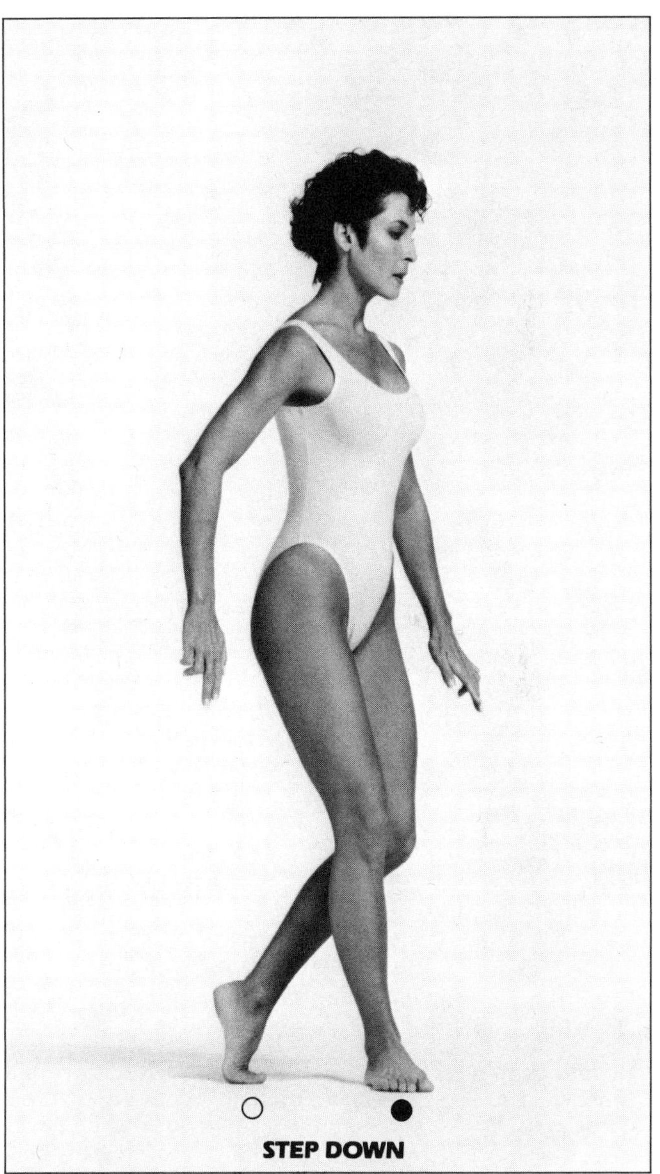

STEP DOWN

Step back down with your left foot and out with your right foot to your *A* stance. Repeat to the other side and alternate for a total of 16 on each side, counting 1–2 through center, 3 for the cross and lift, and 4 for the step back down.

Thigh Trimmer

BENEFITS: To strengthen and tone your thighs, calves, hips, buttocks, and upper back, to define and stretch your chest, to firm your abdominals.

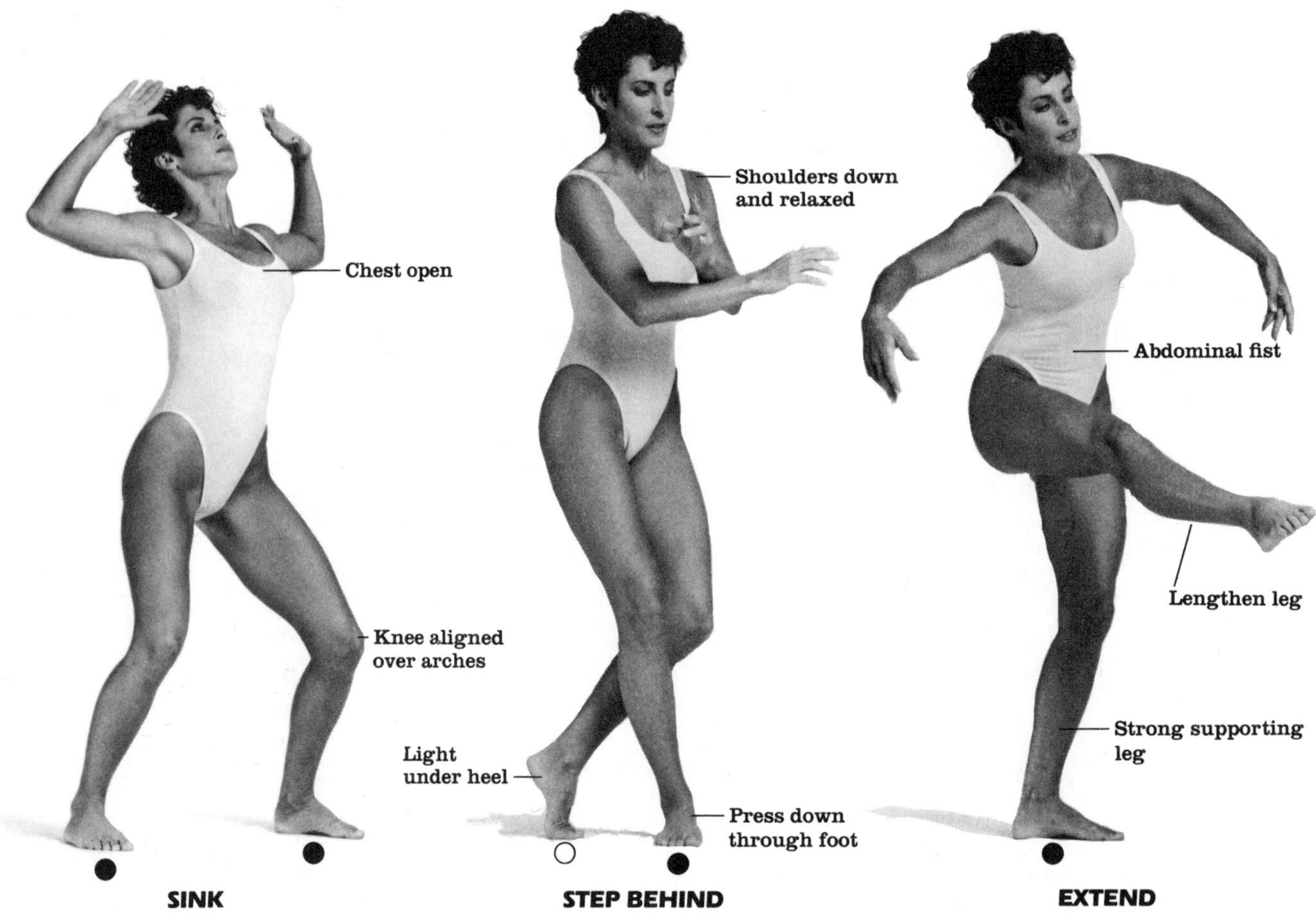

In your *A* stance, sink center as you inhale and draw your elbows back, chest wide.

Shift onto your left leg and cross your right foot behind, drawing your arms down in front of you and crossing at the wrists.

Pressing into the whole of your right foot, exhale and contract your abdomen to protect your lower back as you gracefully extend your left leg up in front, squeezing your thigh bone with your muscles and using the support of your back leg to generate the movement. As your leg comes up, sweep your arms elegantly out and back.

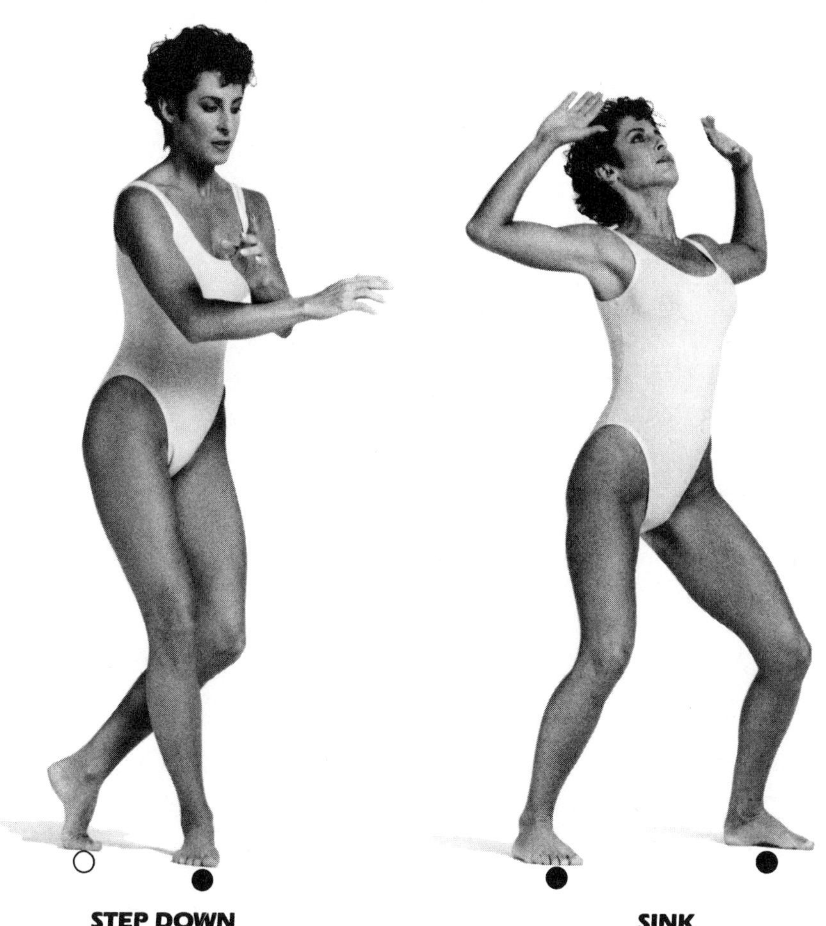

STEP DOWN

SINK

Step back down and then out to your *A* stance. Repeat on the other side. Continue for a total of 16 on each side.

RECHARGE
JAZZ WALK

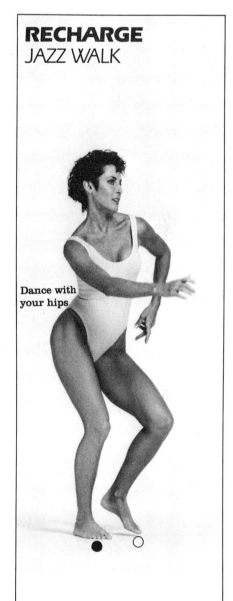

Repeat the Jazz Walk 16 to 24 times with your arms hanging loosely at your sides.
Body Check: Ease up or put more into your motion at this point. Breathe.

Leg Leaner

BENEFITS: To increase your ankle flexibility and strength, to tone your calves, to trim your thighs and buttocks, to enhance your coordination, to stretch your Achilles tendon, to define your shoulders, upper back, and chest.

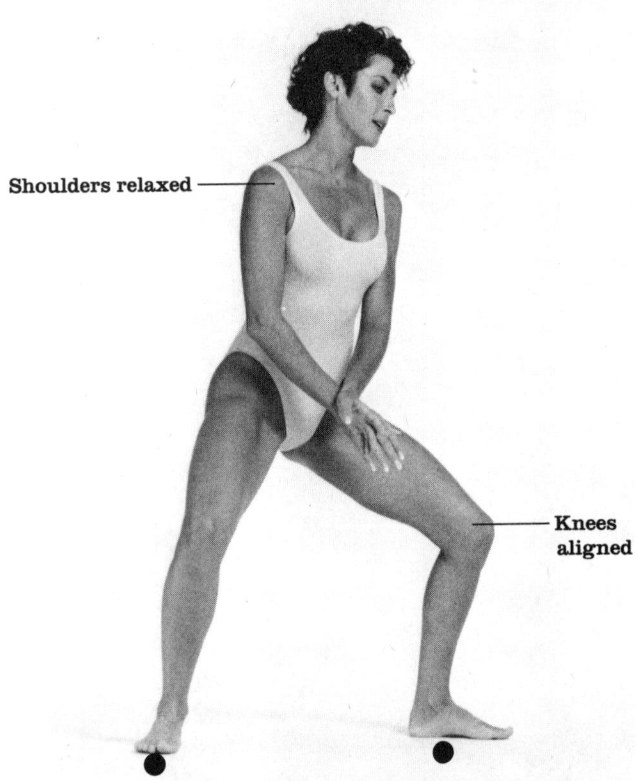

In your *A* stance, sink slightly, your weight evenly distributed through your feet as your arms relax down and cross at the wrists.

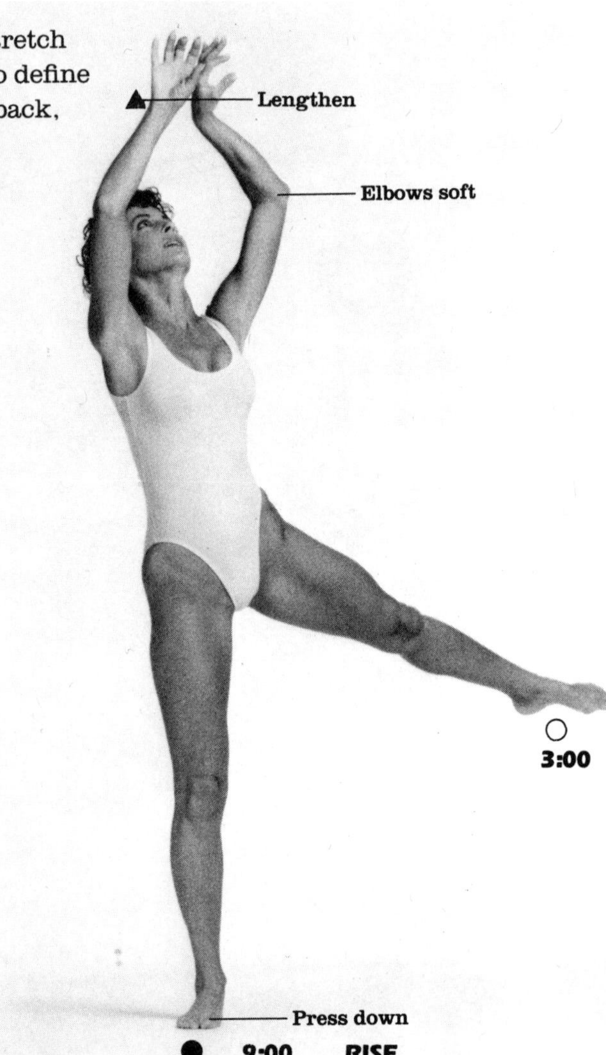

Shift your weight into your left leg at 9:00. Press down through your foot and rise up tall as you inhale and lift your right leg up over 3:00, sweeping your arms out wide to either side and tapping your wrists high above your head. Let your arms be willowy and loose.

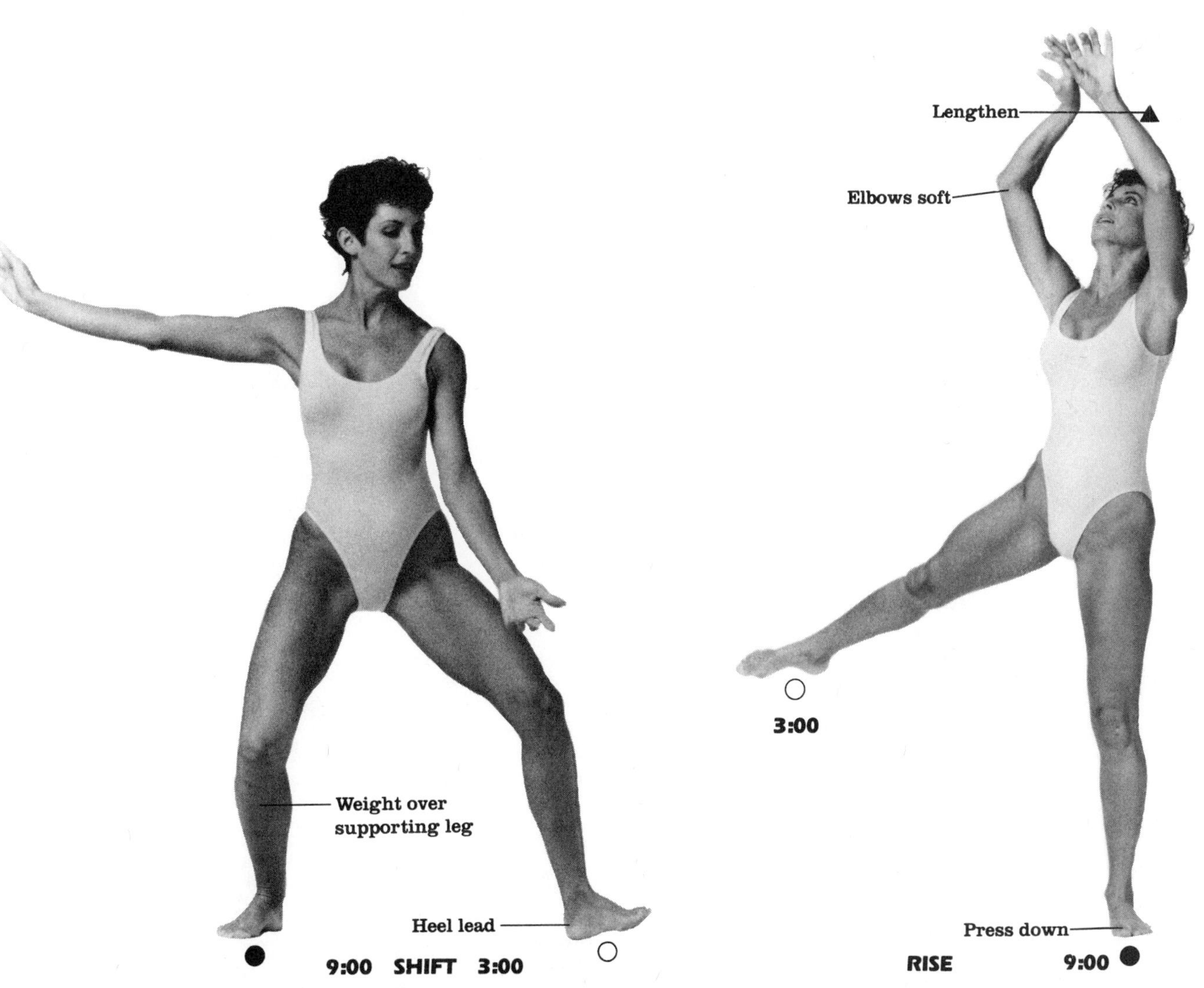

Exhale a rich sound as you sink and shift back fully through center. Inhale as you rise up over your right leg at 3:00, lengthen and lift your leg over 9:00. When rising, don't jerk, but really use the power of your feet and legs to push away from the floor. Rise and sink at an even pace to ensure muscle balance. To keep your knees from thrusting forward when you sink, imagine sitting on a high stool and make sure you can lift your toes. The power of the motion starts in your feet and is generated by the strength of your thighs and buttocks; it should not be felt in your knees. Repeat 16 times, alternating left and right, counting 2 beats down and 2 beats up. To lighten, tap your free leg to the side instead of lifting.

Shift your weight into your right leg at 3:00. Press down through your foot and rise up tall as you inhale and lift your left leg up over 9:00, sweeping your arms out wide to either side and tapping your wrists high above your head. Let your arms be willowy and loose.

The Whole-Body Slimmer

BENEFITS: To stretch the sides of your body, to trim your waist, to tone your shoulders and chest, to tone and trim your calves, thighs, abdominals, and buttocks, to strengthen and increase the flexibility of your feet and ankles, to enhance your balance.

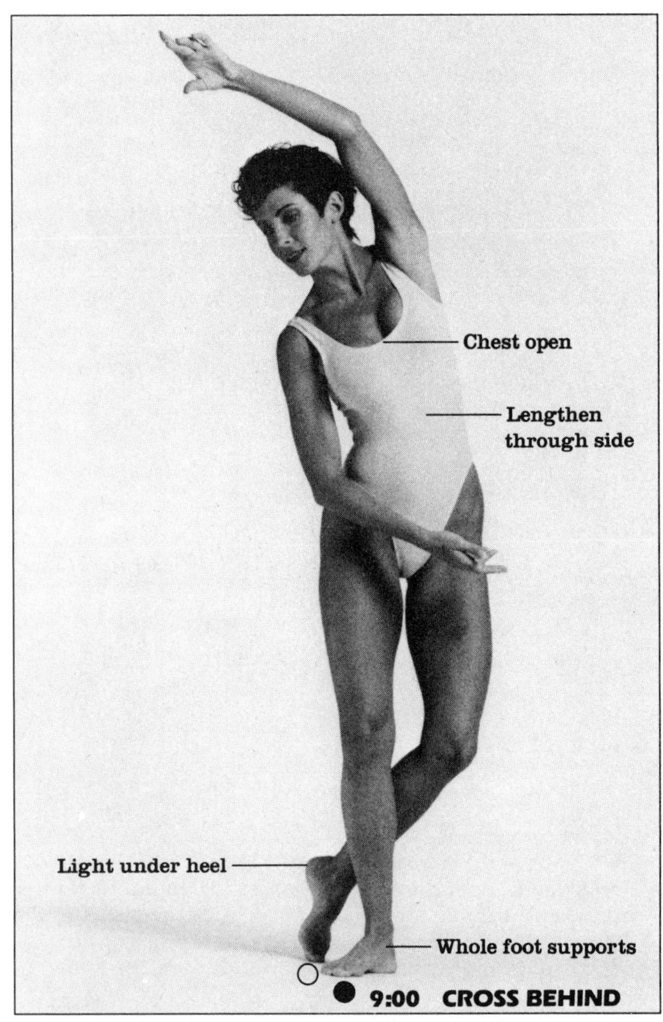

9:00 CROSS BEHIND

Still rising and sinking in one continuous, fluid motion, inhale, rise up at 9:00, and cross your right foot closely behind your left. To add the arms, imagine wiping your hands along the inside edges of a large hula hoop suspended directly in front of you. As you cross your right foot behind, your right arm wipes up and your left arm wipes down.

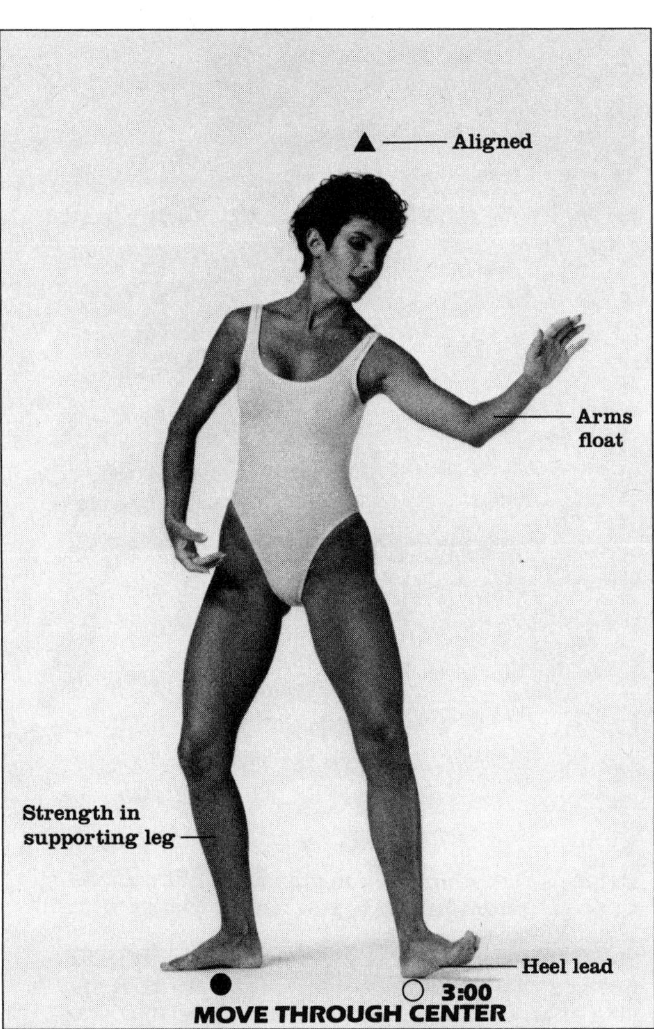

3:00 MOVE THROUGH CENTER

Exhaling a deep sound and scooping in your abdomen, sink back through center leading with your heel and step out at 3:00, your right arm wiping down, your left arm wiping up.

RECHARGE
JAZZ WALK

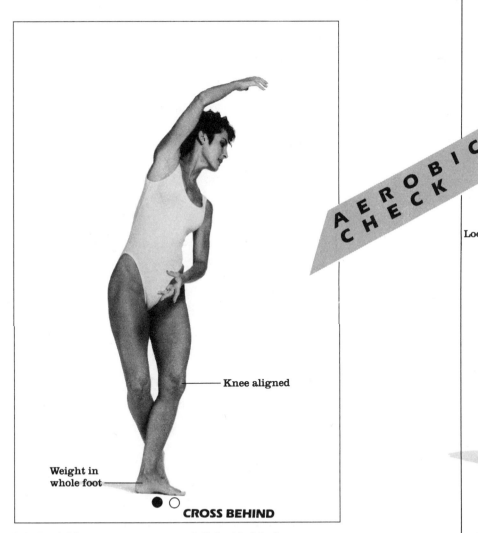

CROSS BEHIND

Inhale richly as you cross your left foot behind your right. Now your left arm wipes all the way up and your right arm wipes all the way down. Alternate left and right, really using your deep exhalation to tone your abdomen, your inhalation to recharge your body with oxygen. Repeat 16 times altogether.

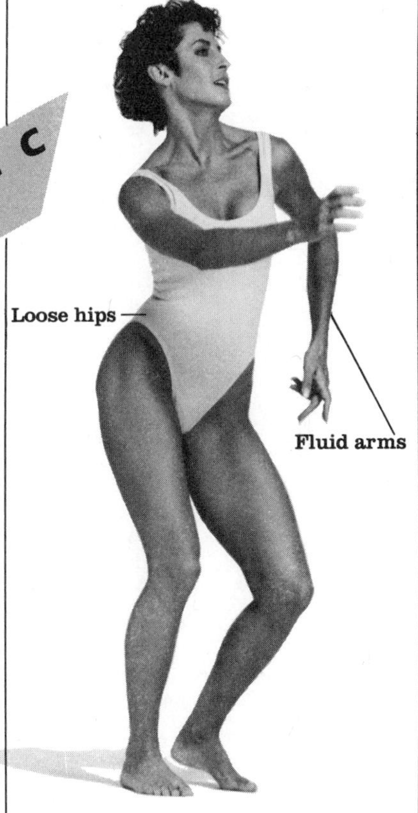

Repeat 16 to 24 times, counting 1-2-3-one, 1-2-3-two, and so on and letting your arms sway naturally. **Body Check:** Are you breathing? Breath is a wonderful recharge.

The Karate Dance

BENEFITS: To enhance your coordination, to stretch and strengthen your back, to tighten your abdominals, to firm and stretch your buttocks and hamstrings.

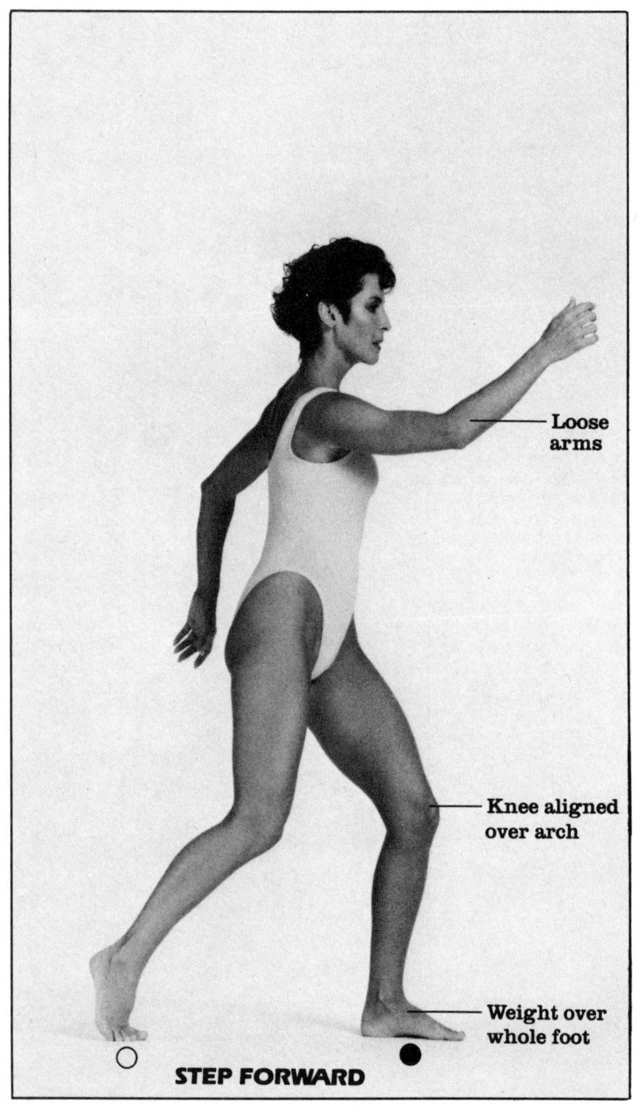

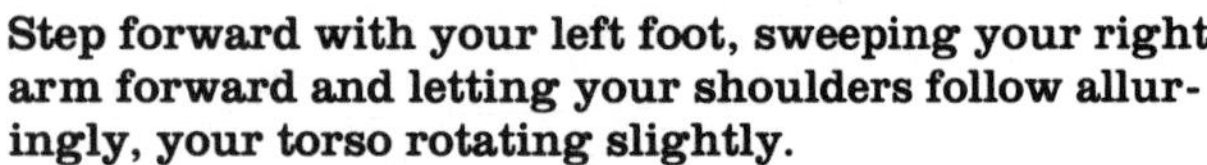

Step forward with your left foot, sweeping your right arm forward and letting your shoulders follow alluringly, your torso rotating slightly.

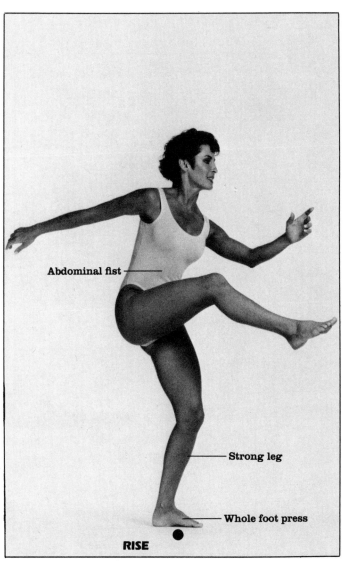

Draw your right knee up toward your chest as you exhale "Yeet!" and sweep your left arm forward.

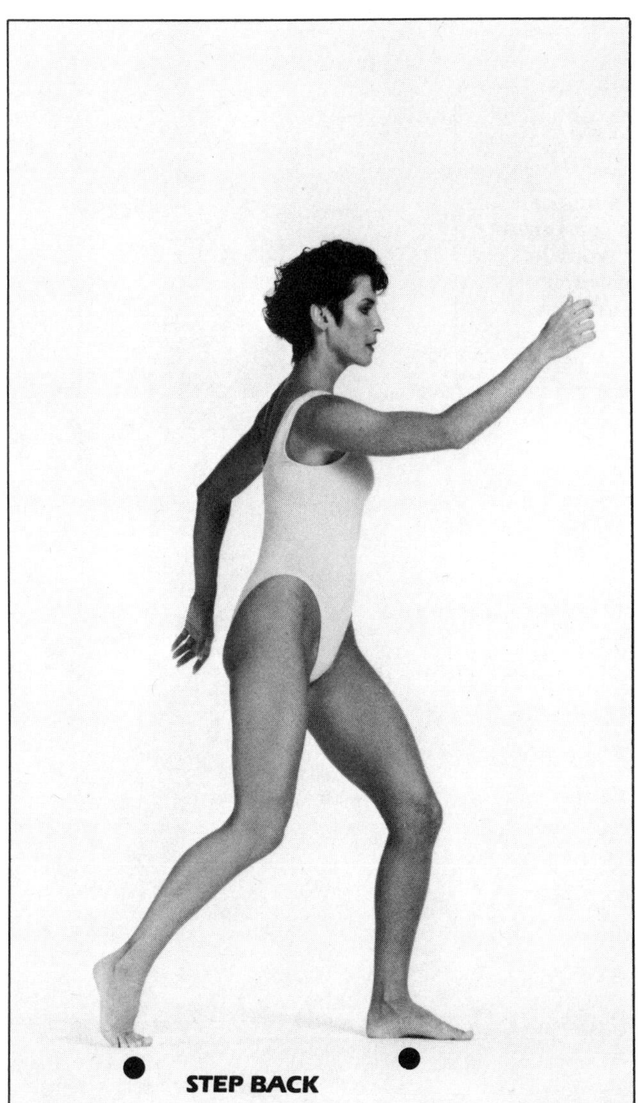

Step back to center with your right leg, changing arms—

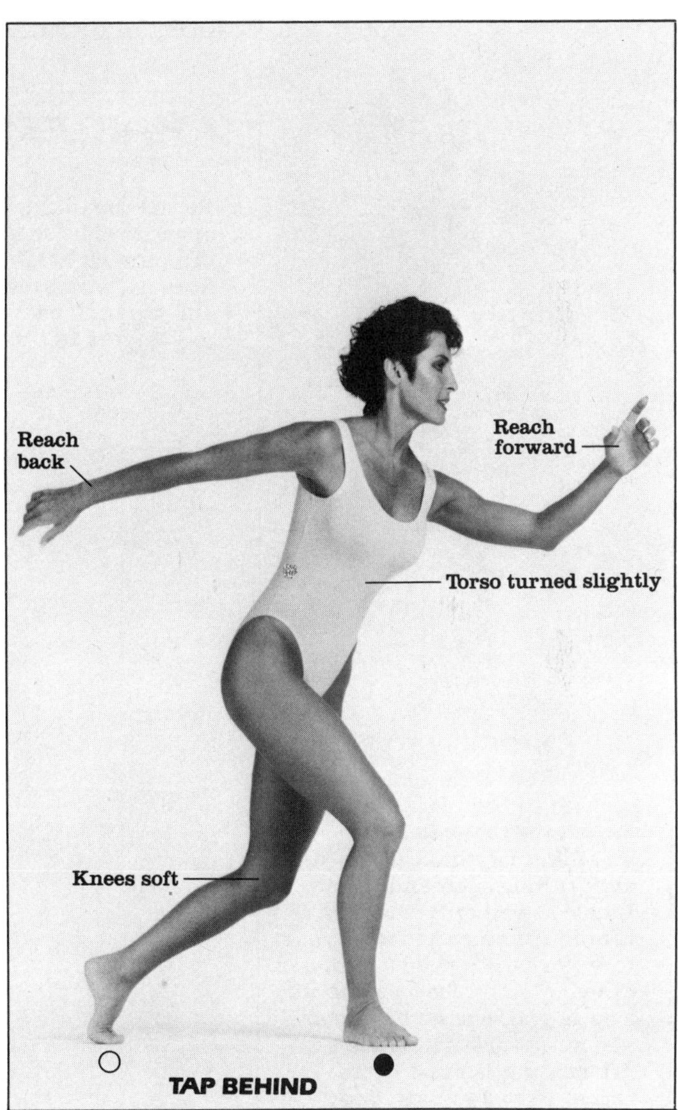

—and tap behind with your left toes, reaching out with your left arm.

Step forward again with your left foot, repeat the knee lift, and continue. Once you settle into the rhythm of the movement, let yourself dance back and powerhouse forward. Repeat front and back for a total of 16 times, more if you feel snappy.

Fun Firmer

BENEFITS: To tone your hips, buttocks, thighs, back, and chest, to increase your spine flexibility, to enhance your balance and coordination.

RECHARGE
CROSS BEHIND

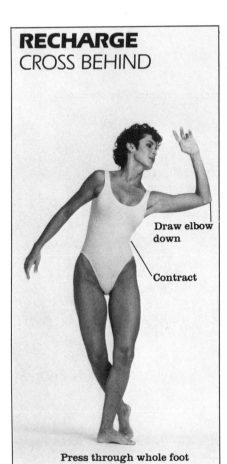

Draw elbow down

Contract

Press through whole foot

Repeat the Cross Behind, breathing rhythmically as you shift through left and right. Inhale as you cross one foot behind the other and wipe your forearm across your forehead, drawing your elbows out to the side as you release. Exhale as you move through center. Alternating left and right, repeat 16 to 24 times. **Body Check:** If your legs are tired, lighten up and put more into your arm and torso movement. Breathe. Then transit fluidly into the Charleston.

CHARLESTON

Repeat the Charleston on the opposite side, so that you begin stepping right. Draw your left knee up, step back to center, and tap back with your right toe. Repeat 16 times.

A

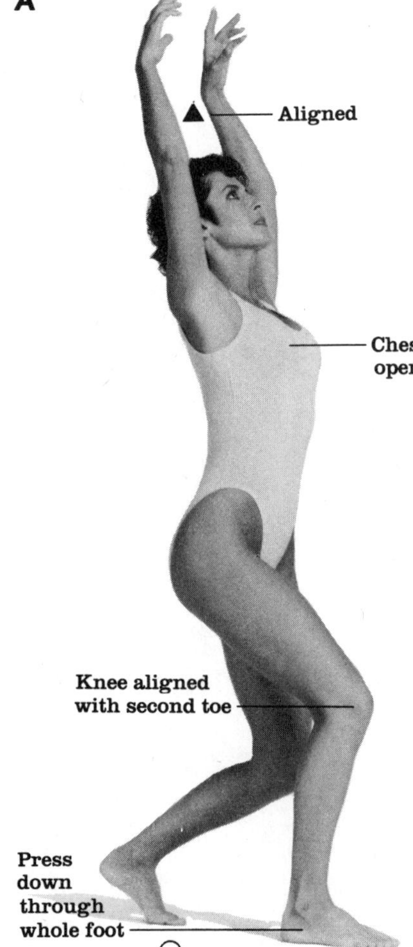

STEP FRONT 1:00

Step out through your right heel to 1:00 and sink slightly into your right leg, inhaling and scooping your arms up above your head.

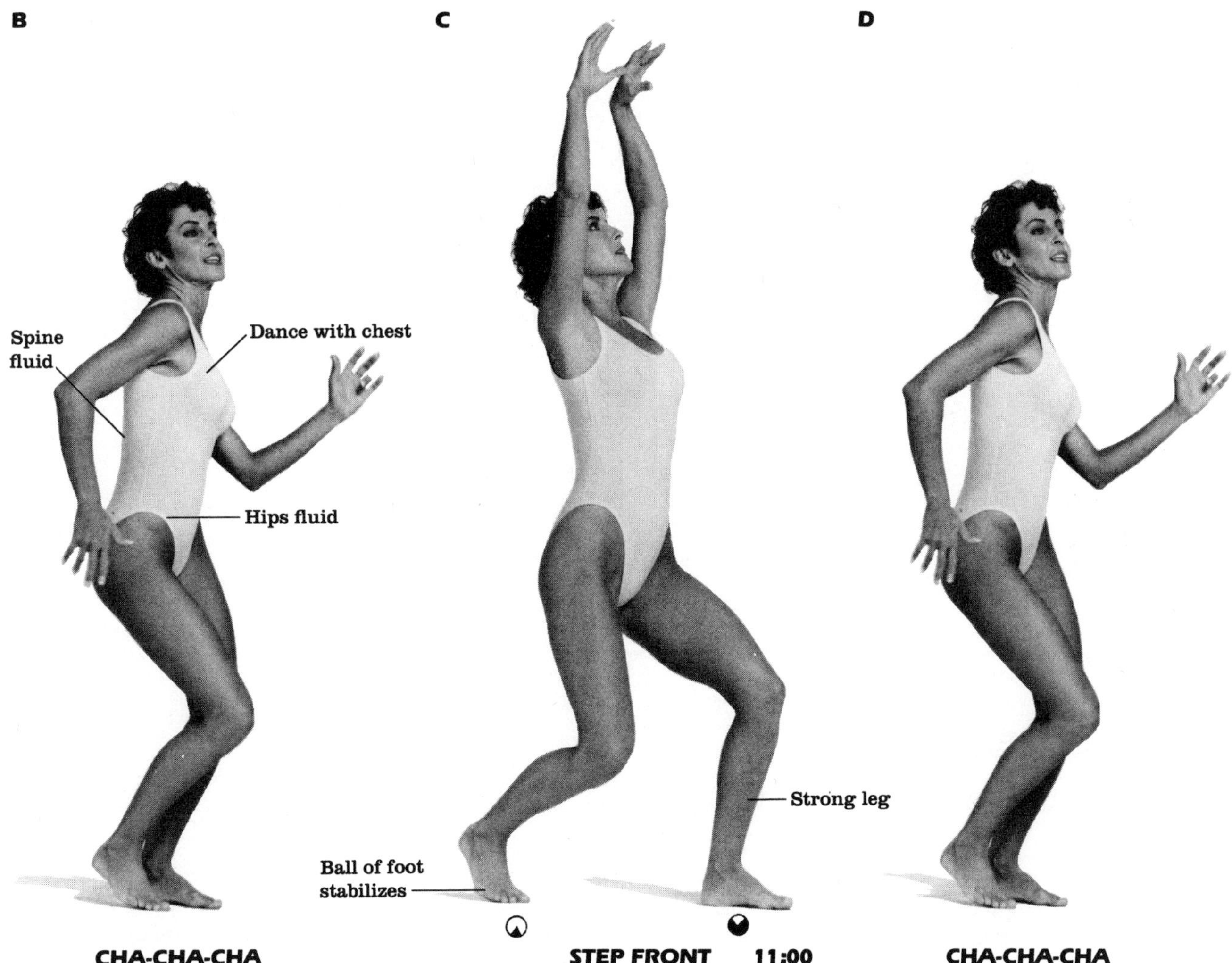

CHA-CHA-CHA

Then push away and scoop your arms down as you step back to center and then cha-cha-cha, walking in place, right, left, right, and letting your hips swish, your arms sway as you exhale.

STEP FRONT 11:00

Step out through your left heel to 11:00 and inhale and scoop your arms up as you sink slightly into your left leg—

CHA-CHA-CHA

—push away and step back to center and then cha-cha-cha, left, right, left. Repeat 8 times on each side and then continue, stepping right to 3:00, center cha-cha-cha, stepping left to 9:00, center cha-cha-cha, for another 8 times on each side.

RECHARGE
SINK 'N' RISE

Shifting side to side and moving through center, lift your free leg back on a diagonal on the rise, pointing over 7:00 with your left toes and then over 5:00 with your right toes. Let your arms smoothly follow the motion, reaching left, then lowering, and reaching right. Inhale on the rise; exhale on the sink. Repeat 16 to 24 times on each side.

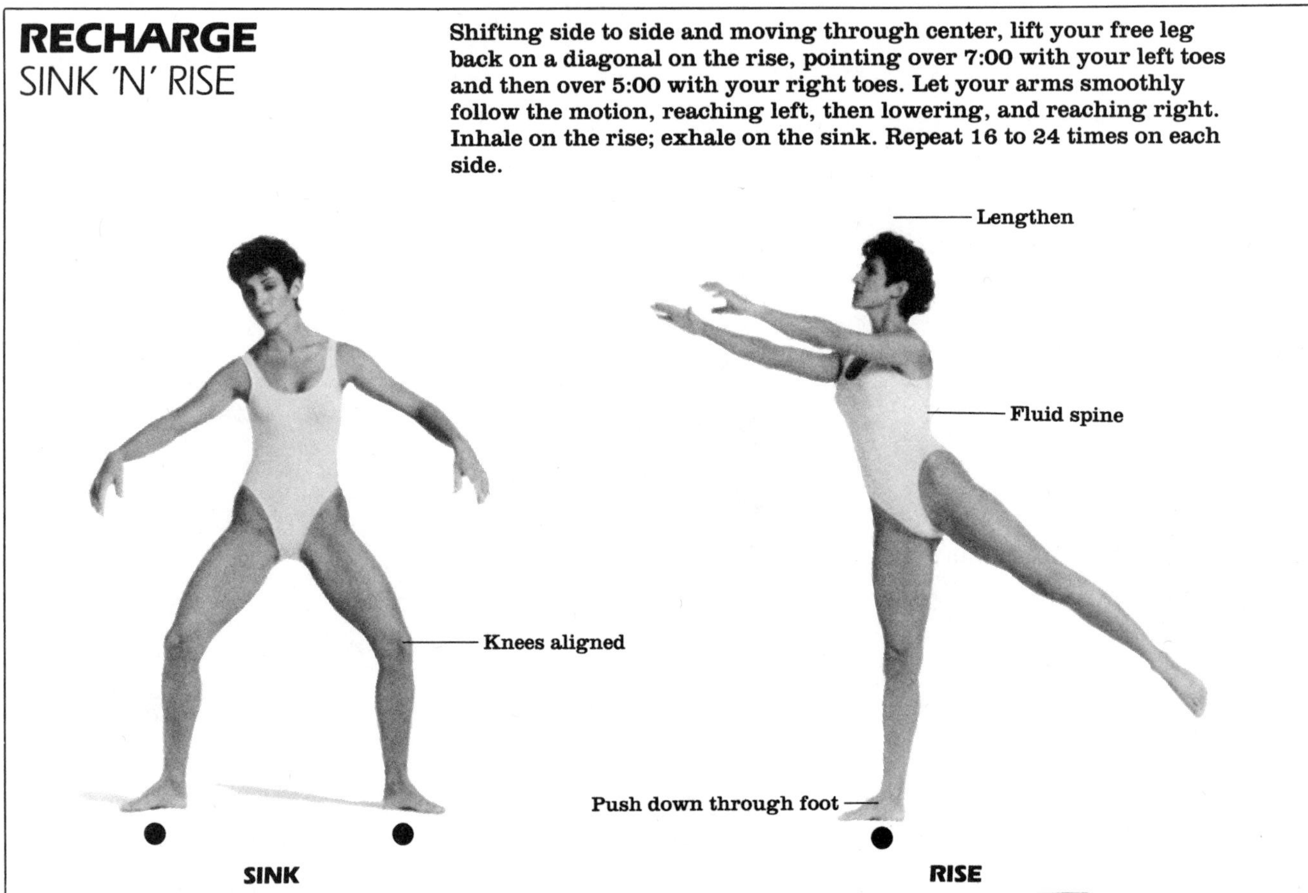

Design Options

CONGRATULATIONS! YOU'VE DONE A GREAT JOB!

- If you're new to exercise and feel like you've done enough work for today, skip over to the Aerobic Check, page 108, and Ease-Out.
- If you want just a little more work, but not a whole lot, go back and repeat, starting with the Step-Back/Touchdown. After the Charleston, go to the Aerobic Check and Ease-Out. If you can, work a little deeper on the rerun, sinking a bit lower, rising a bit higher, reaching a bit farther.
- If you're still feeling pretty snappy, come along for the next part.
- If you feel like you're just getting started and have a whole lot left, go back to the Step-Back/Touchdown and rework the first part as deeply as possible while still staying within your comfort zone. Then finish up by joining us for the next part.

Whatever your choice, give yourself a mental pat on the back for the work you've done. It makes all the difference in training your mind to want to come back tomorrow.

RECHARGE
CROSS BEHIND

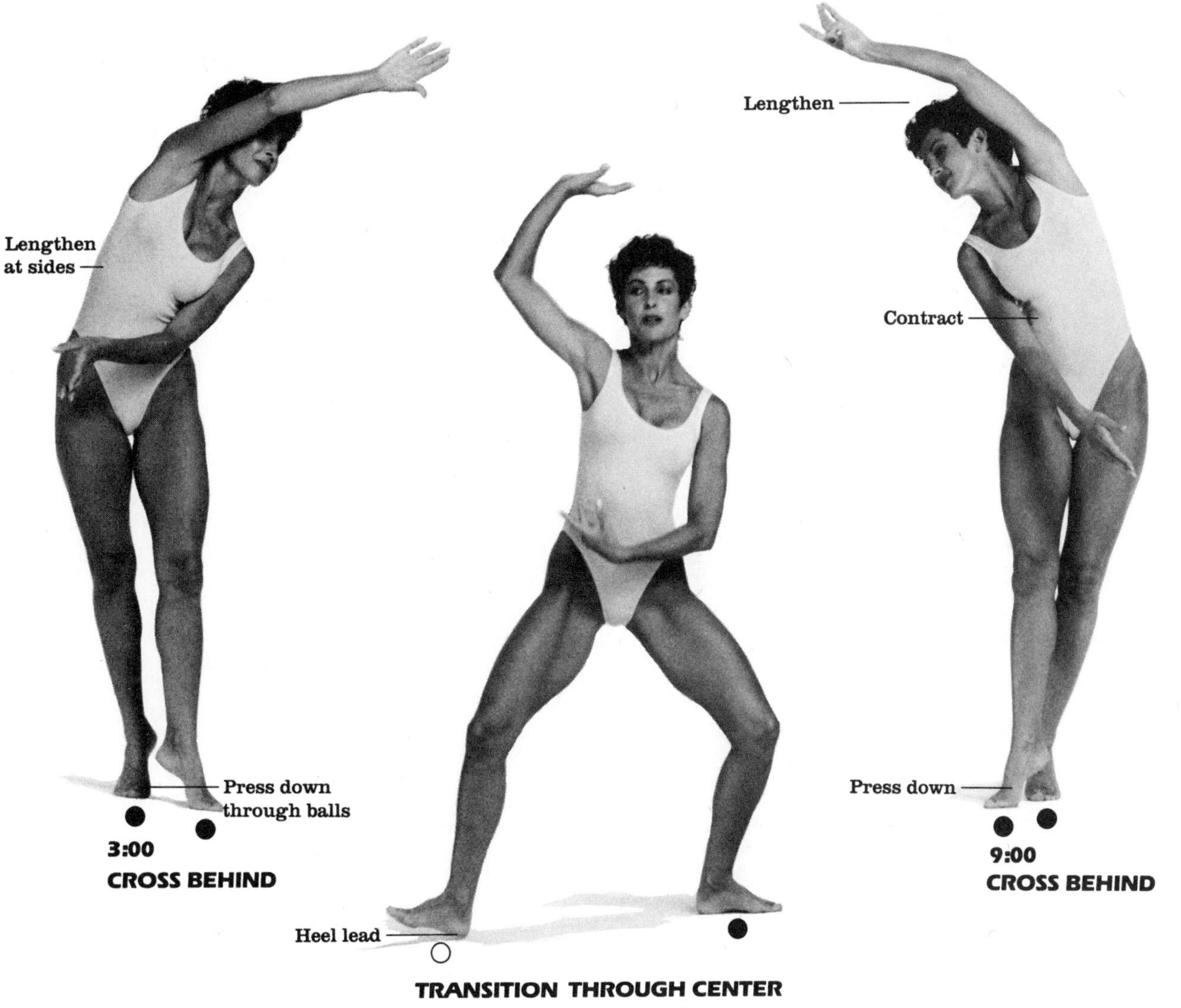

Lengthen

Lengthen at sides

Contract

Press down through balls

Press down

3:00
CROSS BEHIND

9:00
CROSS BEHIND

Heel lead

TRANSITION THROUGH CENTER

Repeat the Cross Behind 8 times in a rhythmic fashion, with a Hula Hoop Wipe, rising high on the balls of your feet. Exhale through center, inhale on the cross behind. **Body Check:** If your arms are tired, work in a smaller range, closer to your body. Breathe.

Abs Away

BENEFITS: To firm and flatten your abdominals, to tone your arms and chest, to strengthen and stretch your torso, to increase your spine flexibility, to trim and strengthen your thighs and buttocks, to stretch your calves and Achilles tendon, to strengthen your legs.

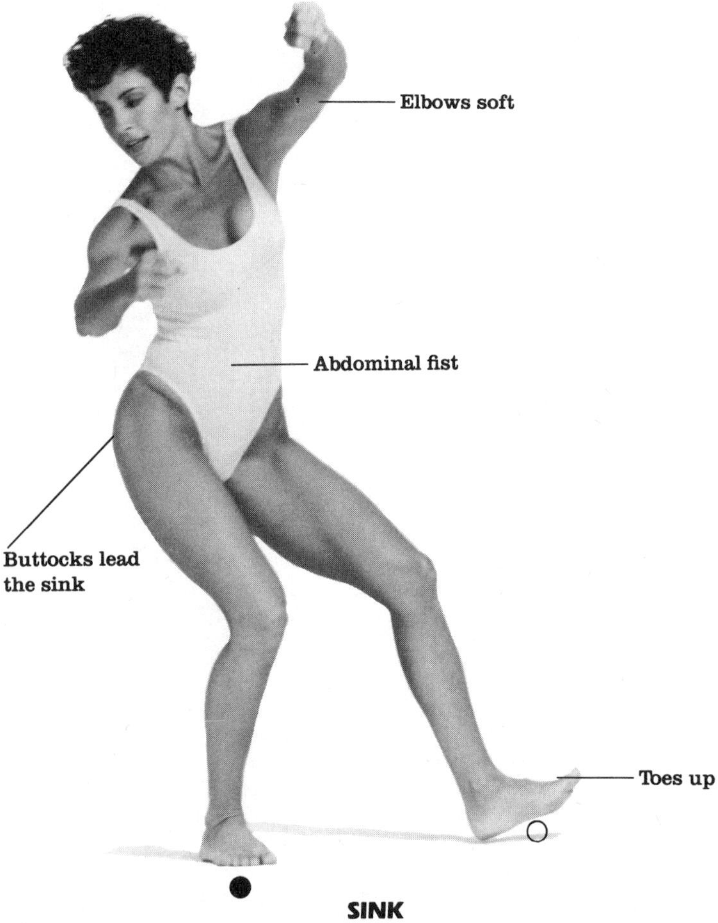

Elbows soft

Abdominal fist

Buttocks lead the sink

Toes up

SINK

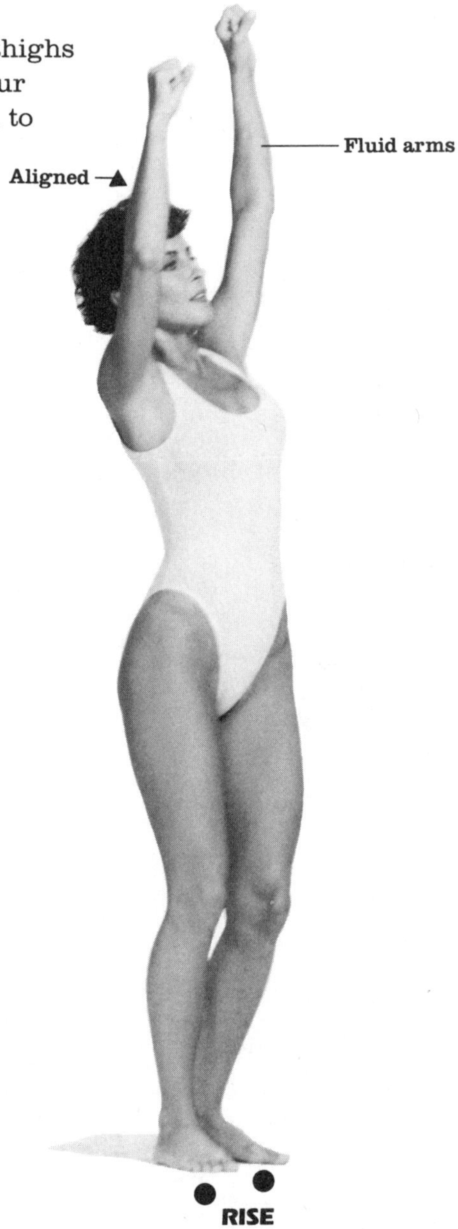

Aligned

Fluid arms

RISE

Still shifting lyrically side to side, alternately touch your left heel to 11:00 and your right heel to 1:00. Inhale and rise fully through center; exhale as you sink and touch with your heel. Repeat, touching left and right, feeling the continuity of your movement, and when you've got the rhythm down, add the arms. Pretend that you're holding a long paddle and imagine tracing figure eights—

—as you sweep it up—

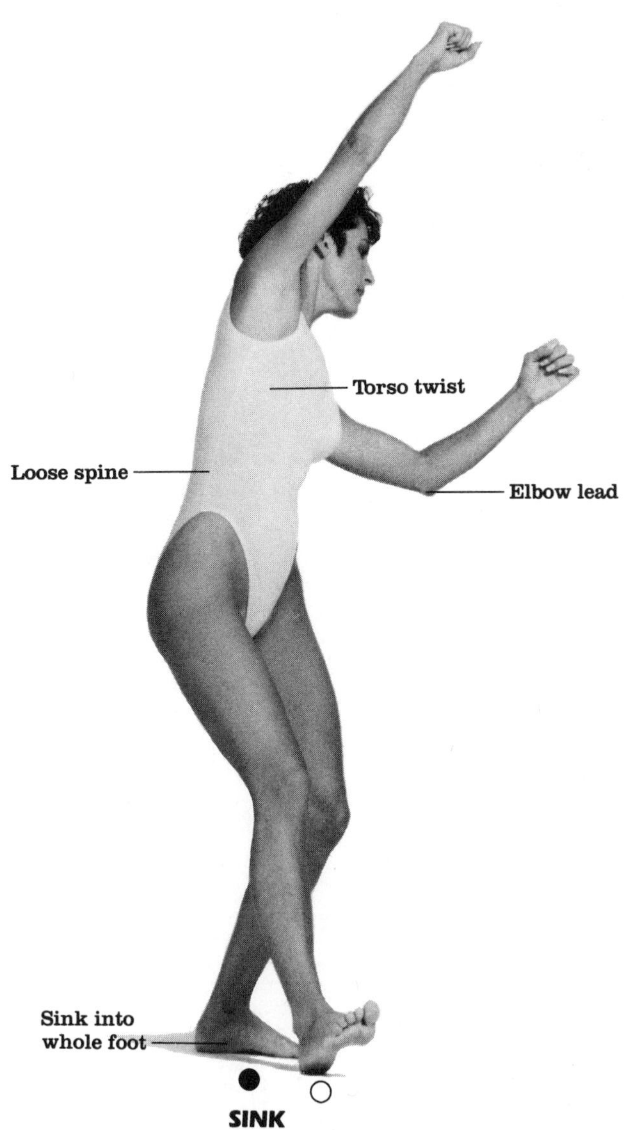

SINK

—and then scoop down so that it's next to your hip as you sink into your supporting leg. Let your torso lead the movement, gently twisting at your waist (not your hips!). By keeping the rotation in your waist, you'll protect your knees from the torquing that can occur if you push through with your hips. Your right shoulder rotates forward as your right foot touches front—and vice versa. Repeat 16 times on each side.

RECHARGE
JAZZ WALK

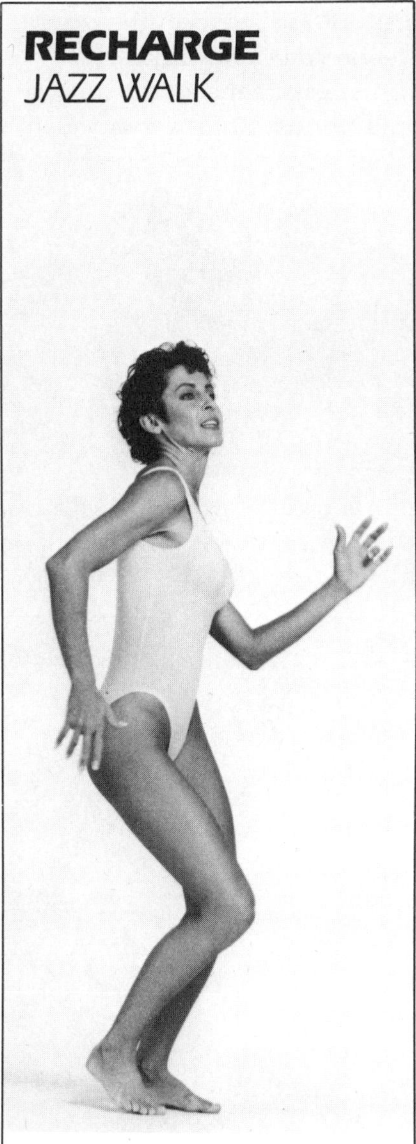

Walk lightly and loosely to a count of 16 to 24, leading with the ball of your foot and letting your hips sway fluidly.

Body Check: If your lower back feels tight, breathe, use your abdominals to round your spine, and soften your waist. Feel the motion of your pelvis.

1-2-3-CURL/HIDE

Definitely Definition

BENEFITS: To strengthen and define your abdominals, to stretch and tone your buttocks and thighs, to trim your waist, to enhance your balance.

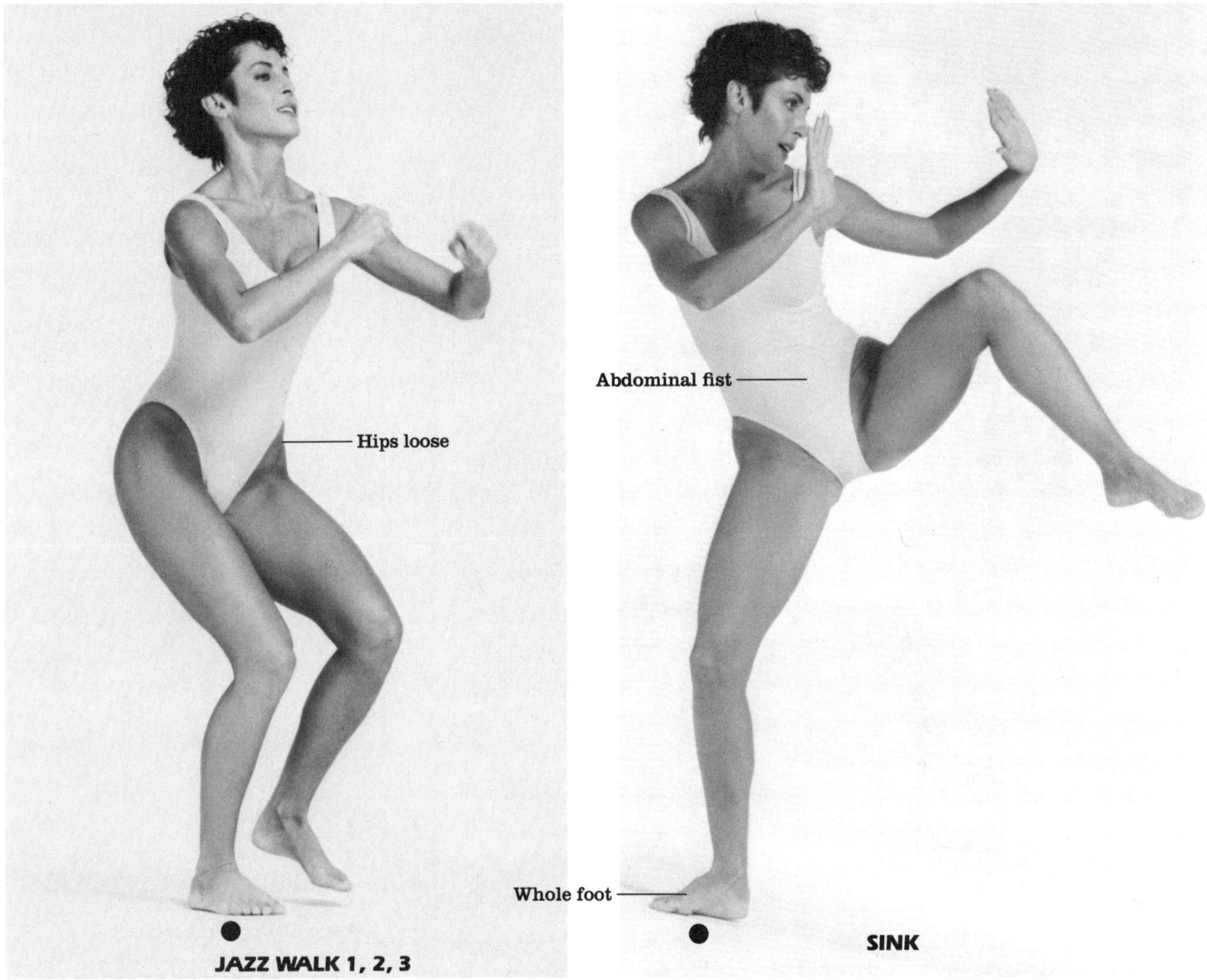

JAZZ WALK 1, 2, 3

Rolling your forearms tightly around each other, jazz walk loosely, left, right, left, to the count of 3—

SINK

—and on 4, sink into your left leg as you draw your right knee up toward your chest with a burst of *"Yeet!"* feeling the press on your abdominal muscles. At the same time, scoop your arms out and up in front of your face as if you're hiding behind them and really stretch out through all five fingers for more definition in your forearm.

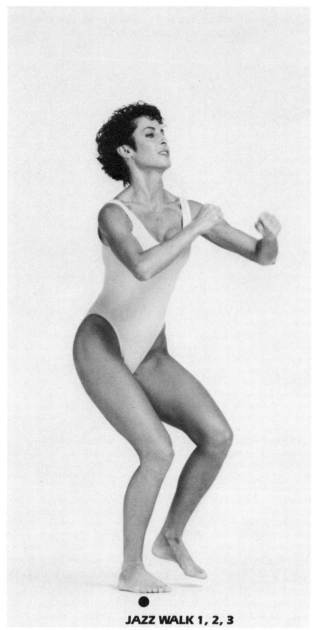

JAZZ WALK 1, 2, 3

Return to jazz walk in place, right, left, right, inhaling richly and rolling your arms, then—

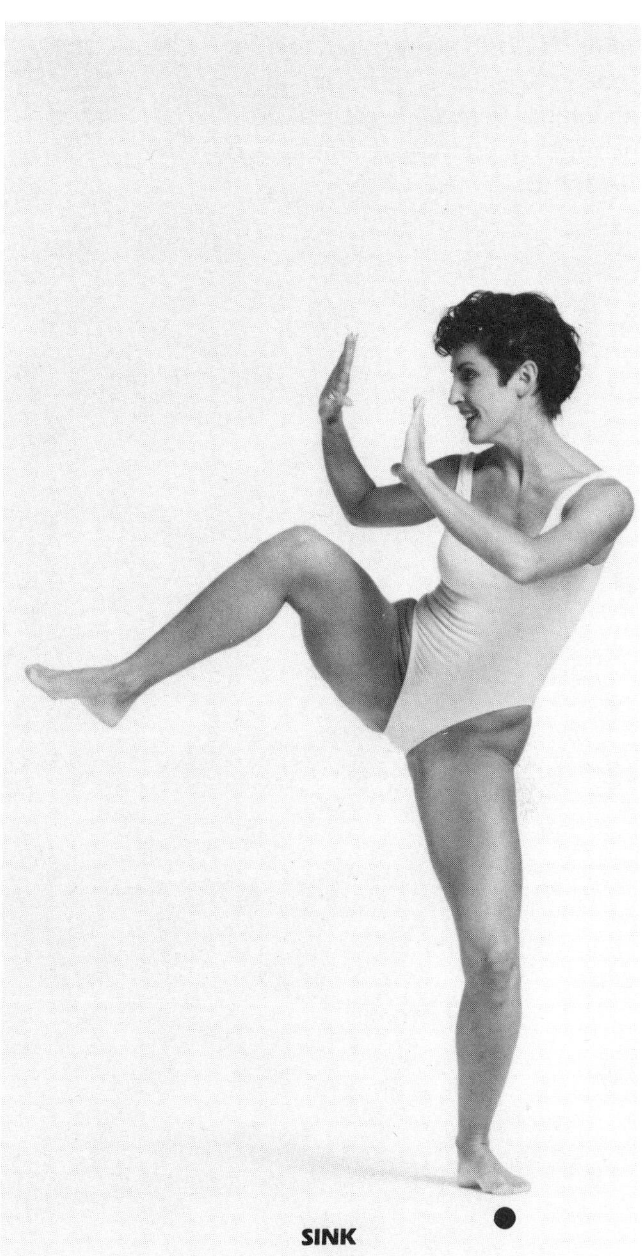

SINK

—on 4, sink into your right leg as you scoop your arms, draw up your left knee, and exhale "Yeet" with an abdominal fist. Repeat 8 times on each side.

1-2-3-KICK/BOW & ARROW

Tension Buster

BENEFITS: To strengthen and tone your thighs, buttocks, and abdomen, to stretch your hamstrings, to increase strength and flexibility of your arms.

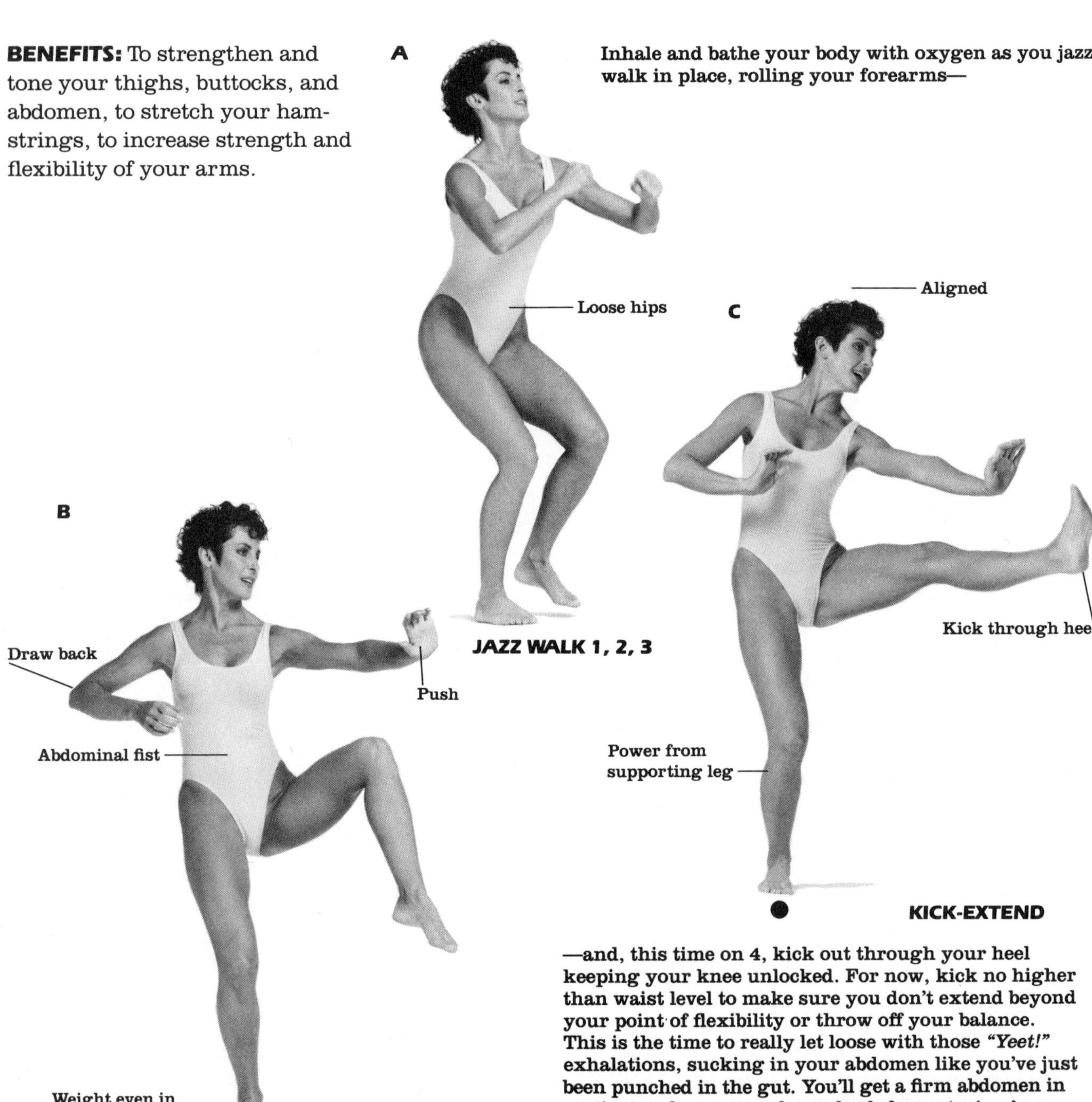

Inhale and bathe your body with oxygen as you jazz walk in place, rolling your forearms—

—and on the count of 3, sink into your supporting leg, drawing your opposite knee toward your chest—

—and, this time on 4, kick out through your heel keeping your knee unlocked. For now, kick no higher than waist level to make sure you don't extend beyond your point of flexibility or throw off your balance. This is the time to really let loose with those *"Yeet!"* exhalations, sucking in your abdomen like you've just been punched in the gut. You'll get a firm abdomen in no time and save your lower back from strain. As you kick with *"Yeet!"* imagine that you're holding a bow and arrow, your right arm extending straight over your right leg, and pull back on the string, take aim, and fire, letting a little more stress shoot out with each arrow. Repeat 8 times on each side.

RECHARGE
PADDLE

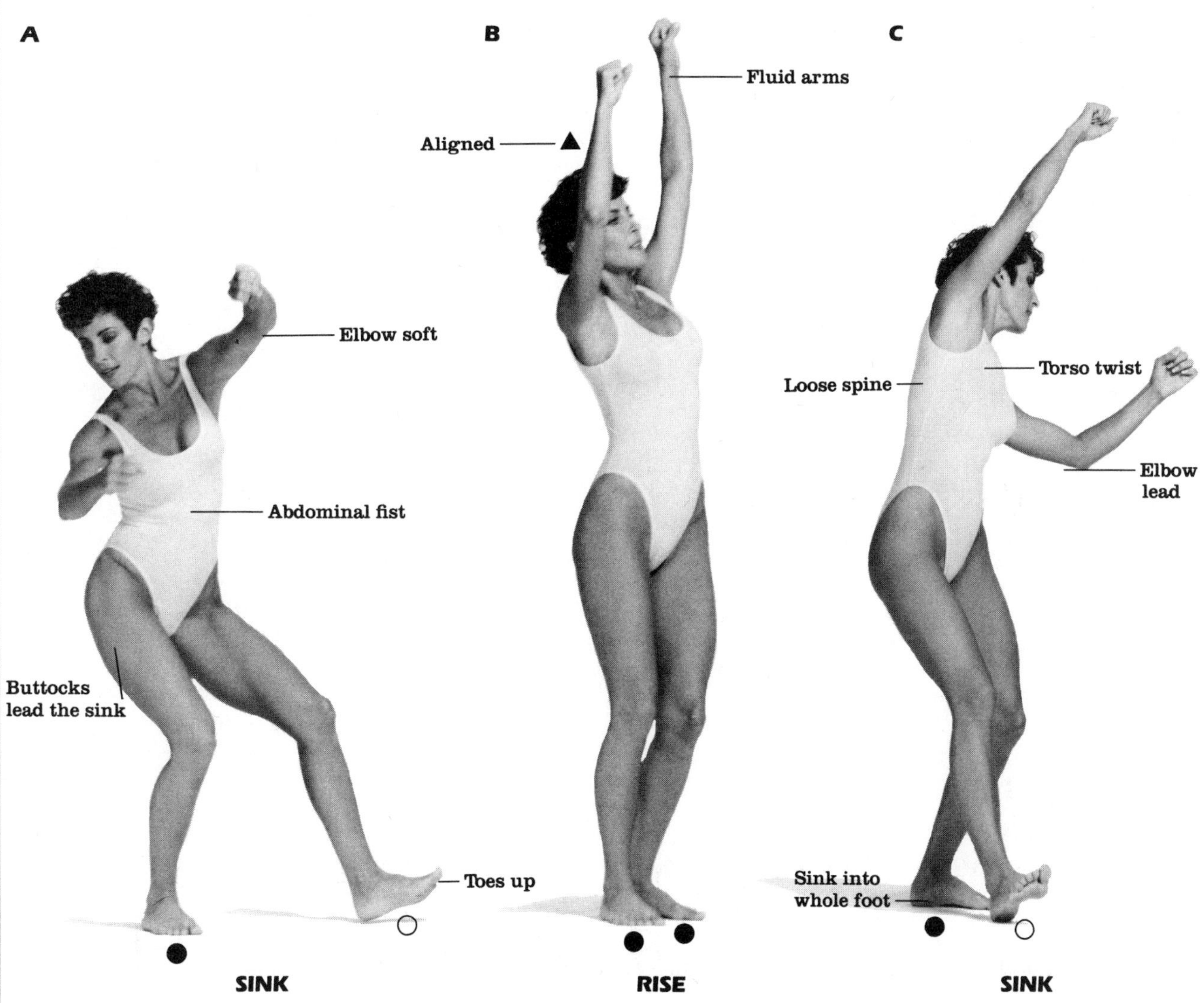

Walk loosely in place to the count of 3 and touch front on 4, sweeping an imaginary paddle in broad horizontal figure eights from your left to your right side. Repeat 16 to 24 times on each side. **Body Check:** Listen to your body signals and adjust accordingly.

Thigh Tamer

BENEFITS: To firm your inner and outer thighs, to increase flexibility of your hip socket, to tone your abdominal muscles, to enhance your balance and coordination.

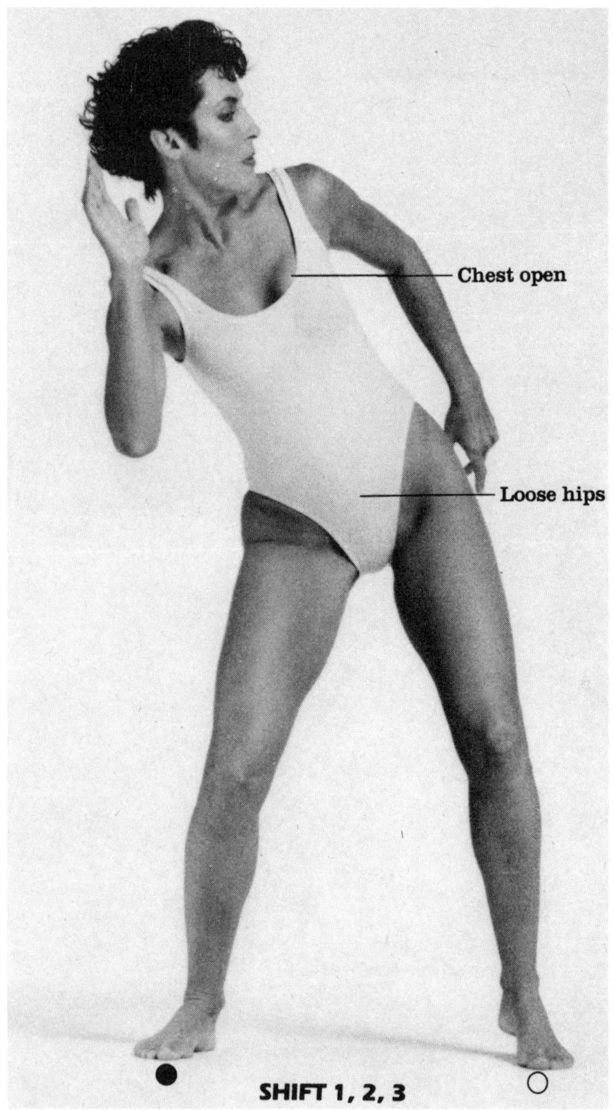

Shift left, right, left, and—

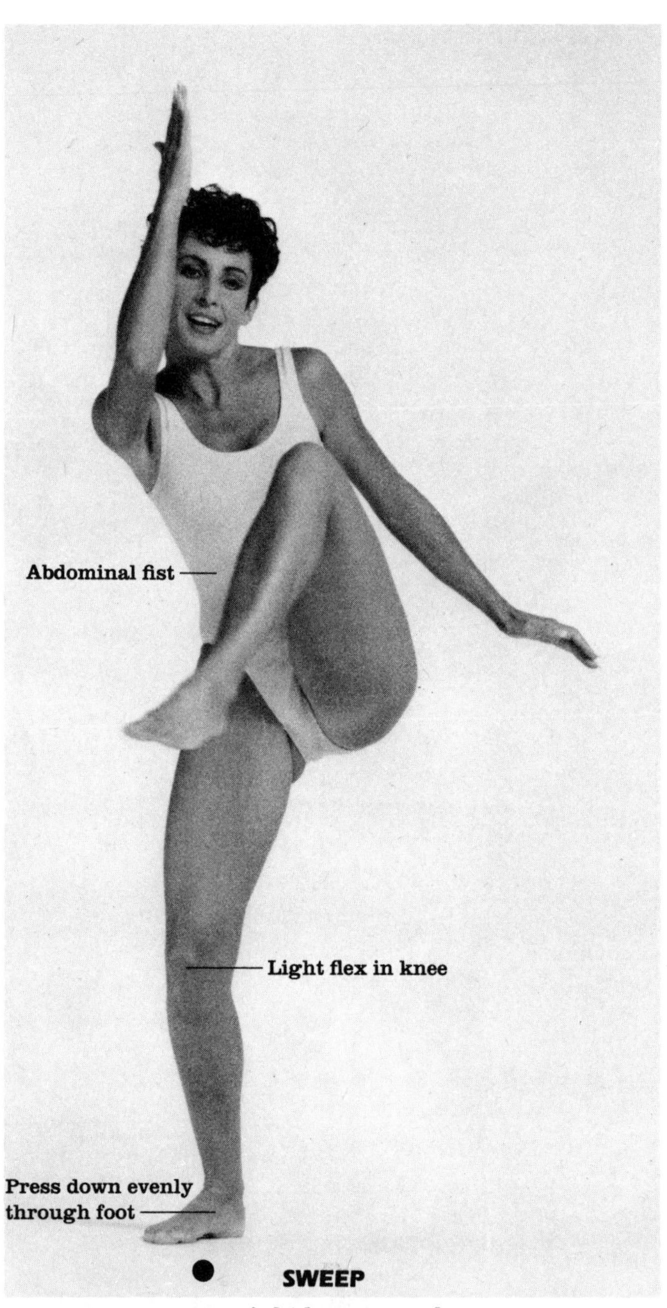

—on 4, sweep your right knee up and across your body to lightly slap across the inside of your knee with your left hand. Then sweep back out and down to the right side—

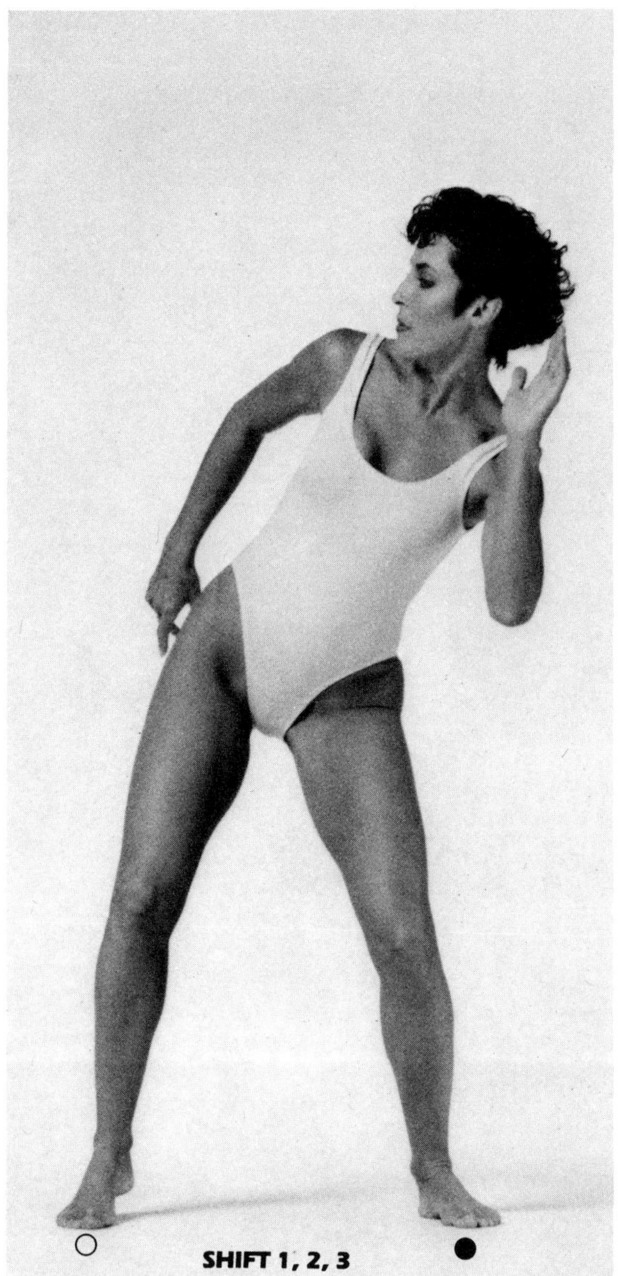

SHIFT 1, 2, 3

—and pick up the count as you step down and shift right, left, right—

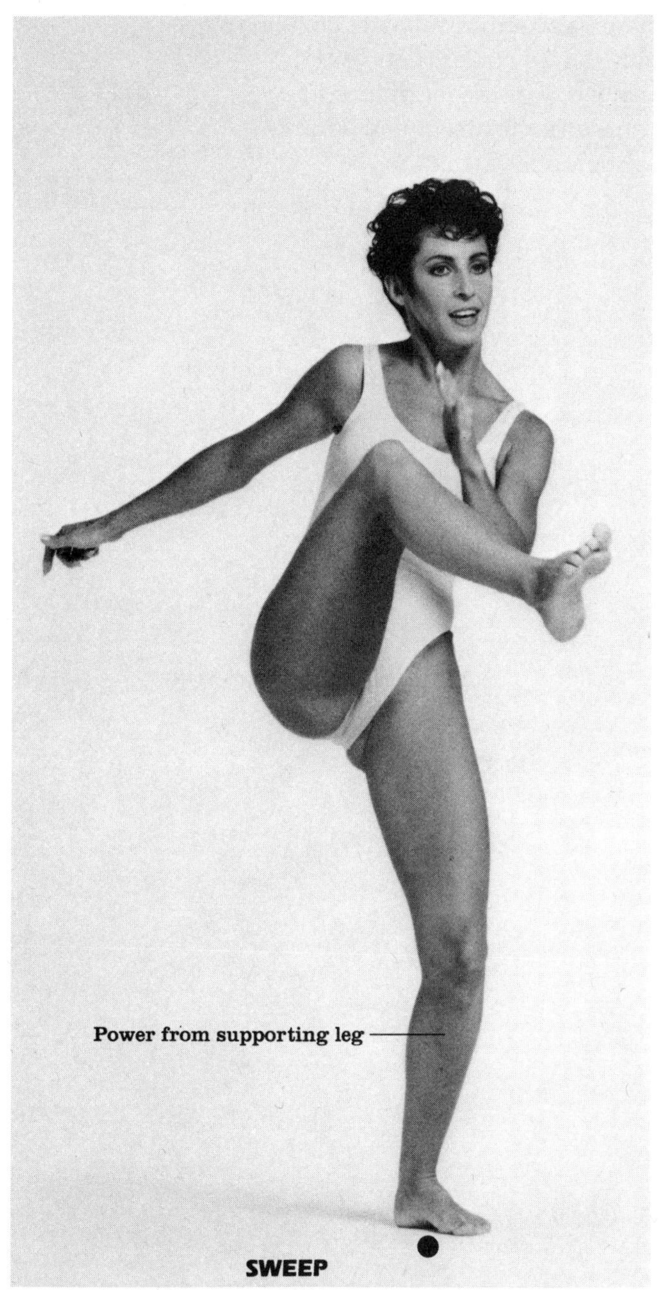

SWEEP

—and on 4, sweep your left knee up and slap. The rhythm is shift, shift, shift, sweep. Be solid on your supporting leg as you sweep. Repeat 8 times on each side.

The Power Pack

BENEFITS: To firm and trim your abdominals, buttocks, and thighs, to strengthen your calves, to increase your spine and torso flexibility, to define your upper arms.

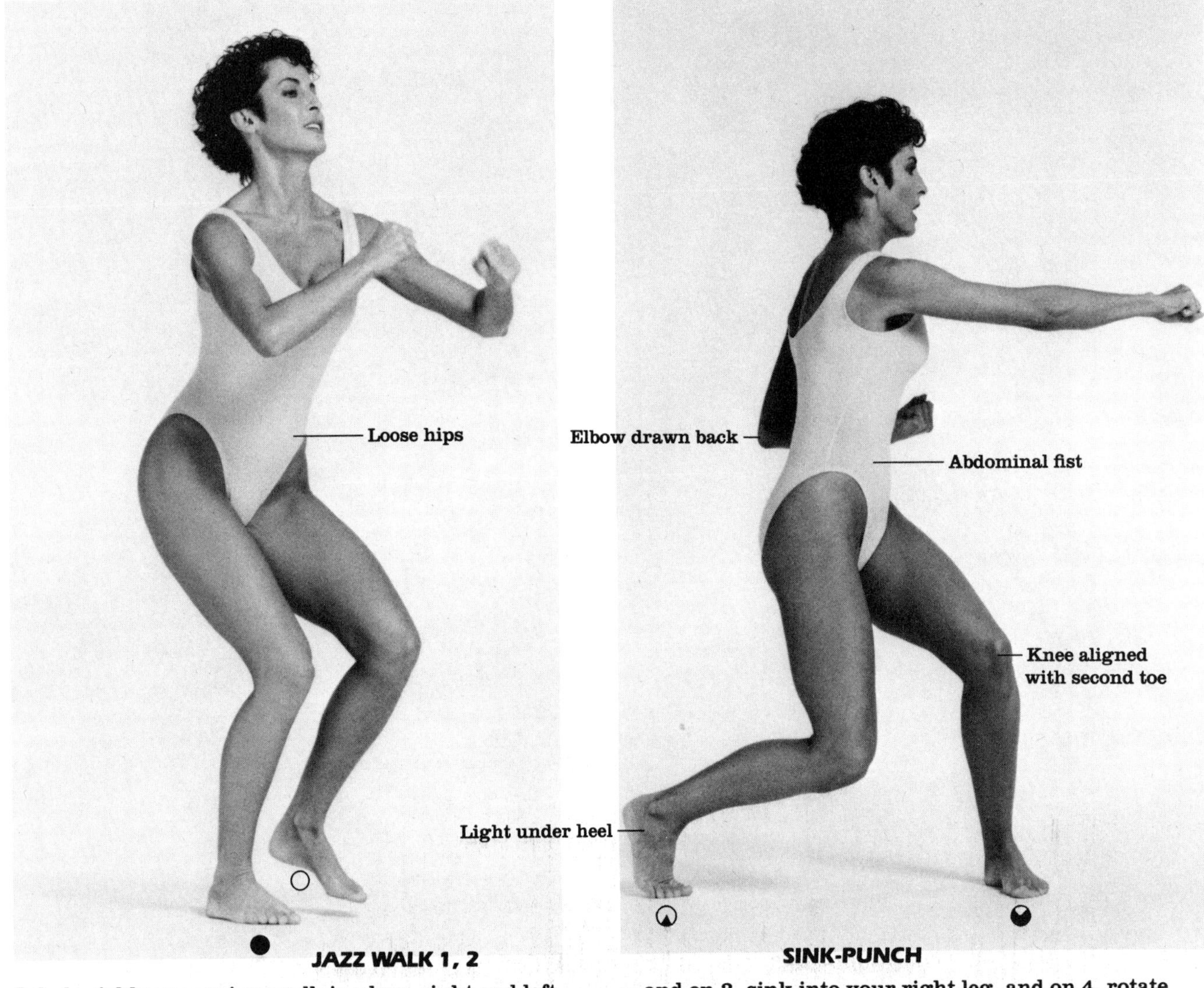

JAZZ WALK 1, 2

Inhale richly as you jazz walk in place, right and left, rolling your forearms—

SINK-PUNCH

—and on 3, sink into your right leg, and on 4, rotate your left leg inward, placing the ball of your foot firmly on the floor as you give a powerful karate punch right with a forceful *"Yeet!"* and abdominal fist. Sink. Don't be thrown forward by your punch.

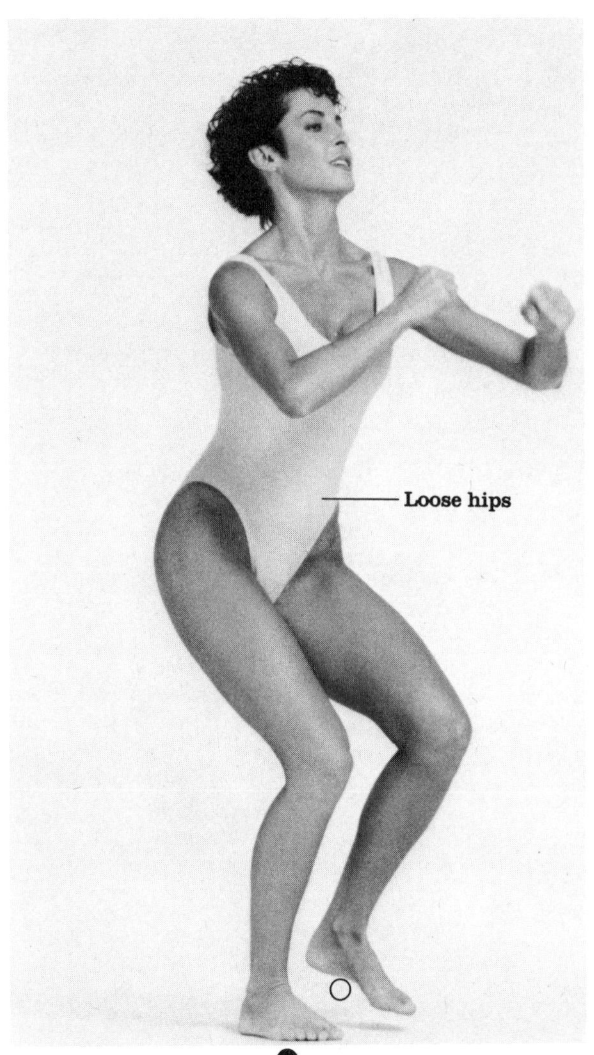

JAZZ WALK 1, 2

Inhaling and recharging in center, walk left and right. Feel your feet and calves working for you—

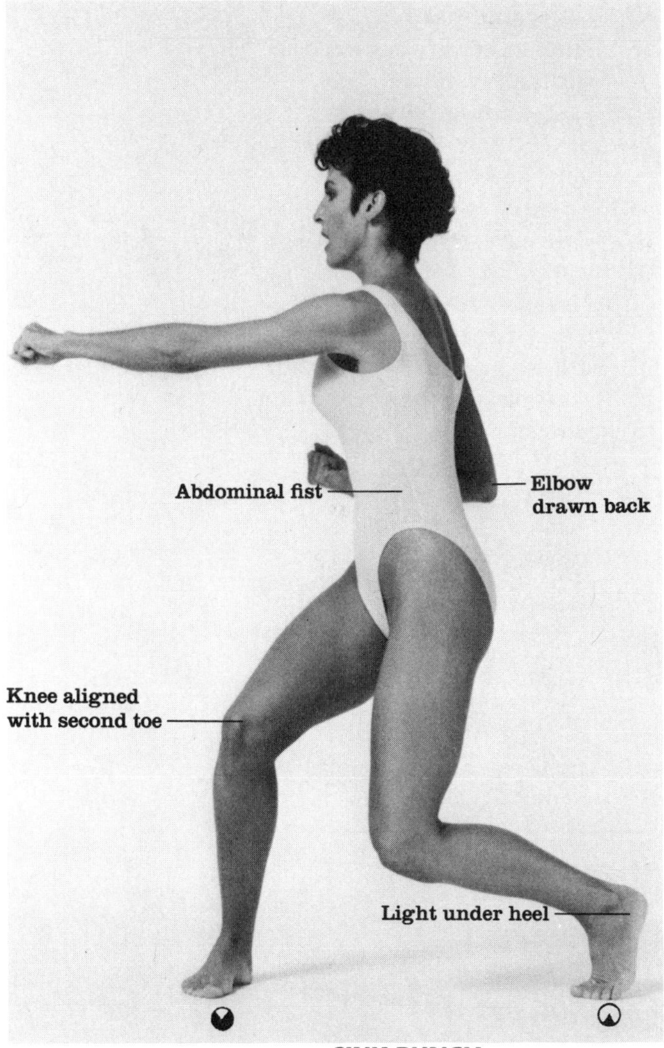

SINK-PUNCH

—and on 3, sink left, and on 4, pivot your right leg and punch left. Repeat 8 times on each side.

AEROBIC CHECK

Shifting easily side to side and keeping your legs in motion, check your heart rate by placing two fingers on either side of your Adam's apple at the carotid artery or the thumb side of your wrist at the radial artery, finding your pulse, and counting the beats for ten seconds. Multiply by six to determine your heart rate. Are you within your aerobic target zone? If you're not sure, refer back to the aerobic formula (page 35. It may take a few practice runs to get the design and pace of your workout just right so that you work within your zone, but please be careful not to exceed your target.

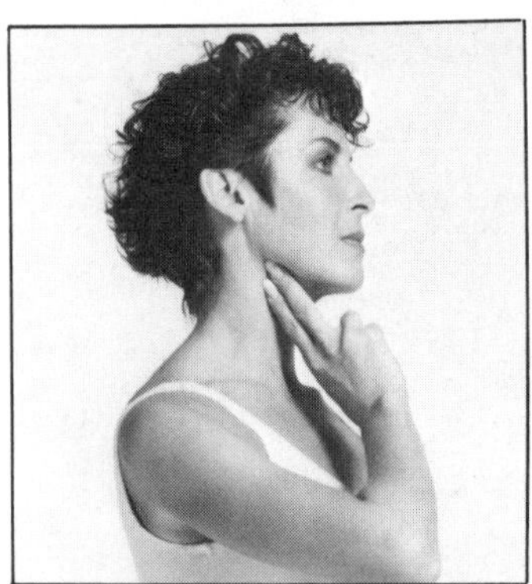

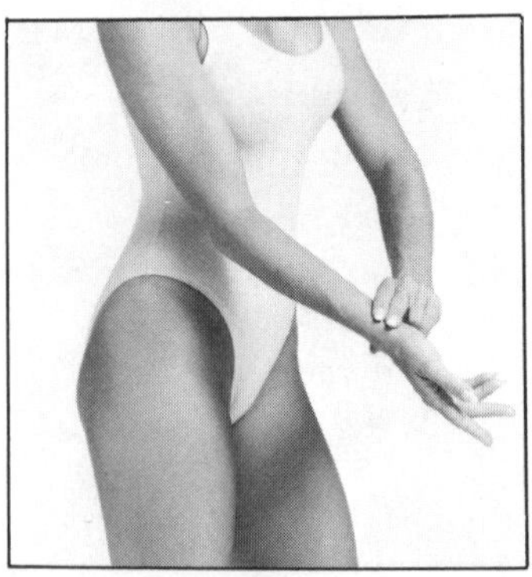

EASE-OUT

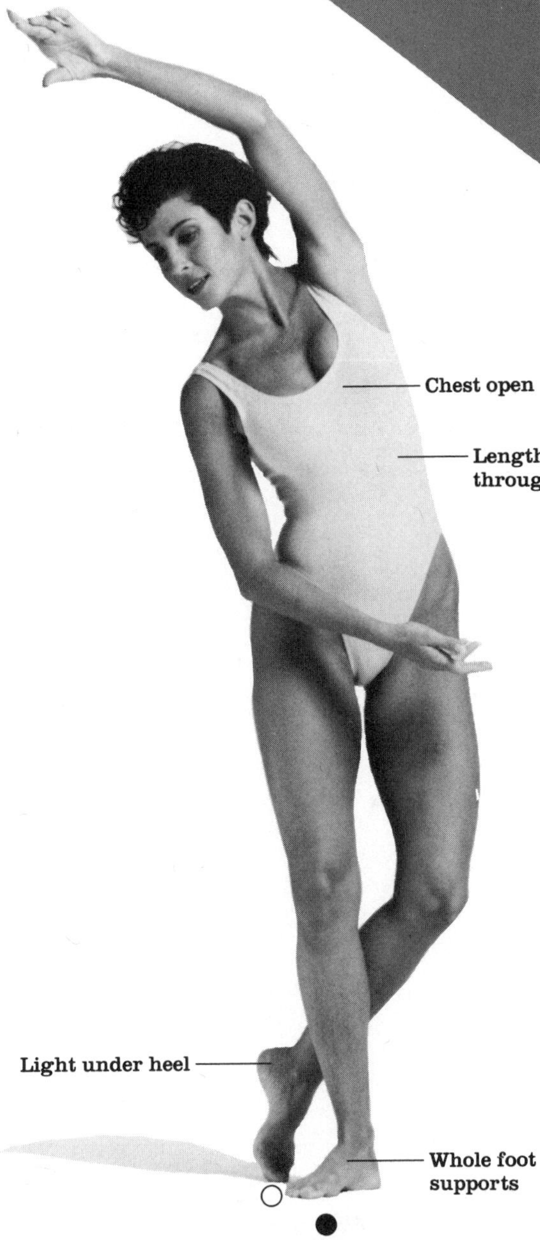

Chest open

Lengthen through side

Light under heel

Whole foot supports

CROSS BEHIND

Your whole body should be surging with vibrant new energy. Now let's ride that exhilaration through the Ease-Out to a sweet finale. Focus on the smooth, velvety ease of your movements, the slow, sensual stretch in each motion.

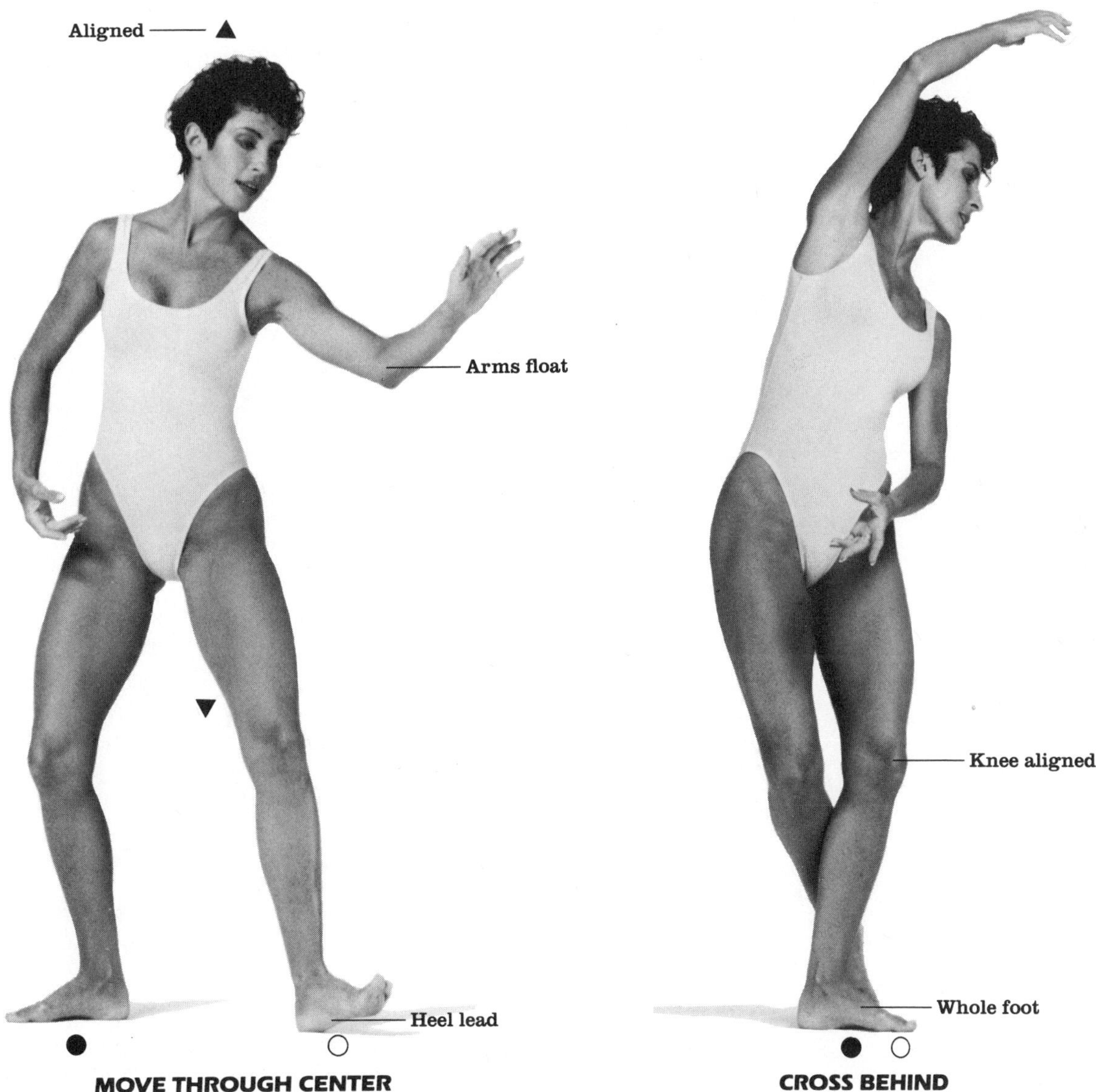

MOVE THROUGH CENTER

CROSS BEHIND

Easily cross one foot behind the other as you continue shifting side to side, your arms comfortably tracing the inside of the hoop. Feel the stretch along the sides of your torso. Shift back and forth 8 times to each side.

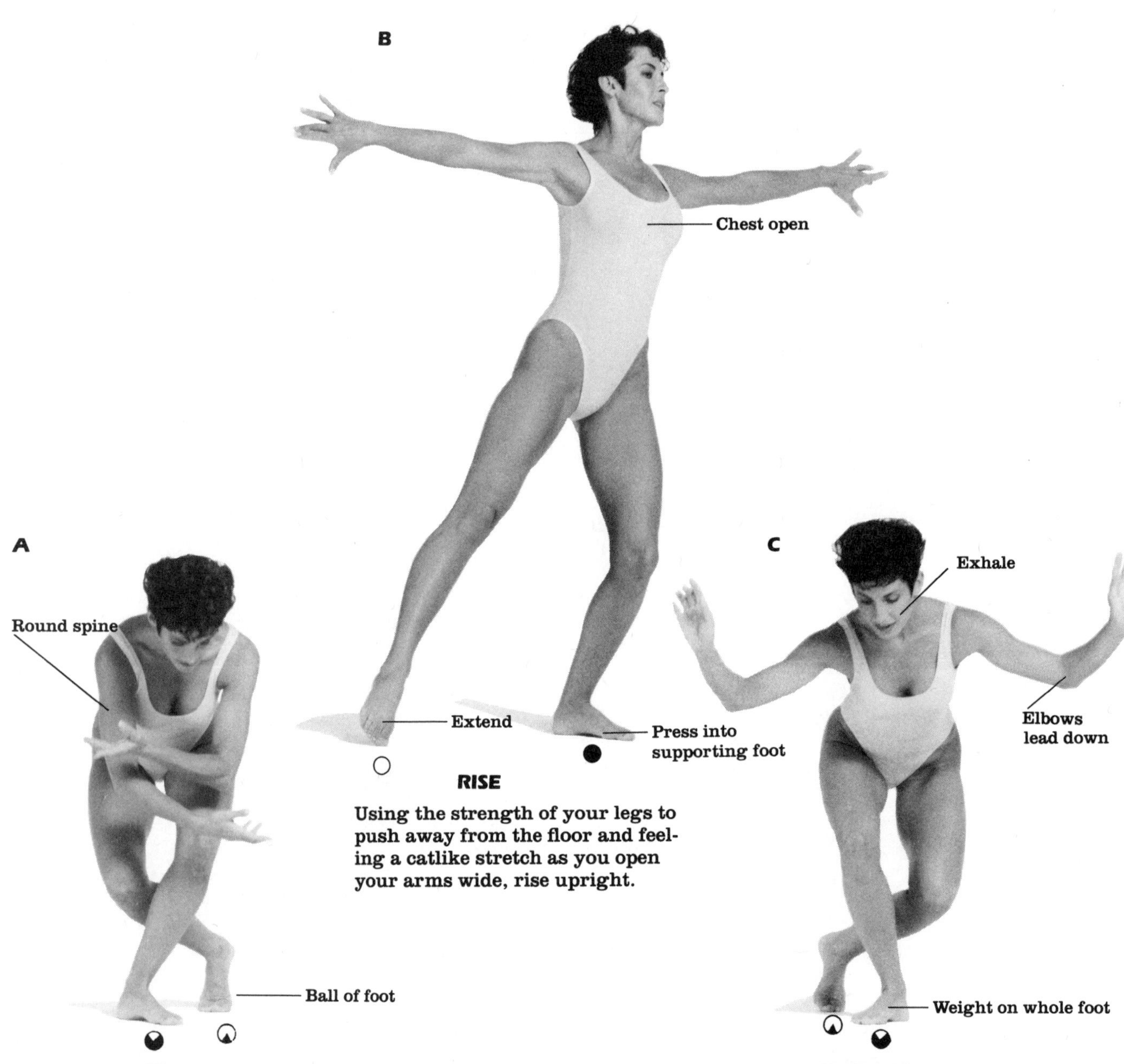

RISE

Using the strength of your legs to push away from the floor and feeling a catlike stretch as you open your arms wide, rise upright.

CROSS-SINK

As you cross behind, slowly sink, exhaling fully and drooping over as if you're scooping flowers from the floor, feeling a warm stretch in your buttocks, along your spine, and through your hips.

CROSS-SINK

Inhale, shift through center and slowly sink, rounding down on the other side, letting your buttocks lower first. Repeat 8 times on each side.

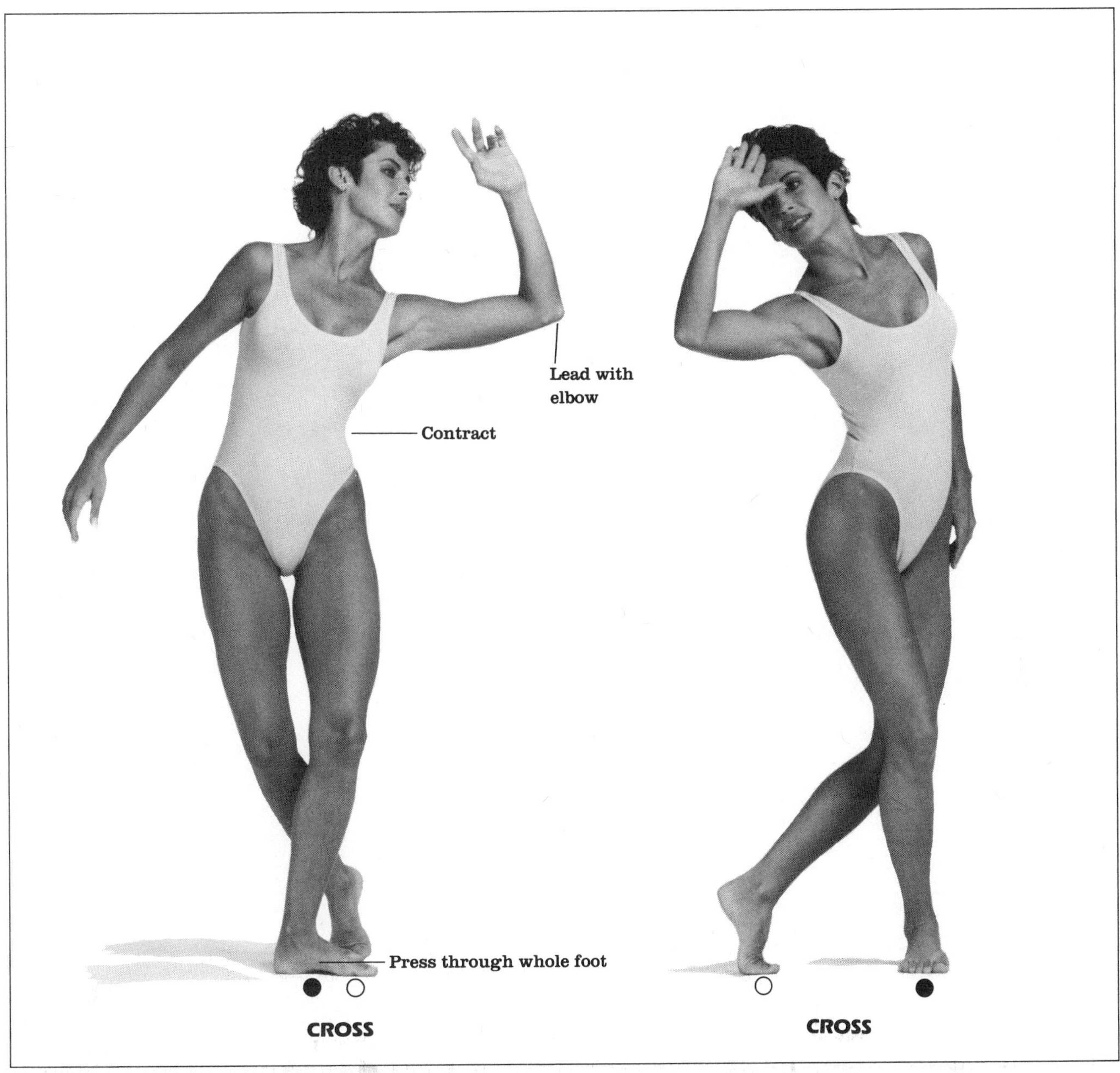

Return to a simple Cross Behind, slowing down now and shifting side to side. This time, barely brush the back of your forearm across your forehead, feeling the silky tickle of your hair against your skin, the stretch through your chest, as you let your arms flow sensually with the movement. Take time to extend your entire arm after you wipe for greater flexibility. Repeat 8 times to each side.

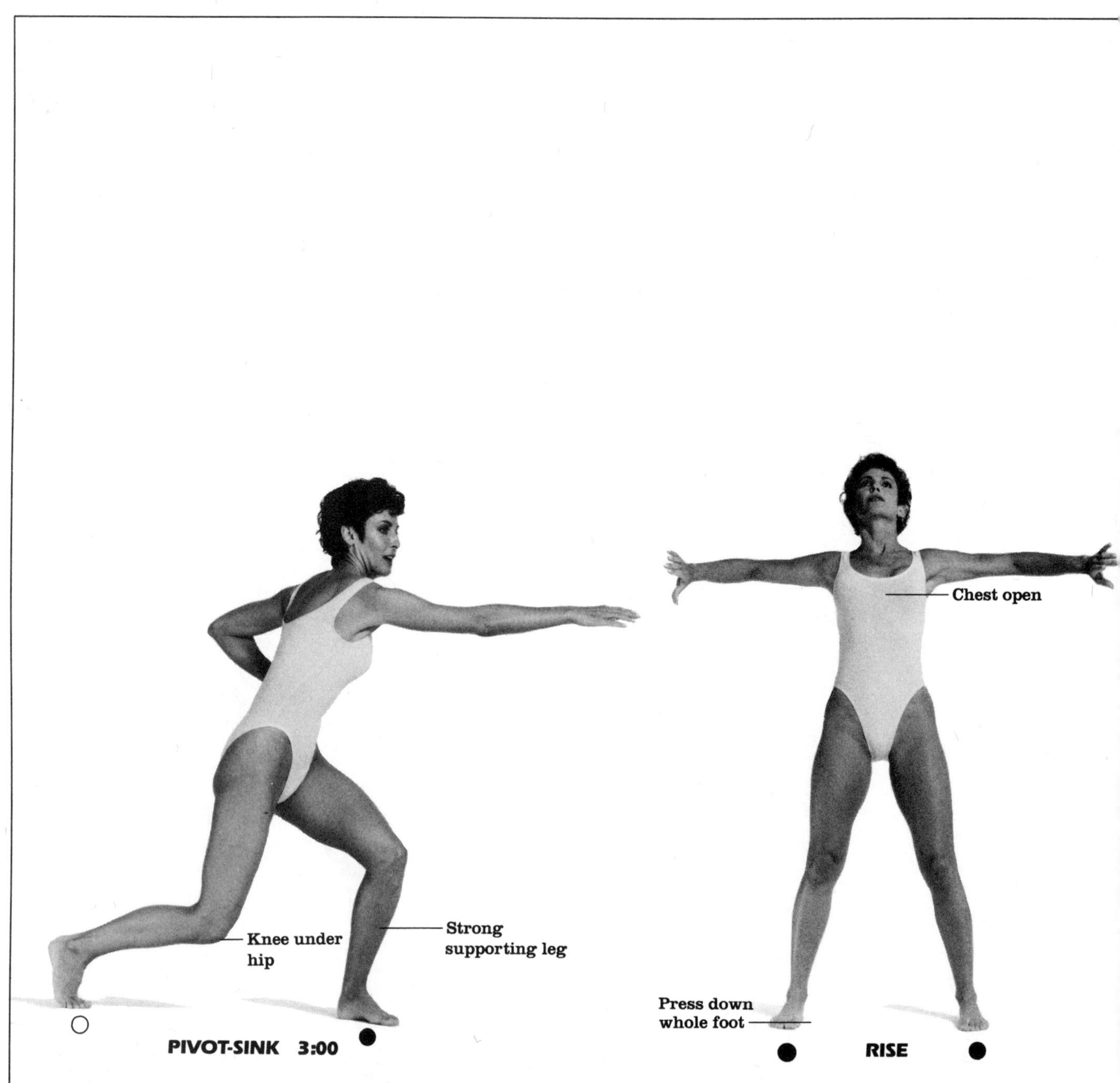

Still shifting side to side, pretend to wipe your hand across a chest-level table, exhaling as you pivot and feeling the long stretch across your back. Rise through center, inhaling and feeling the stretch radiate from the core of your body. Repeat 8 times each side.

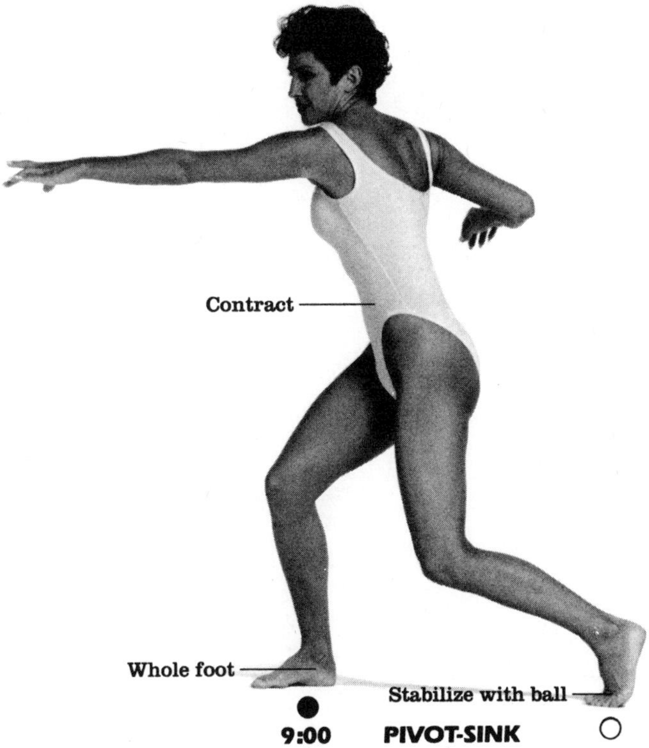

Contract

Whole foot

Stabilize with ball

9:00 PIVOT-SINK

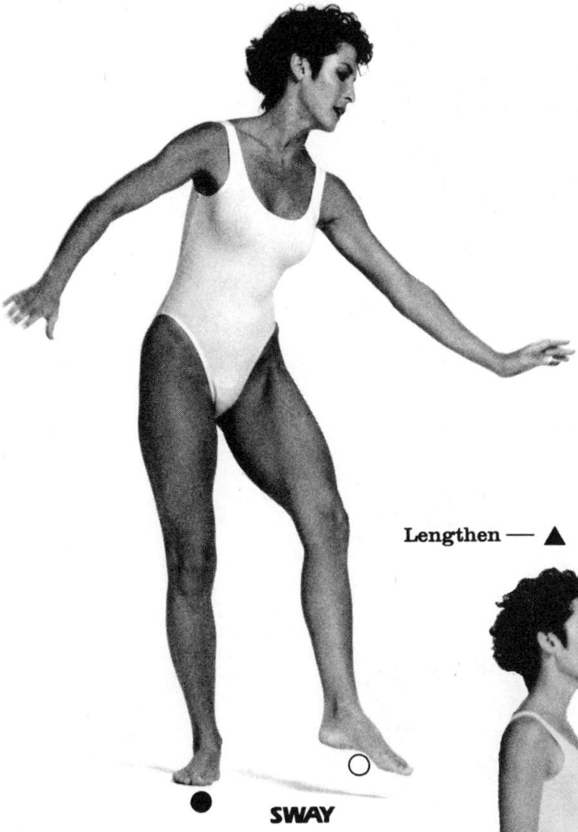

SWAY

Let your arms float languidly at your sides as you gently sway side to side, slowing your movement down until you come to—

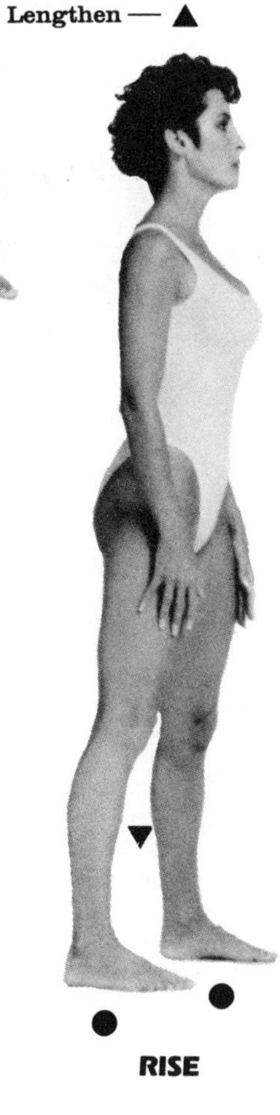

Lengthen

—a quiet center. Pause. Feel for a loose, relaxed body.

RISE

SPINE ROLL

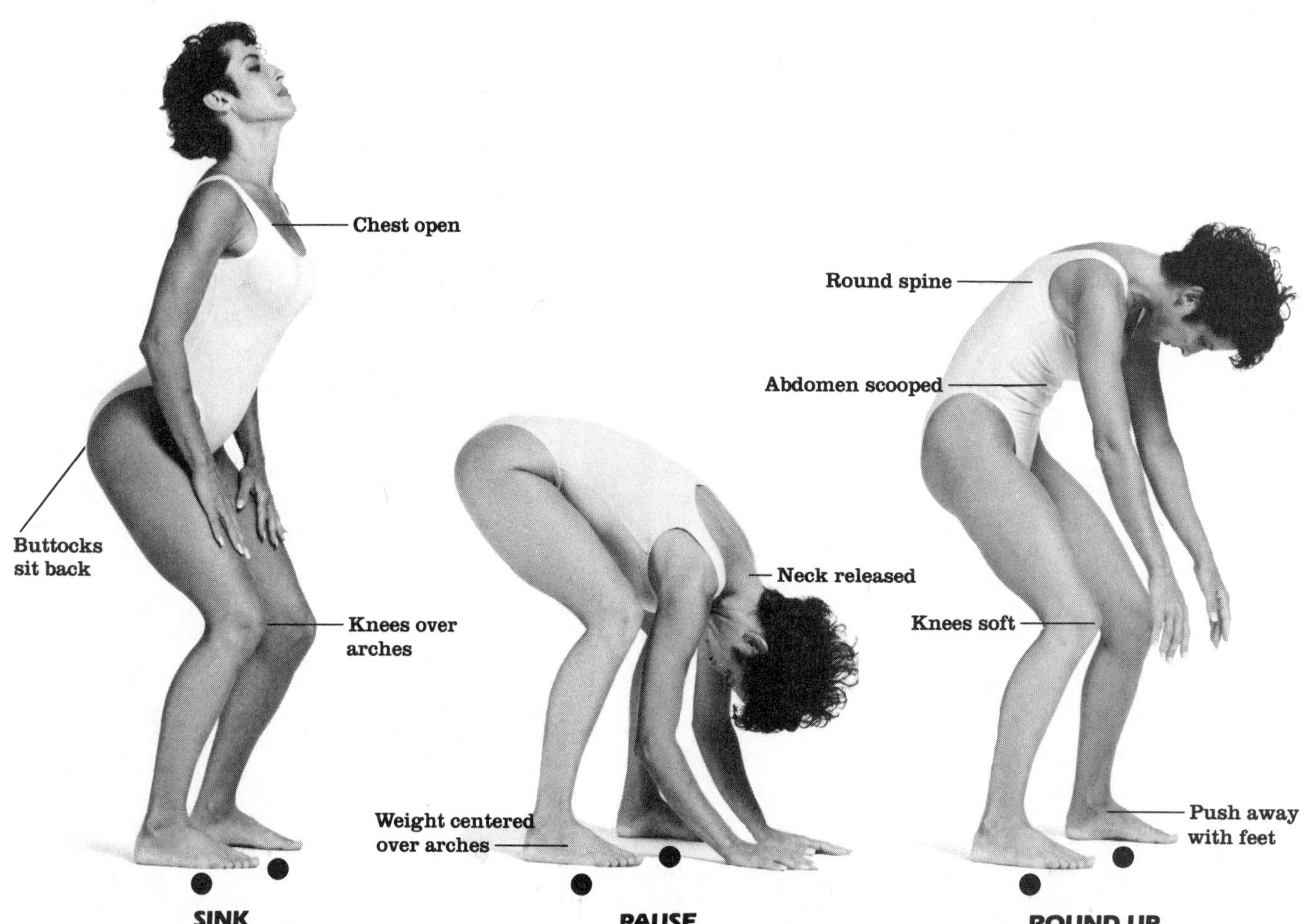

SINK

Standing in a hip or *A* stance, your feet parallel, inhale deeply as you place your hands softly on your thighs and, stretching your chest open, sink your buttocks, chest, and head, rounding over at a comfortable depth. You're coming out of your workout. Ebb gently and quietly.

PAUSE

Pause and just hang for a moment, feeling that feline stretch along your spine. Acknowledge your good work, your healthier body.

ROUND UP

Then, using the strength of your legs to push away, exhale fully and unroll your vertebrae, slowly, smoothly, one at a time, letting the weight of your body massage your back as you come upright. Come up very slowly, especially if you hang over for a while, and breathe in new energy. Repeat 4 times, ending rounded over.

ALL-FOURS CIRCLING

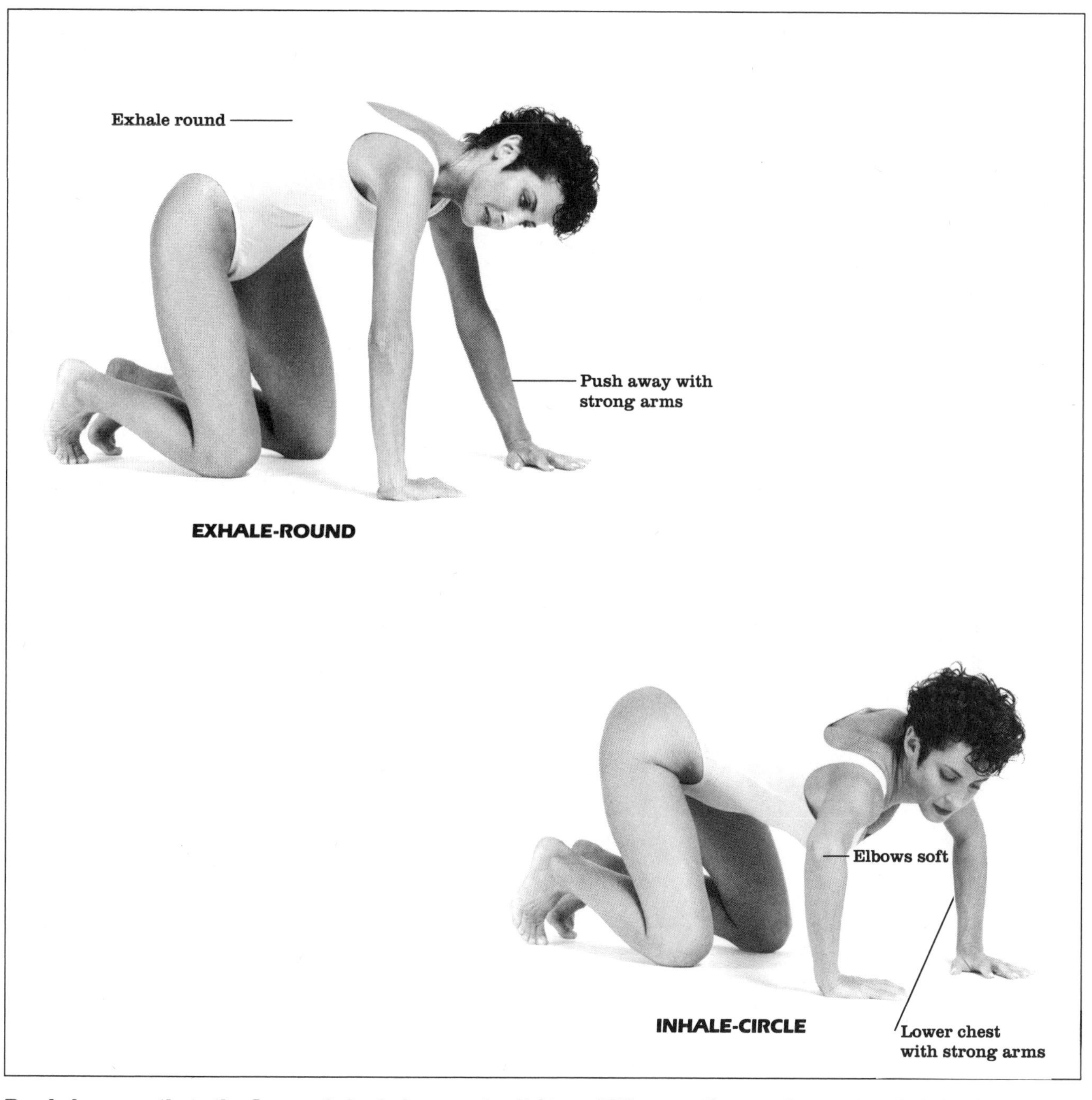
Exhale round
Push away with strong arms
EXHALE-ROUND
Elbows soft
Lower chest with strong arms
INHALE-CIRCLE

Reach down gently to the floor and slowly lower onto all fours. With your elbows soft, your hands below your shoulders, your knees under your hips, sensually circle your hips and torso 8 times in each direction, keeping your circles small at first. Exhale as your spine rounds to the ceiling. Feel a release in your entire spine, letting the muscle contractions massage you.

Without moving your hands, slowly lower your buttocks back onto your heels and feel the long stretch through your spine. If this isn't comfortable, place a pillow between your calves and thighs. Hold for 8 counts, breathing naturally. Rest. Feel at peace, calm.

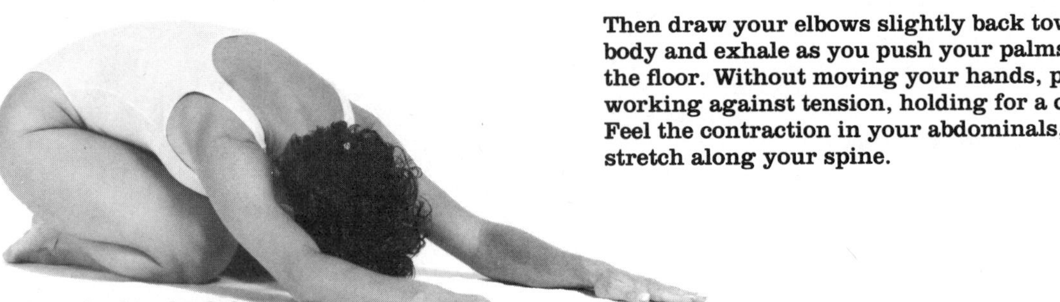

Then draw your elbows slightly back toward your body and exhale as you push your palms firmly into the floor. Without moving your hands, pull back, working against tension, holding for a count of 4. Feel the contraction in your abdominals, the added stretch along your spine.

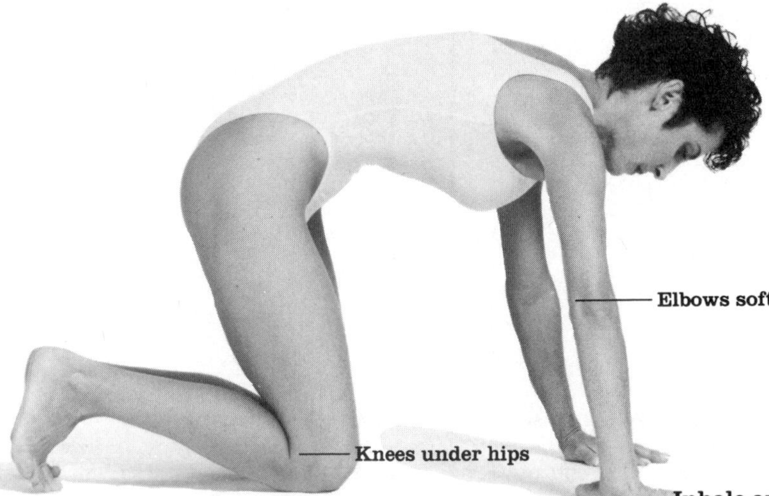

Inhale and rise back up onto all fours. Pause. Breathe.

HIP STRETCH

Now exhale and sit back on your heels slightly, your knees apart if it's more comfortable. Using your arm strength for support, lower yourself down to the left and slide your right hand out diagonally, reaching long through your right hand. Pause, hold for 8 counts, breathing naturally, and feel the stretch in your left hip. Imagine the floor responding to your touch with a smooth caress. Then, using the strength of your arms, exhale and gently push yourself back up to center. Repeat on the other side.

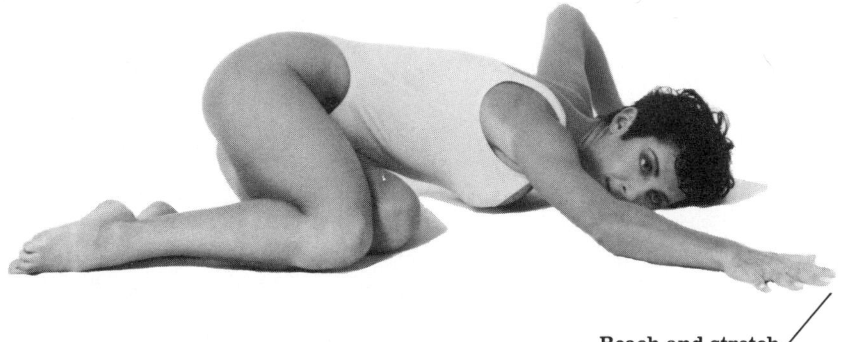

SPINAL TWIST

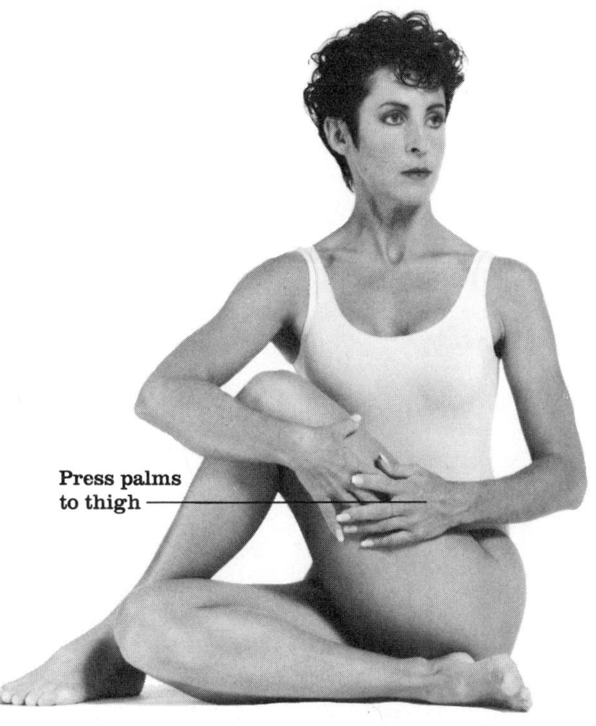

Using the strength of your arms, press your chest away from the floor so that you're sitting up tall over your right hip. Wrap your left leg over your right leg, your buttocks resting evenly on the floor. If your left buttock lifts up, extend your right leg comfortably out in front of you. Now lengthen through your spine and hug your left knee close into your chest, turning your torso slightly and feeling the stretch through your outside hip and entire torso. Hold for a count of 8, breathing naturally. As you come back out of the twist, lead with your head first to release, your torso following. Pause. Breathe.

THIGH STRETCH

Your left leg still wrapped over your right, slowly lower your torso down to the right and rest on your right elbow and forearm. Be sure your elbow is comfortably under your shoulder. With your left hand, take hold of your left ankle and slowly draw your knee back, feeling a comfortable thigh stretch. If you feel pain in your knee, release your hold. Do not arch your back, but lengthen the front of your body. Hold for 8 counts, breathing naturally, and then release gently.

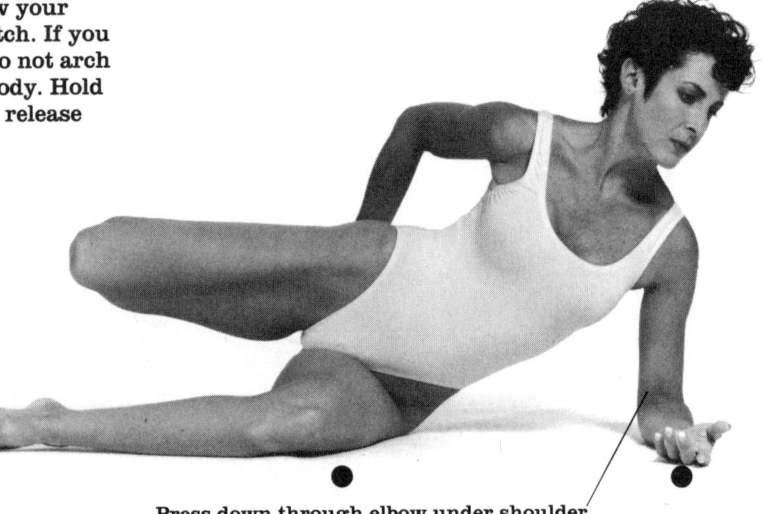

SIDE STRETCH

Now extend your left leg comfortably back as you reach diagonally with your left arm, stretching into a full, long extension that ripples all along the left side of your body. To modify, keep your elbow and knee slightly bent. Hold for 8 counts, breathing naturally and feeling your breath expand your chest, increasing your spine flexibility.

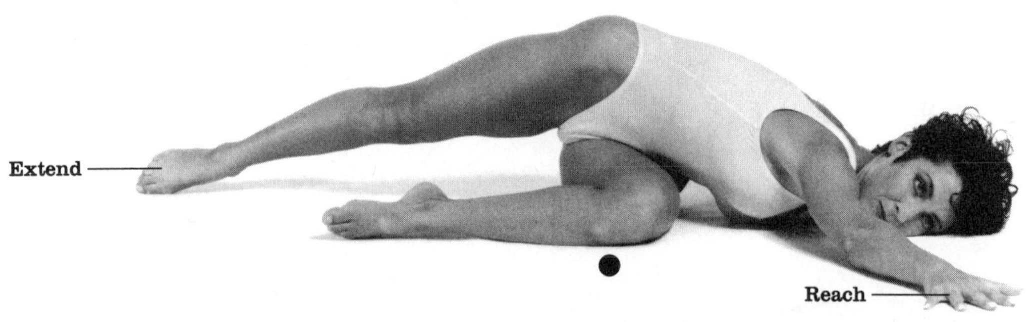

Then soften both knees, drawing them closer to you, and bring your hands under your chest. Using the strength of your arms, push away from the floor to rise as you exhale.

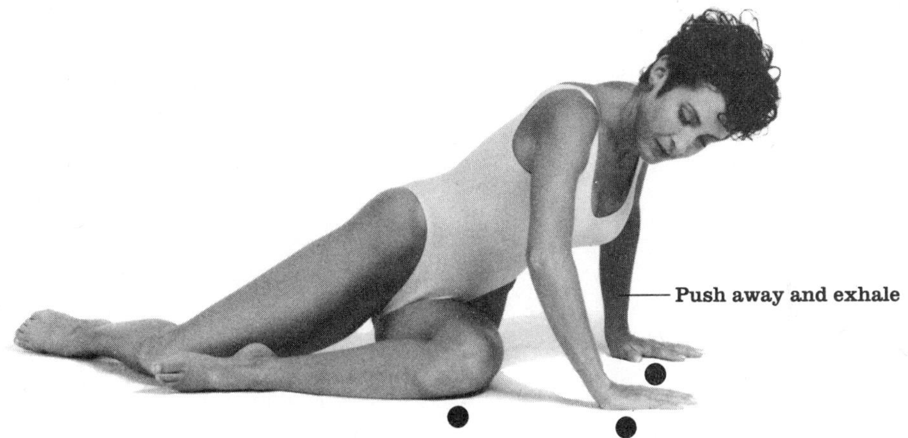

KNEE HUG

Sitting onto your buttocks, hug both knees into your chest. To modify, keep your knees farther away from your chest and round over less. Pause and prepare to nourish the other side of your body with the stretches.

Muscle Balancer

Repeat the Spinal Twist, Thigh Stretch, and Side Stretch to the opposite side and end in a Knee Hug. Then lower to the right and walk your hands out in front of you so that you're on all fours. Repeat All-Fours Circling.

PUSH AWAY

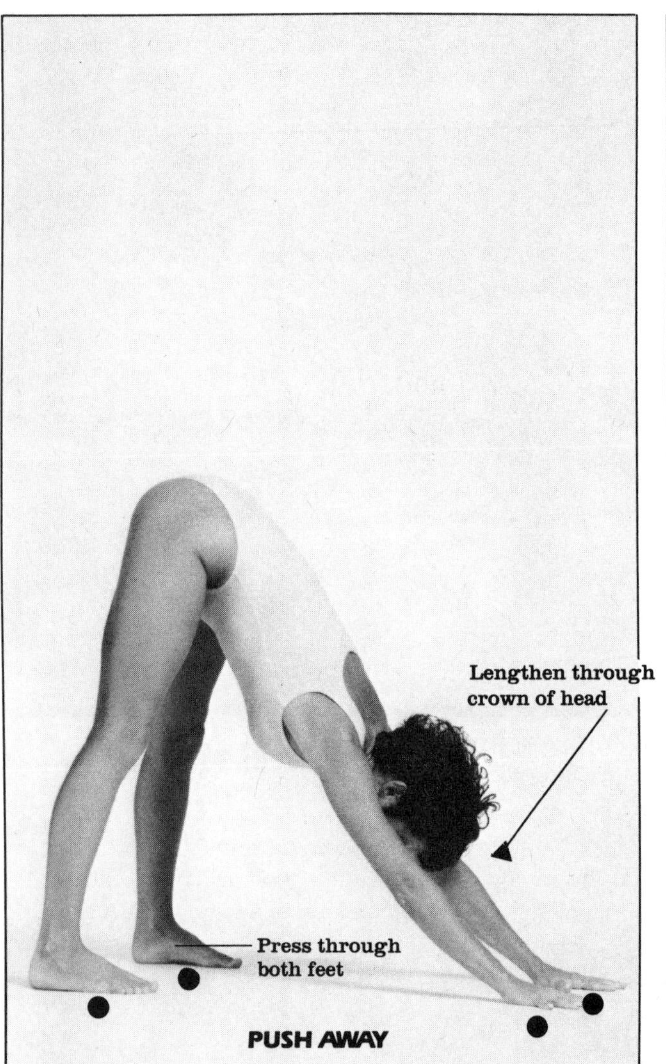

PUSH AWAY

With your toes curled under, your feet wider than your hips, and your hands below your shoulders, use the strength of your arms to push away from the floor, feeling your buttocks rise, your heels lowering into the floor. If this is too difficult, keep your knees bent and walk your hands closer to your feet. Now walk your hands back until you feel your pelvis above your arches, and pushing your fingertips forward, feel for a nice stretch through the back of your legs, your neck lengthened. Breathe naturally as you hold for 8 counts, adding new energy with each breath, new comfort with the stretch.

ROUND-UP

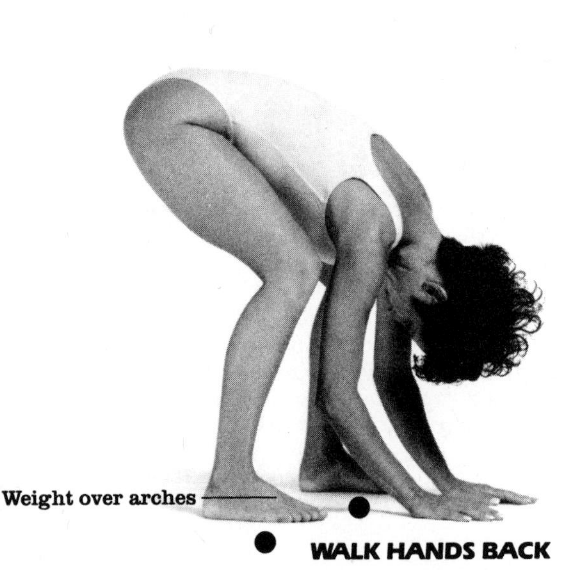

WALK HANDS BACK

Walk your hands slowly back to your feet, lower your buttocks a few inches, and using the strength of your legs, exhale and slowly round up.

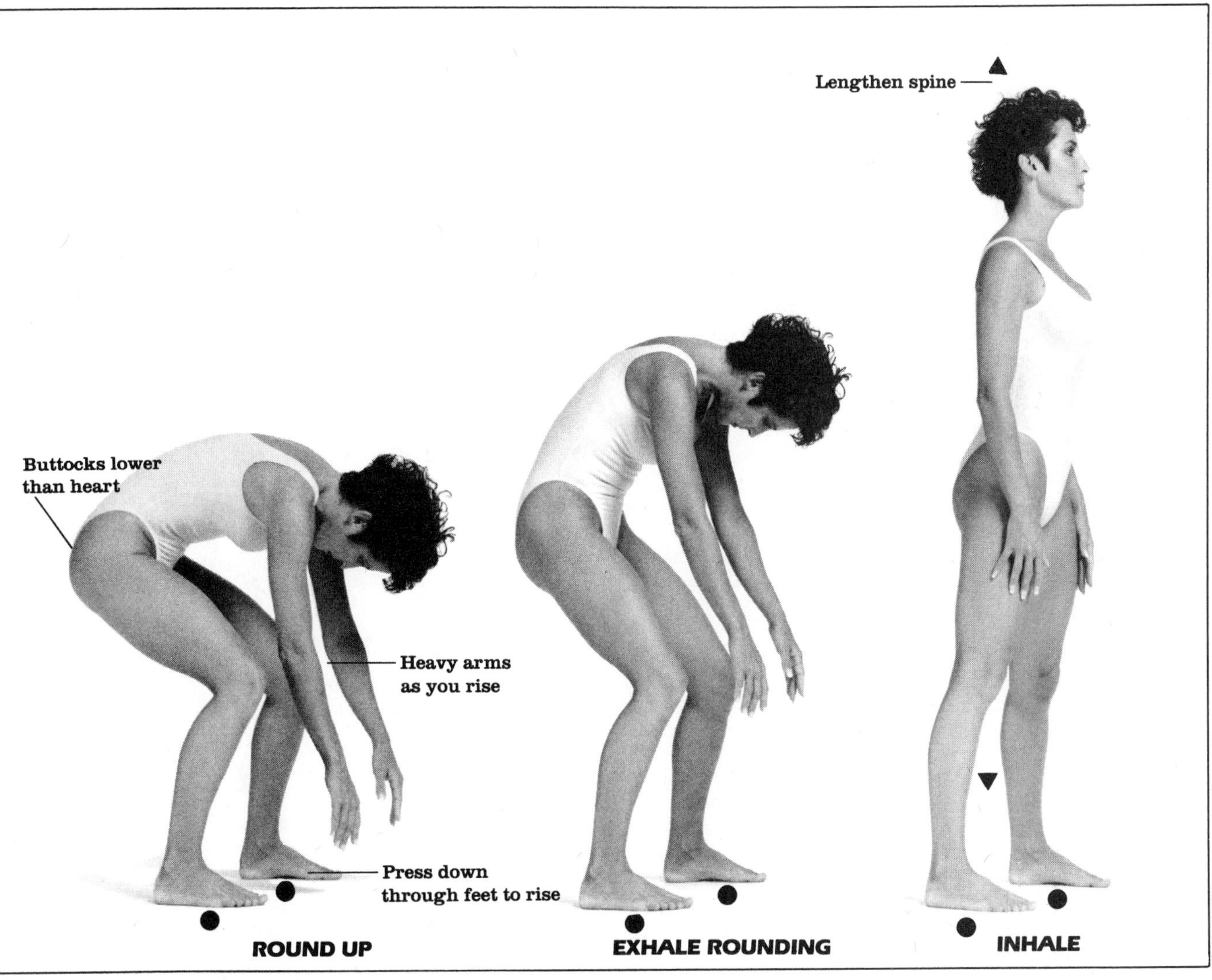

Stacking one vertebra at a time until your head is the last part of your body to become upright. Feel aligned. Breathe. Remember, you can come up slowly, pausing at your knees for an instant and continuing up little by little to avoid dizziness.

1. Inhale richly, feeling the new expanse of your lungs, and float your arms out to either side, drawing them up above your head. Now press your palms together and lift up through the crown of your head, lengthening your entire torso. Reach high, feeling the stretch run down from your fingertips through your arms, along the curve of your upper back and down your spine, imagining that you have roots growing out of the soles of your feet as the stretch pours down through your legs and out your feet.

2. With your palms pressed together, exhale, bend your elbows, and lower your thumbs to the nape of your neck, softening your knees. Feel the stretch along the underside of your upper arms. Inhale and reach, lengthening tall and ending in a high reach again. Repeat 4 times, ending in a reach.

3. Now exhale as you lower your arms straight down in front, slightly below shoulder level. Feel the stretch across your upper back. Open your hands so your palms face away from you, your thumbs and first fingers touching to form your Triangle. Pause. Breathe.

4. Inhale, breathing in new energy as you bend your elbows and draw your Triangle toward your face so that your first fingers touch the tip of your nose. Then exhale, releasing and relaxing as you push your Triangle away, gazing through its center and feeling the relaxation take hold. Repeat 3 times.

5. Now briskly rub your palms together, building up a good heat.

6. Open your palms, feeling that heat spread outward. Pause for a moment, feeling yourself at peace, in harmony with your life. Then close your hands and make a fist, keeping enough of that heat and energy for yourself today.

7. Inhale, drawing your elbows back by your sides and bringing that energy into your body. Open your chest and feel a wave of renewal course through every cell of your body.

8. Exhale and push your palms straight down by your sides, affirming that renewal. Jiggle, letting it reverberate through you.

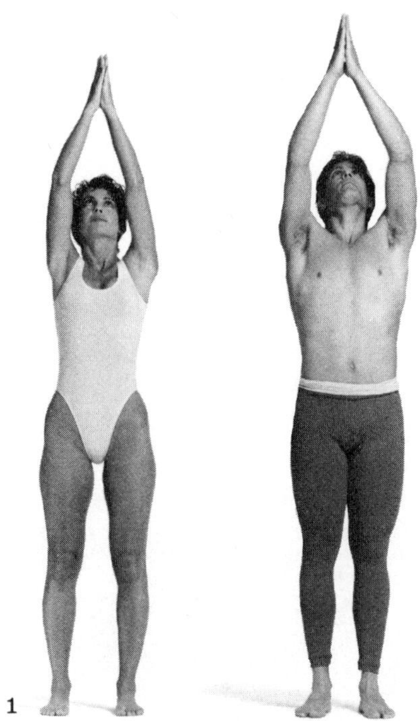

1

INHALE NEW ENERGY

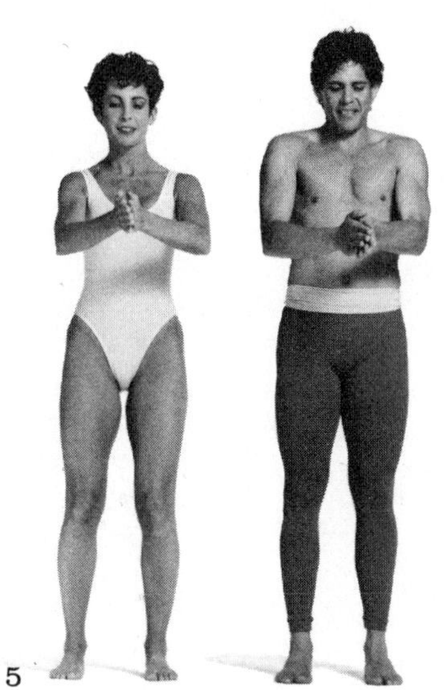

5

GENERATING WARMTH

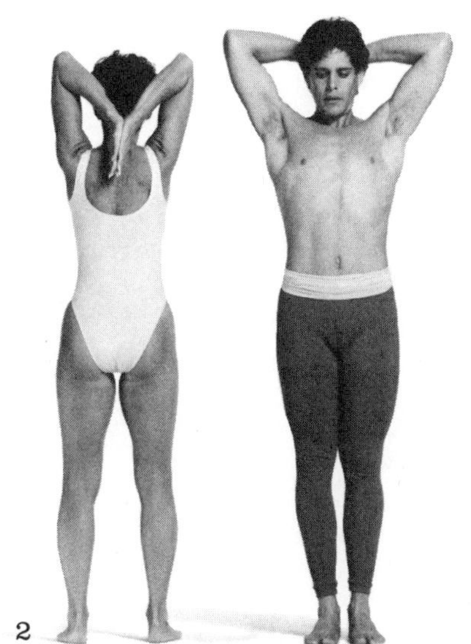
2

EXHALE, LET GO

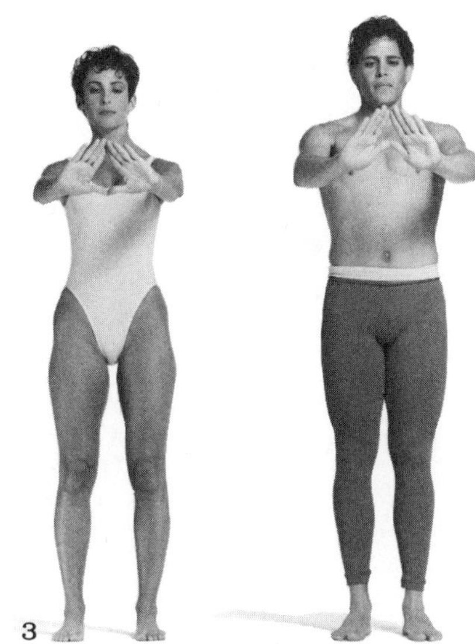
3

FOCUS AND FEEL

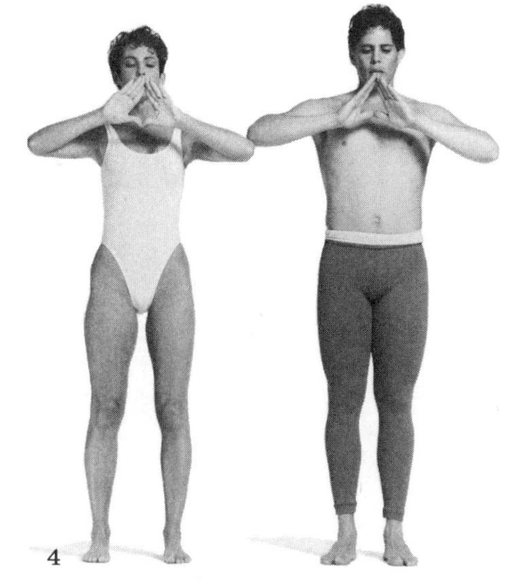
4

INHALE NEW ENERGY
EXHALE, RELEASE

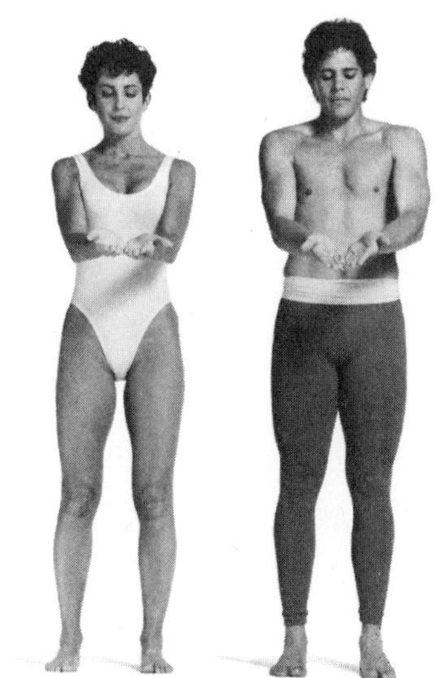
6

OPEN PALMS, FEEL

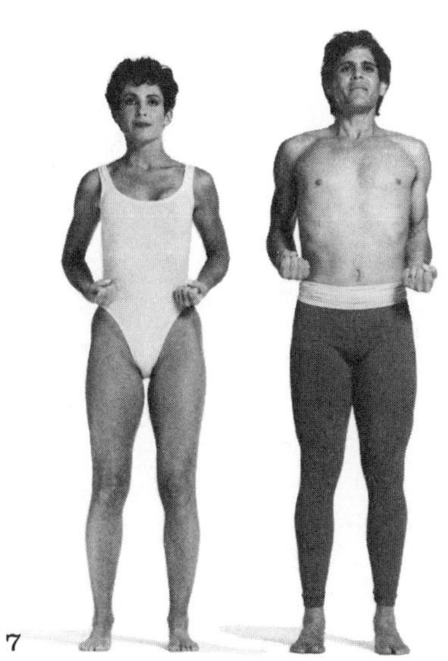
7

INHALE A NEW YOU

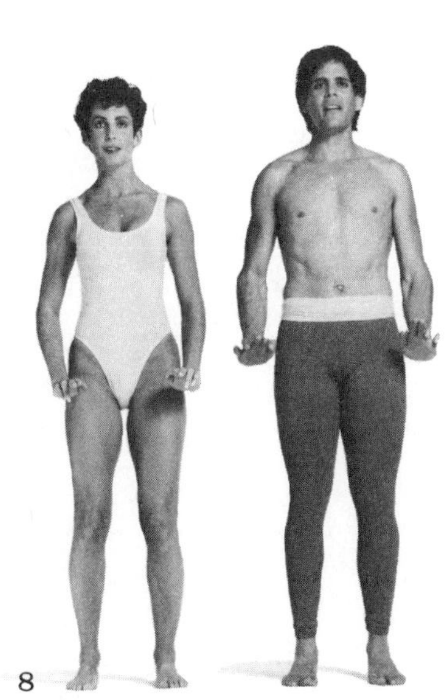
8

EXHALE INTO A NEW DAY

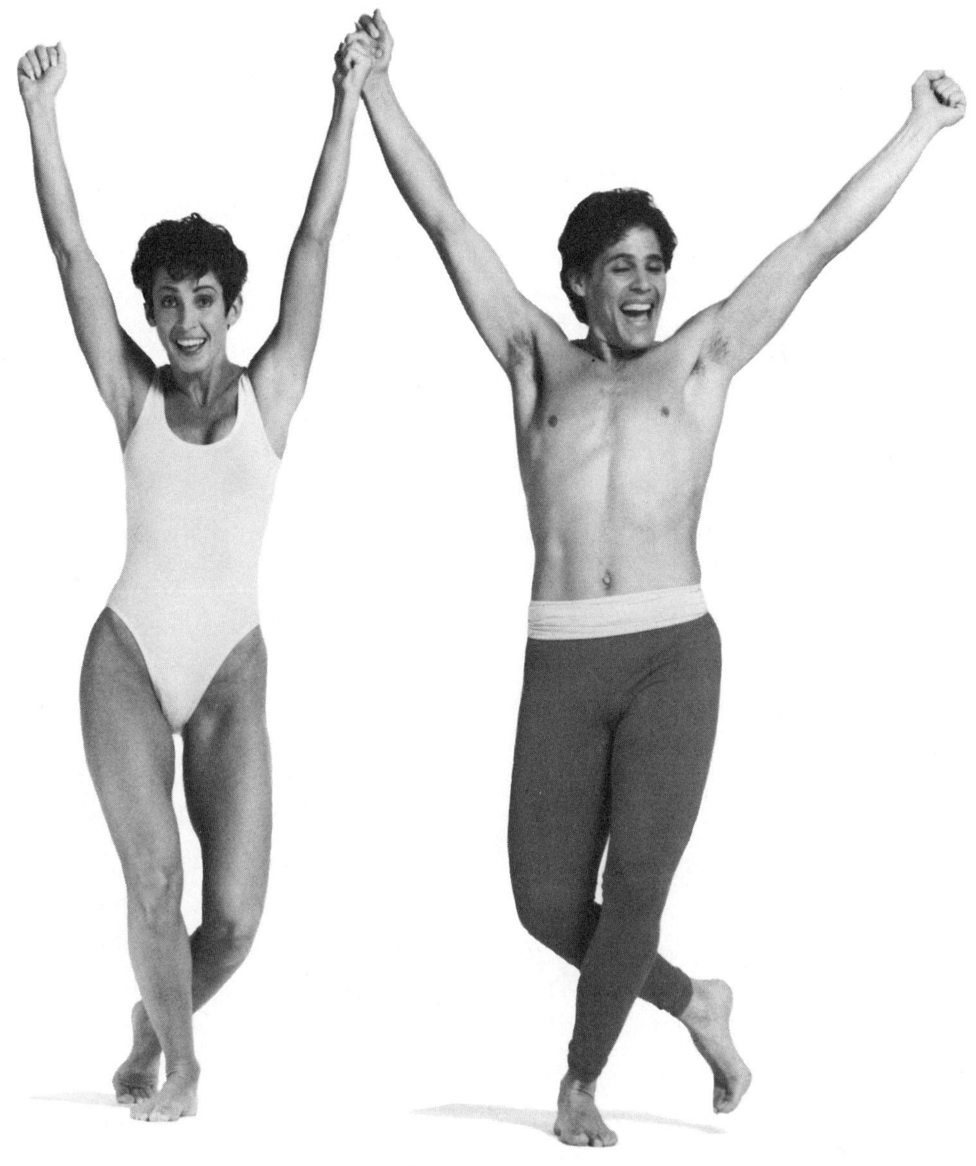

Take two purposeful steps gently back, stepping into a new body, a new you, a new day.

6/WORKOUT II

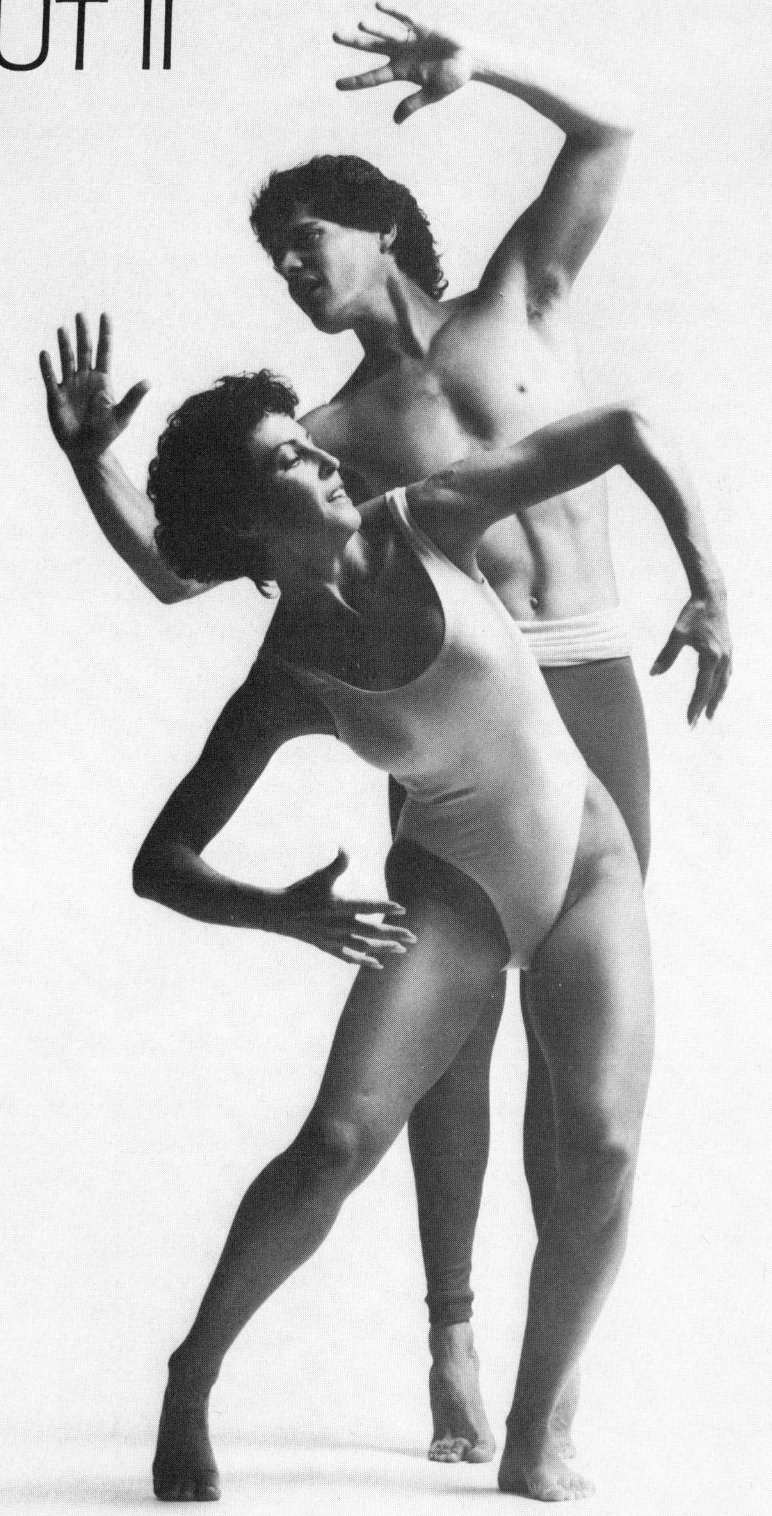

Now that you've mastered Workout I, you should be—

- completely familiar with the movements and how to tailor them
- comfortable with your pace, range of motion, and intensity of work
- in sync with your own rhythm
- adept at sinking and rising, shifting your weight, and aligning your body properly.

Your challenge now is—

- increasing the depth of your work
- adding variations that use even more muscle groups
- focusing more on the fluid dance of your workout
- traveling your movements
- customizing for more refined sculpting
- moving visually instead of technically

Your move into Workout II should be smooth and easy and gradual. You don't want to make a dramatic leap to a new level of intensity; continue building off Workout I and slowly increase the challenge of Workout II. Remember, each new step means new acclimation within your body, which needs time to adapt. Carlos is demonstrating some top-of-the-line movements. Don't try to imitate them right away. Give yourself plenty of time to refine and strengthen and progress toward a peak workout.

Making it Easy

Page through Workout II to get an idea of how the movements are extended. Once again get a mental image of yourself doing the movements. Then slowly move through the workout without music to feel the difference in the movements. Don't try to get a workout yet; just aim to become familiar with the changes. Remind yourself to relax—often—and use the imagery to enhance your movement, to create full, systemic conditioning.

When you're ready, put on an easy piece of music and focus on new balance and muscle work, running through the workout with just the leg movements first and then adding your arms. Once it all feels familiar, use faster, but never frenetic, music, varying your pace from one day to the next. As you become more adept with the workout, you can challenge yourself even more by using interpretive music and moving more with your own evocative, expressive rhythm than with the timed beat of the music.

Repetitions

Remember, the quality of your movements and how you feel doing them are far more important than the quantity of repetitions. We've given you a range of repetitions with each movement; start at the low end and build gradually. Even if you do the same number of repetitions as you did in Workout I, you'll be working harder because of the increased depth of your work. Don't burn out on marathon reps; you'll get more if you focus on—

- attaining greater balance and control
- mastering the intricacies of each movement
- getting the very most out of each movement
- generating a comfortable heat out of each motion

Remember, nobody's watching; nobody's judging your performance. Make it just right for you. Go for feeling good.

Tailoring Workout II

Just as you vary your music, use the lighten and load tailoring tools to vary the intensity of your work. Just because you've reached an advanced level doesn't mean that you should work harder and harder with each passing day. Alternate light and load days so your body has plenty of time to acclimate and gradually become more and more fit. And always listen to what your body wants most. Taking it easy doesn't mean you're slipping behind; it means you're playing it safe and smart. Work within your comfort zone.

The tailoring tools are set out in detail in Workout I, and by now you should have a full grasp of them. We'll recap briefly.

Body Alerts

- Always work in a comfortable range of motion.
- Never let your knees press beyond the arch of your foot.
- Keep your knee aligned with your second toe.
- Feel your work in the belly of your muscles, not your joints, never in your knees.
- Lead with your buttocks as you lower.
- Rise and lower slowly and evenly.
- Inhale fully to recharge your motion.
- When you step behind, stay on the ball of your foot so you make lots of light under your back heel.
- Always step back onto a soft, not locked, knee.
- Use only the amount of effort necessary for a motion.
- Never force your range of motion.
- Think fluid, lyrical as you move, reaching for both the relaxation and the work in each motion.
- Let your arms evoke and convey feeling with passion.
- Relax: Tension depletes your energy and constricts your breathing.

NO PAIN, MORE GAIN

TO LIGHTEN

Plane Work: Shallower
Work/Recharge: Work less, recharge more
Range of Motion: Closer to body
Muscle Groups: Core of body, plus light arms or light legs
Holds: None
Travel: Forward and backward, small steps

TO LOAD

Plane Work: Deeper
Work/Recharge: Work more, recharge less
Range of Motion: Broader
Muscle Groups: Core of body, plus all extremities down to fingertips and toes
Holds: Two to four beats
Travel: Vary patterns, broad

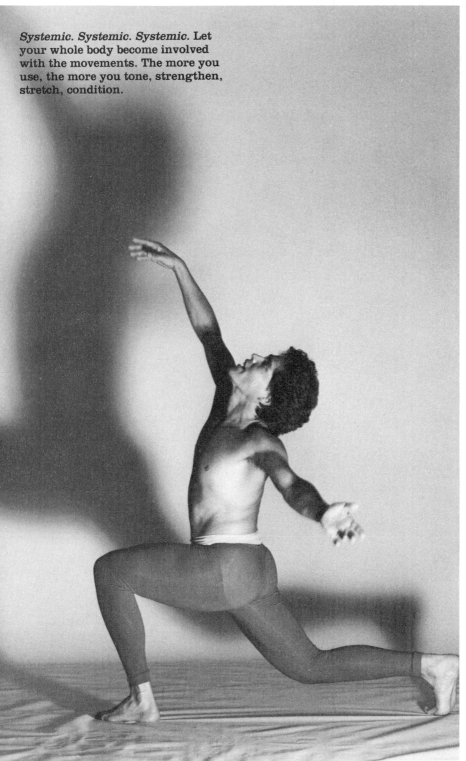

Systemic. Systemic. Systemic. Let your whole body become involved with the movements. The more you use, the more you tone, strengthen, stretch, condition.

Let's Go

Put on your music and let's go. Lightly walk in place, your whole body loose and fluid as you find the rhythm of your music. Remember, your count is 1–2–3–4, and each 4-count equals one repetition. If you can't readily find a 1–2–3–4 beat, pick another piece of music in which the beat is clear and easy to follow. To catch your beat, walk to the count of 3 and clap on 4; keep going until you've done eight repetitions.

The count of 1-and-2 is always an inhalation and 3-and-4 is always an exhalation, except for the Spine Roll, Jazz Walk, Charleston, and Karate kicks. Try out your breathing with another eight repetitions of the walk in place. This is a guide only; if it doesn't feel comfortable, follow your own natural breathing rhythm.

Be sure to read the benefits; they indicate where the changes are taking place in your body and where you should be feeling the movements. Use the customizing tips for more detailed body sculpting.

The NIA Mind Tamer

BENEFITS: To get ready and quiet your mind, to tune in to your body's mood and bring it into unison with your mind, to become balanced, at ease, in sync with the rhythm of your breath, which is the beginning of all movement, to focus on your workout goal.

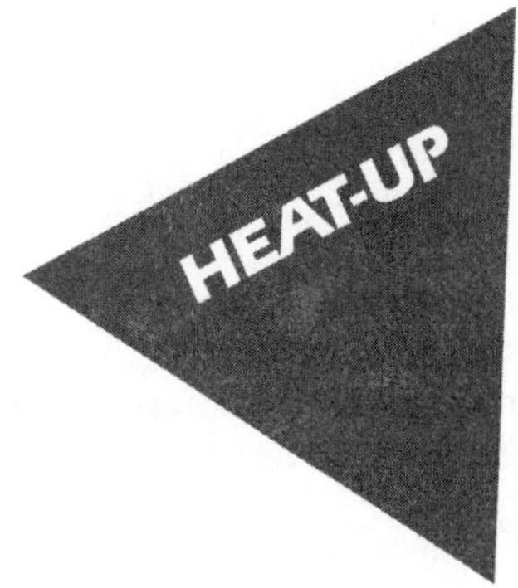

Take two purposeful steps forward into the center of your clock. Do so with feeling, bringing all your good intentions and energy into this one place. Pause . . . feel your body relaxed and centered . . . breathe. . . .

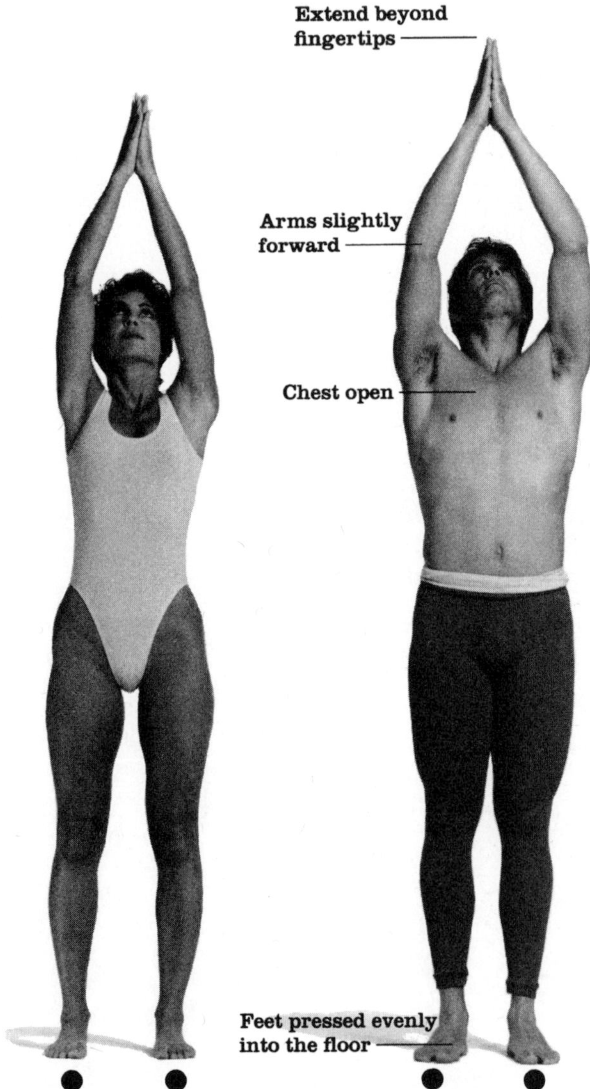
Extend beyond fingertips
Arms slightly forward
Chest open
Feet pressed evenly into the floor

INHALE

Inhale deeply as you draw your arms slowly out from the sides of your body, ending up high above your head with a clap of your hands.

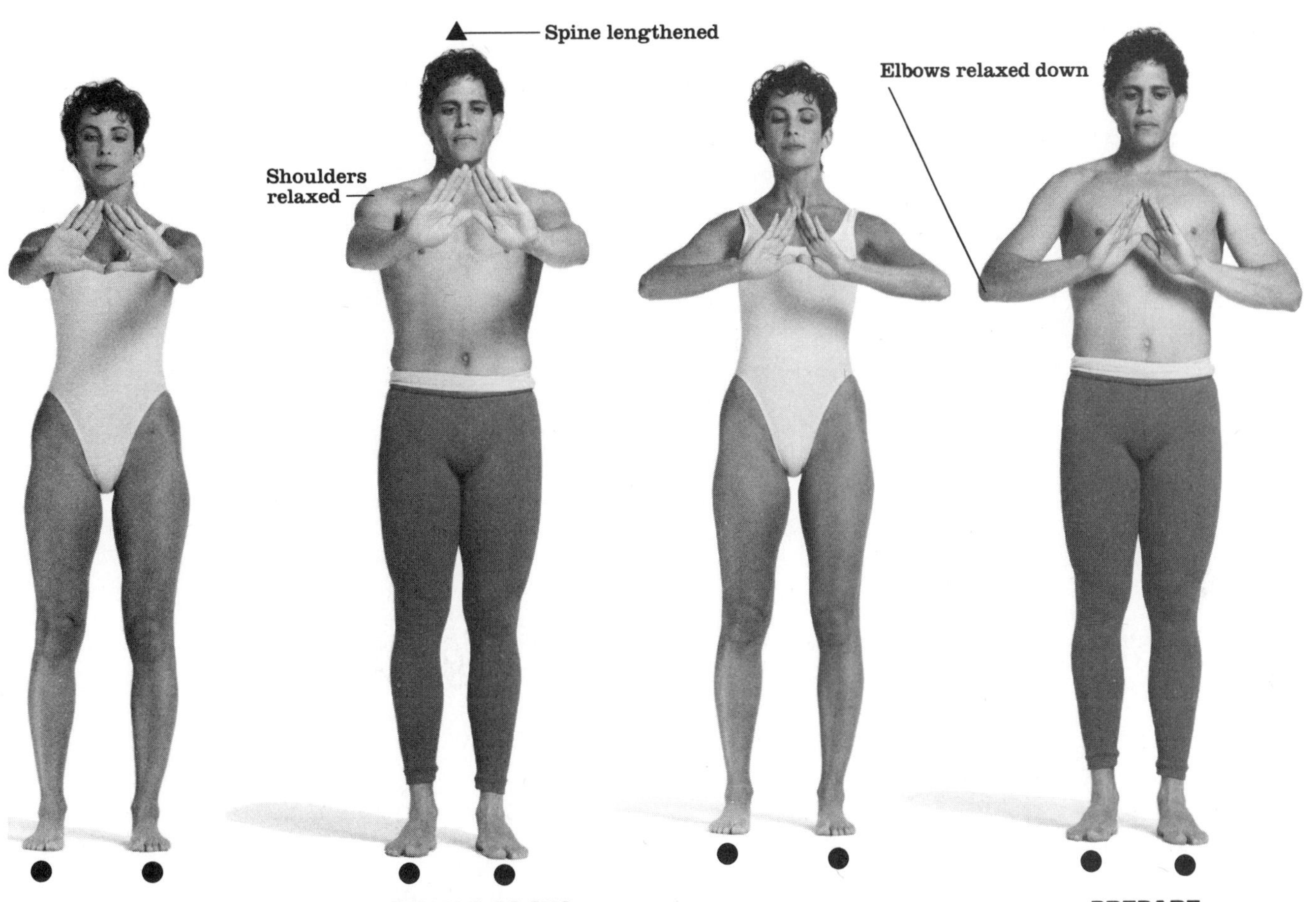

EXHALE-FOCUS

Exhale as you slowly lower your arms, your fingers forming the Triangle. Looking through your Triangle, take a minute to check in with yourself. How are you feeling, mentally, emotionally, physically? Be honest with yourself—and understanding so that you can gear your work toward a rich synergy of mind, body, and spirit. With every workout, take the time to visualize a goal in your Triangle and let it change as you do. Make it as vivid, as colorful, as you can, and hold that image as your point of focus throughout the entire workout.

PREPARE

Slowly draw your hands back toward your chest and let them relax to the sides of your body as you mentally prepare to move.

Muscle Relaxant

BENEFITS: To warm up your body in an unexerciselike way, to loosen through your spine and extremities.

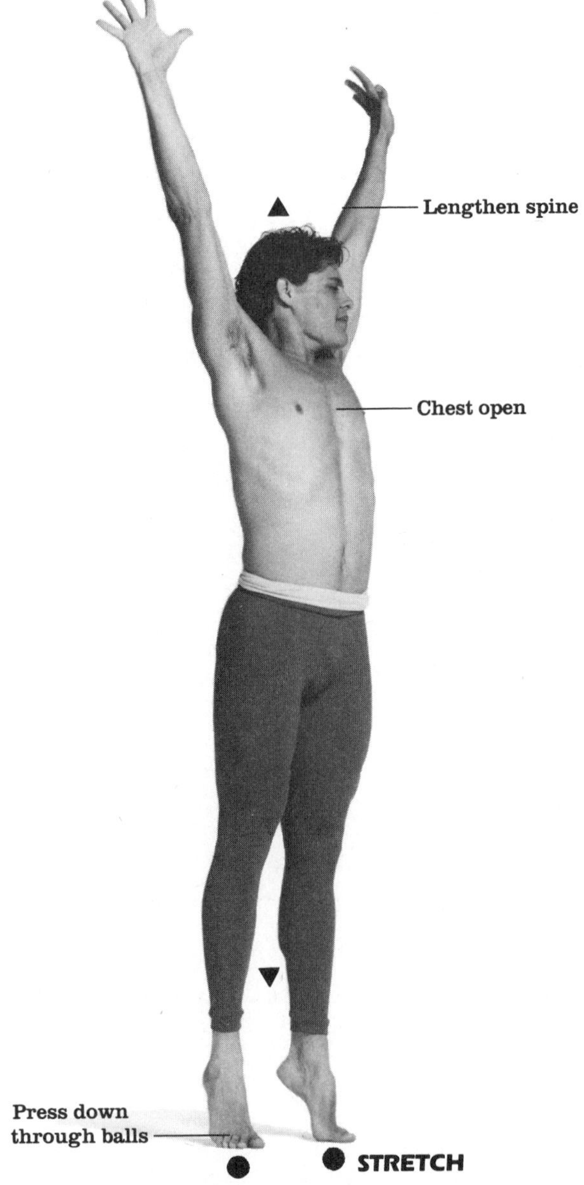

STRETCH

Inhale your arms up high above your head as you rise up onto the balls of your feet. Stretch toward the ceiling as if you're just waking up.

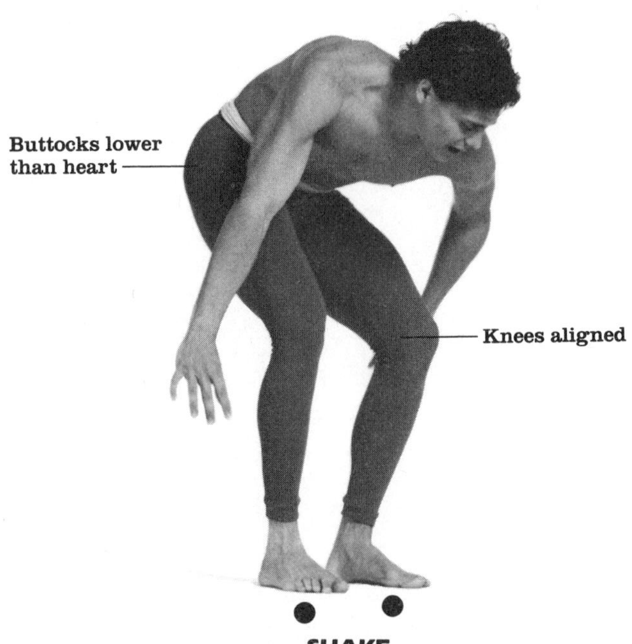

SHAKE

Exhale and sink your buttocks toward the floor, rounding your chest and head over as you let go and shimmy and shake—nothing too wild, just little jiggles—lightly loosening every joint in your body. As you shake, let your head and chest droop a little so the weight of your upper body gently stretches the full length of your spine. Still lightly shaking, press your feet into the floor as you round back up, stacking one vertebra at a time, and continue fluidly through to reach high and stretch again, rising up onto the balls of your feet. Repeat 8 times with feeling. Droop over a little farther each time, waking up more of your body. If you can comfortably and gradually bend all the way down to touch the floor, great. Otherwise, go just as far as you can without forcing the stretch.

Playful Improvisation

BENEFITS: To stimulate your own body language, your imagination.

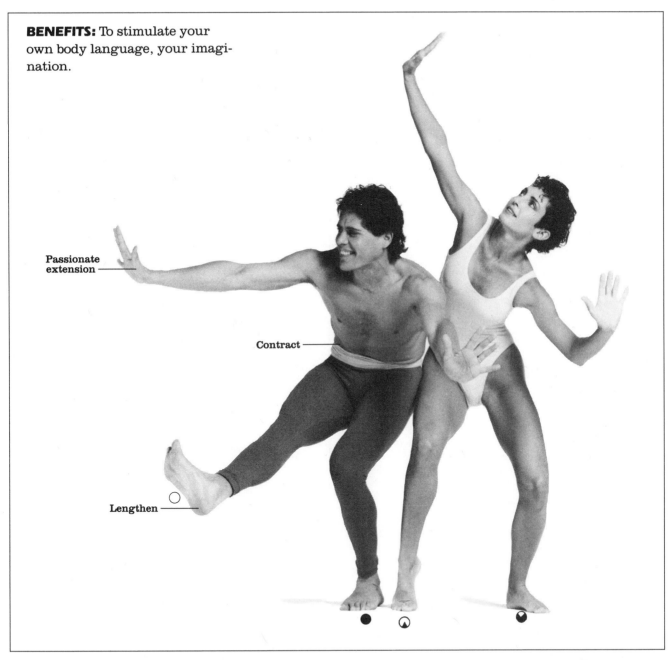

Imagine that you're standing in the center of a large, clear bubble and push on the sides of it with both your palms, your fists, stretching up, down, left, right, working in a broad range of motion by reaching and stretching wide. Work against the light resistance of the filmy, shimmery surface, now sinking deeply to press it with your back, buttocks, knees, shoulders, hips. Inhale when your chest and arms open; exhale when your chest and arms close. Explore, play until you feel ready to go on, at least for a count of 60.

SPINE ROLL

Whole-Body Warm-Up

BENEFITS: To increase your spine, hip, and knee flexibility, to strengthen your legs and buttocks, to warm up your whole body in an undulating fashion.

CUSTOMIZE: Slow down to strengthen your thighs; dig through your heels on the rise to firm your buttocks and the backs of your legs.

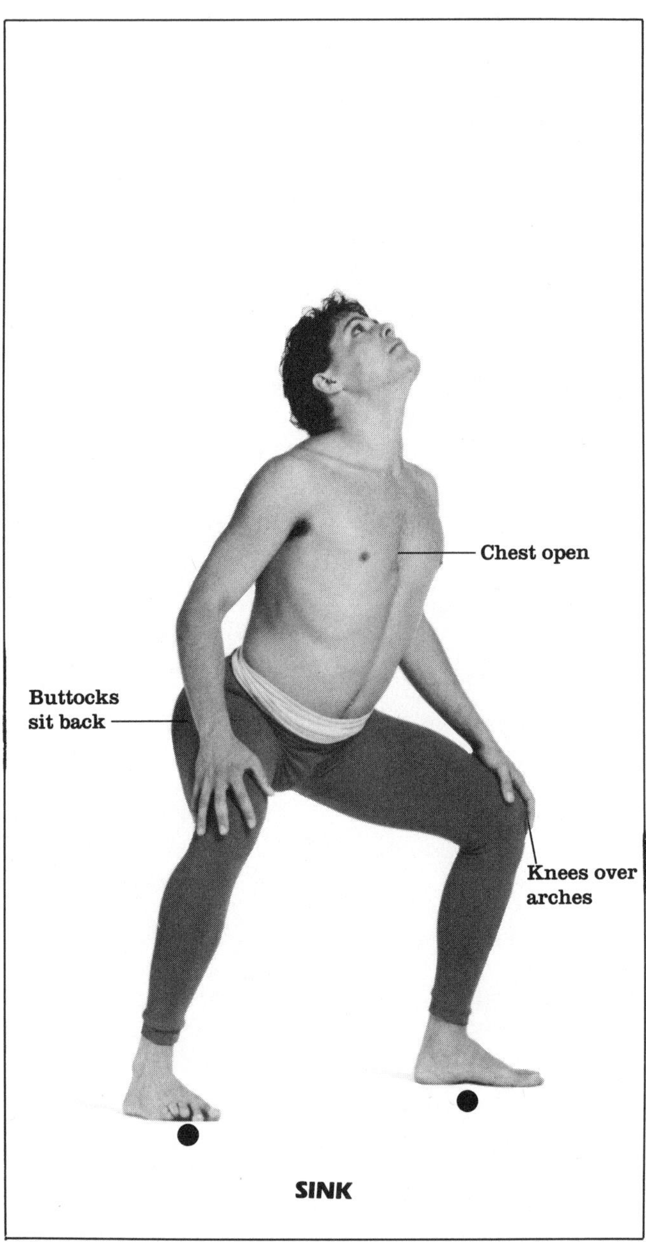

Standing in an *A* or riding stance, sink your buttocks deeply onto an imaginary chair, gently sliding your hands down your thighs toward your knees, inhaling deeply and opening your chest. Stop your hands at your knees and lift your toes to check your alignment and balance. Continue inhaling, lowering your buttocks a little more.

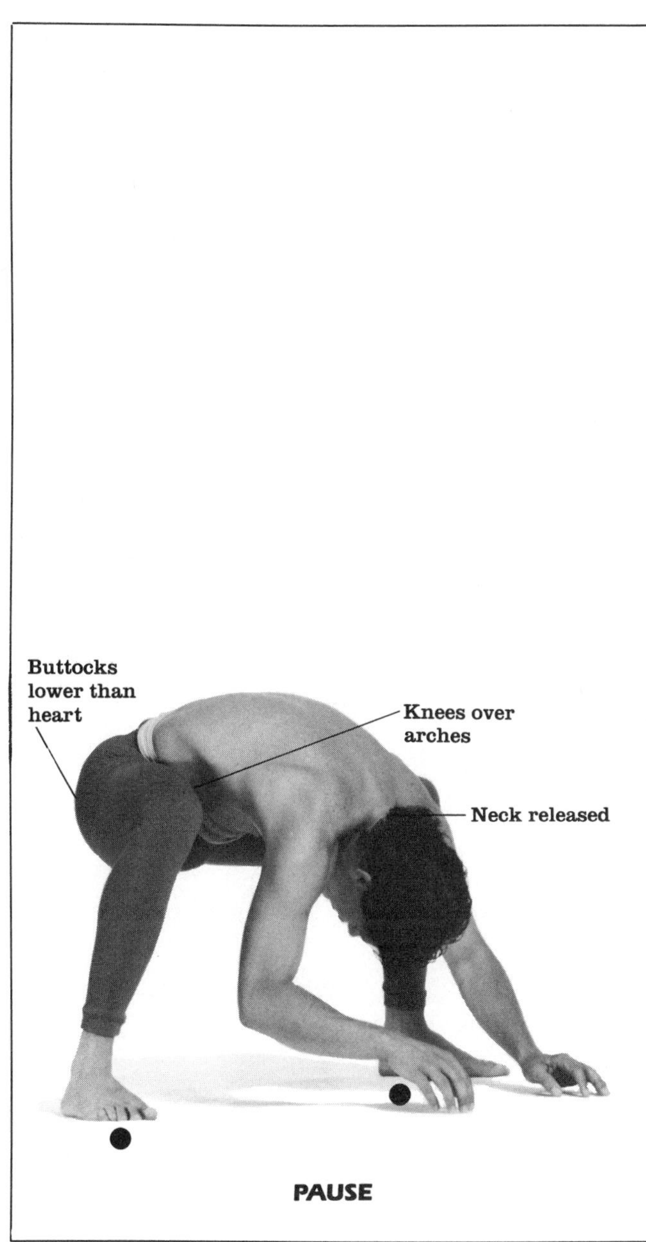

PAUSE

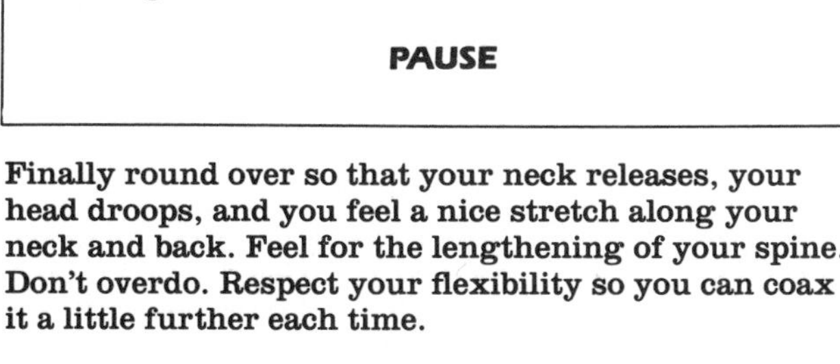

Finally round over so that your neck releases, your head droops, and you feel a nice stretch along your neck and back. Feel for the lengthening of your spine. Don't overdo. Respect your flexibility so you can coax it a little further each time.

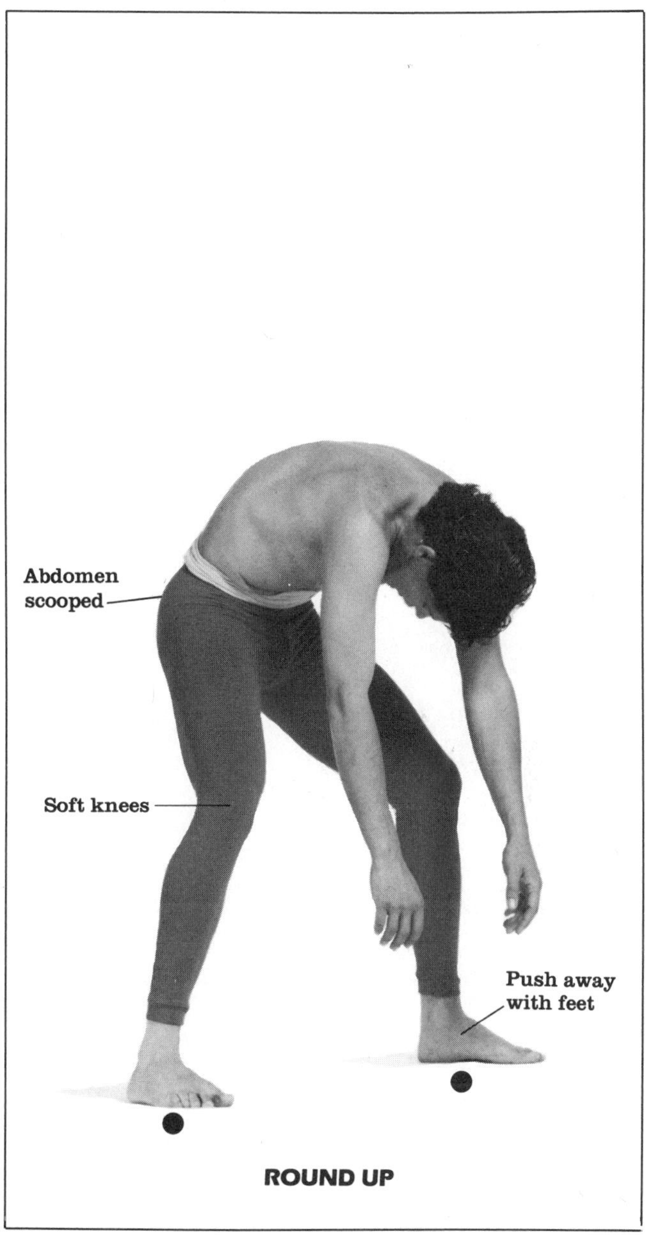

ROUND UP

Really using the strength of your legs to push away, and pressing your feet firmly into the floor, exhale and round slowly back up, stacking each vertebra one at a time, until your head finally tops them all. Roll down and round up 8 times, drooping farther over each time.

Extremity Wake-Up

BENEFITS: To strengthen and define your forearms and lower legs, to increase the circulation, flexibility, and dexterity of your fingers and feet.

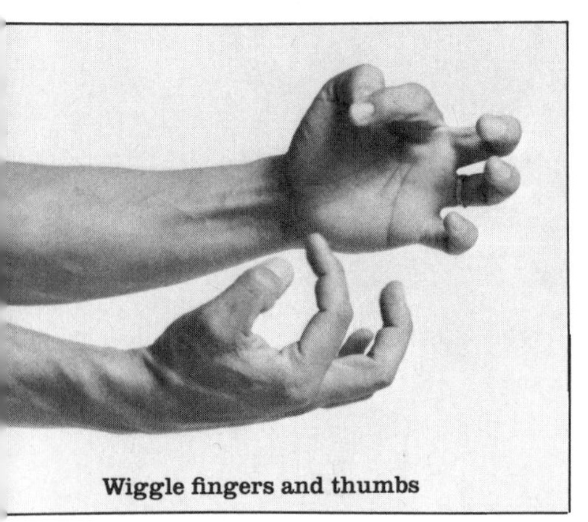

Wiggle fingers and thumbs

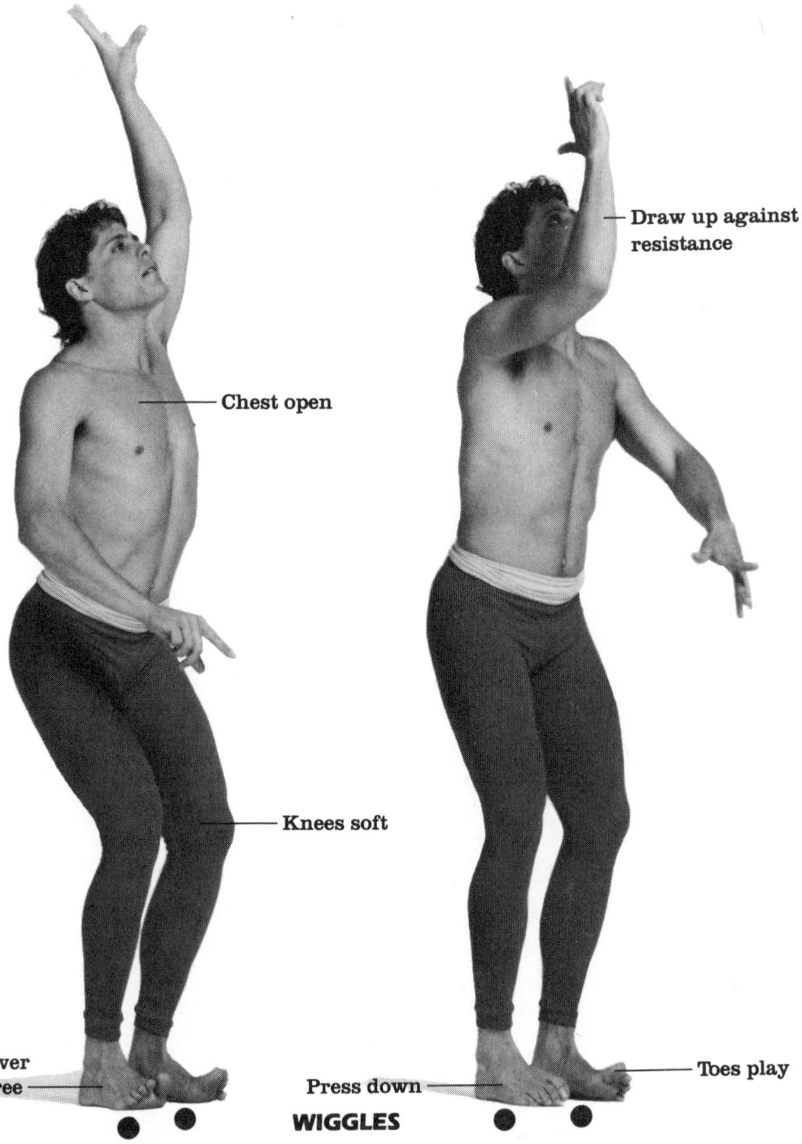

Chest open

Draw up against resistance

Knees soft

Weight back over arches, toes free

Press down

Toes play

WIGGLES

Standing in a closed stance, wiggle your fingers and toes, working all your joints until you feel a nice warmth building up through your arms and rising from your feet into your calves. Imagine being at the beach and squiggling the sand between your toes. Now, still wiggling your fingers, imagine painting a wall, alternating your arms up and down. Repeat for a count of 60.

Shin Strengthener

BENEFITS: To strengthen the muscles along your shins, helping to protect against shin-splints, to stretch your calf muscles and Achilles tendon, to tone and increase the flexibility of your shoulders, arms, and hands.

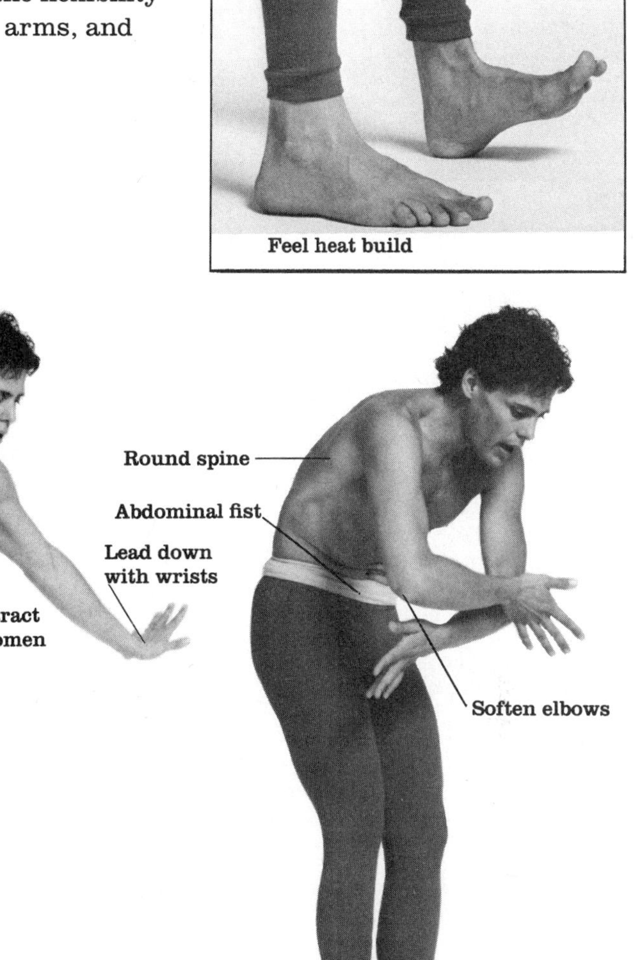

Feel heat build

Three weights aligned

Chest open

Knees soft

Press heels into floor

Contract abdomen

DUCK WALK

FLY

Alternately lift the front of your feet off the floor as high as possible. Don't let your knees snap back or your buttocks thrust behind, but stay soft and feel for the movement through your feet and ankles.

Now fly scuth, drawing your arms up high and sweeping broadly down like wings, your elbows and wrists loose and fluid, your spine undulating. Exaggerate the expansion of your chest as you lift your wings and the contraction of your abdominals as your wings lower and your spine rounds slightly. Imagine you're moving against a gale wind to increase the intensity of your flight. Wiggling your fingers and leading with your elbows, inhale your arms up on a 2-count; exhale your arms down on another 2-count while working your feet. Repeat for a total of 16 to 24, counting 1-2-3-one, 1-2-3-two, and so on.

Circular Balance

BENEFITS: To stabilize your ankles, to lubricate the joints in your toes, ankles, knees, and hips, to strengthen your legs and upper body, to increase your upper body flexibility, to enhance your balance, to get a feeling for circular motion involving your whole body.

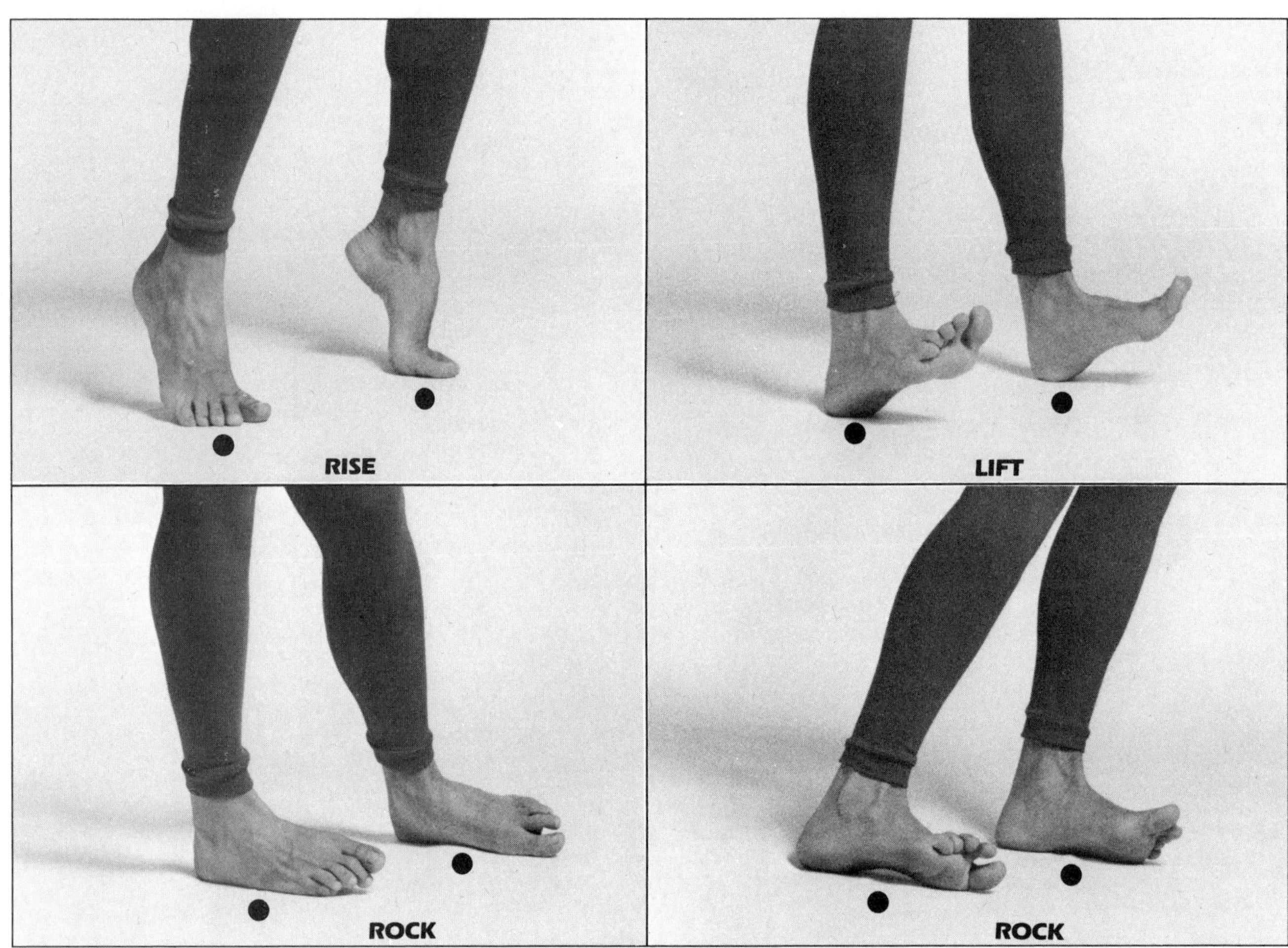

Standing in a closed or *A* stance, rock high onto the balls of your feet and back high onto your heels, moving through the entire length of your feet as you rock back and forth several times. Then rock side to side, pressing deeply into both the inside and outside edges of your feet and feeling the warm massage across the balls of your feet.

Finally, tie the movements together, rocking all around your feet, making broad, full circles, and pressing deeply onto the edges. Circle slowly in one direction several times and then reverse, letting your whole body sway with the motion. Feel the warm massage through your lower back, the heat building in your hips to loosen the ligaments, to melt away any constriction. As your hips sweep front, inhale, rise to the balls of your feet; as your hips sweep back, exhale, rock back onto your heels. Imagine your hips are sweeping around the inside rim of a hula hoop. Repeat 8 times in one direction; then reverse for another 8. And then—

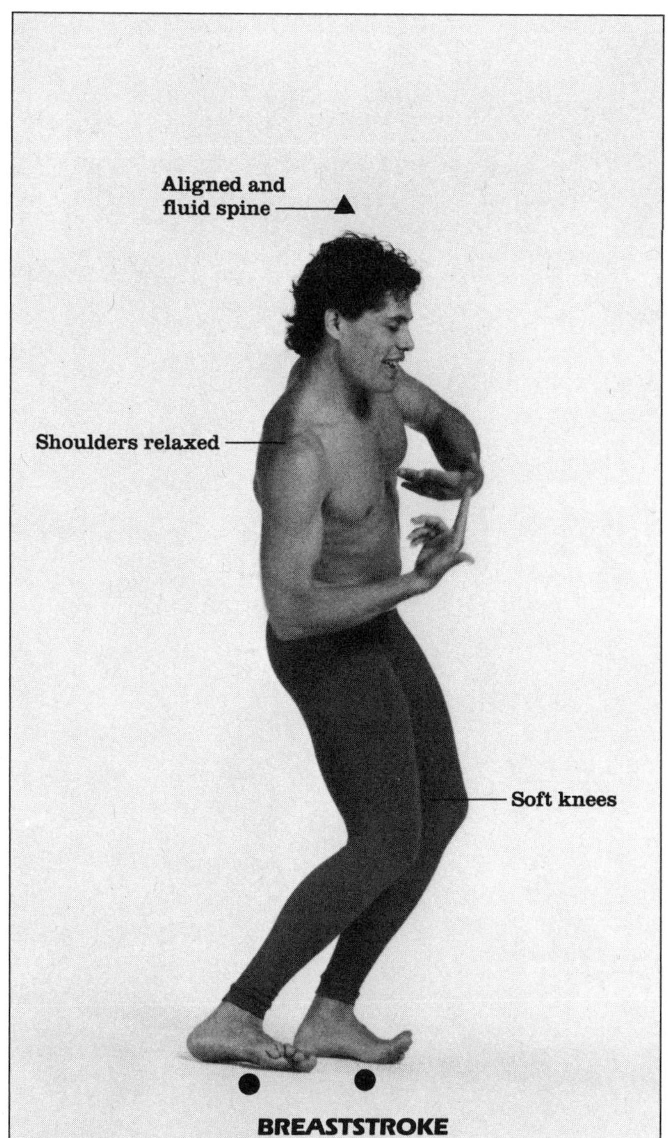

BREASTSTROKE

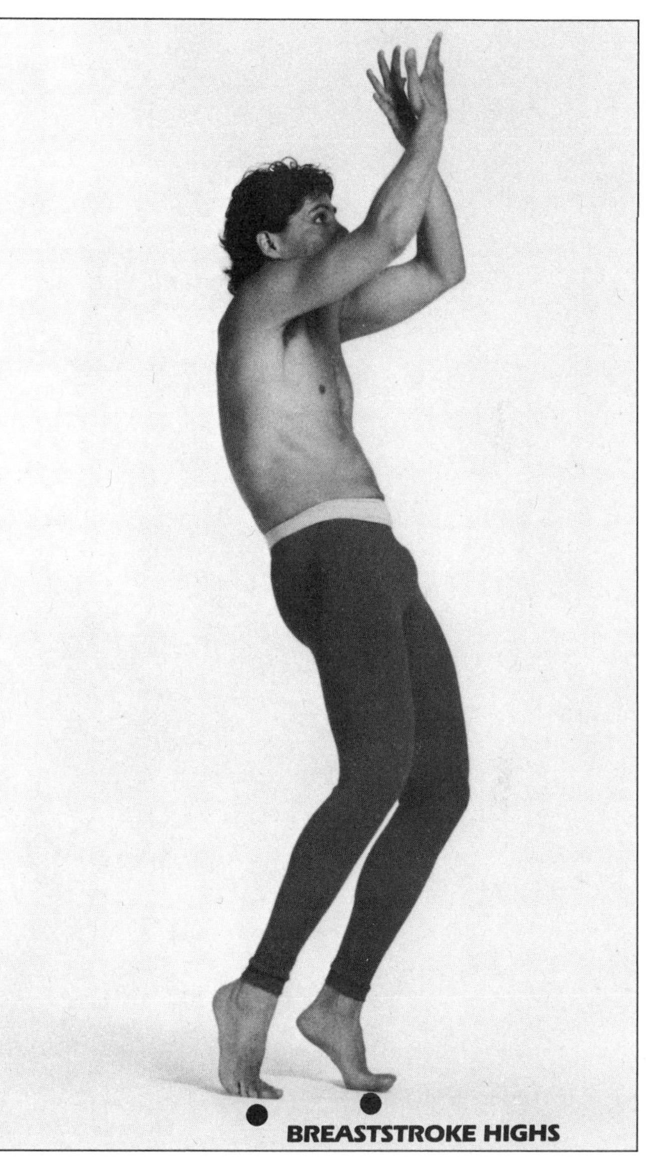
BREASTSTROKE HIGHS

—add a breaststroke in front of your chest, inhaling when your arms are wide open to either side and exhaling as they cross in front of your body, all the while rocking around on your feet. Then add a breaststroke high above your head and alternate high and low breaststrokes with each circle of your hips. Imagine you're swimming and work against the dense resistance of the water. Continue 8 times in one direction and then reverse for another 8, letting your whole body become involved in the motion as you breaststroke. Repeat for another total of 16.

The Whole-Body Press

BENEFITS: To strengthen your feet and calves, to create flexibility in your ankles, chest, and upper back, to give new definition to your calves and shoulders, to enhance your balance.

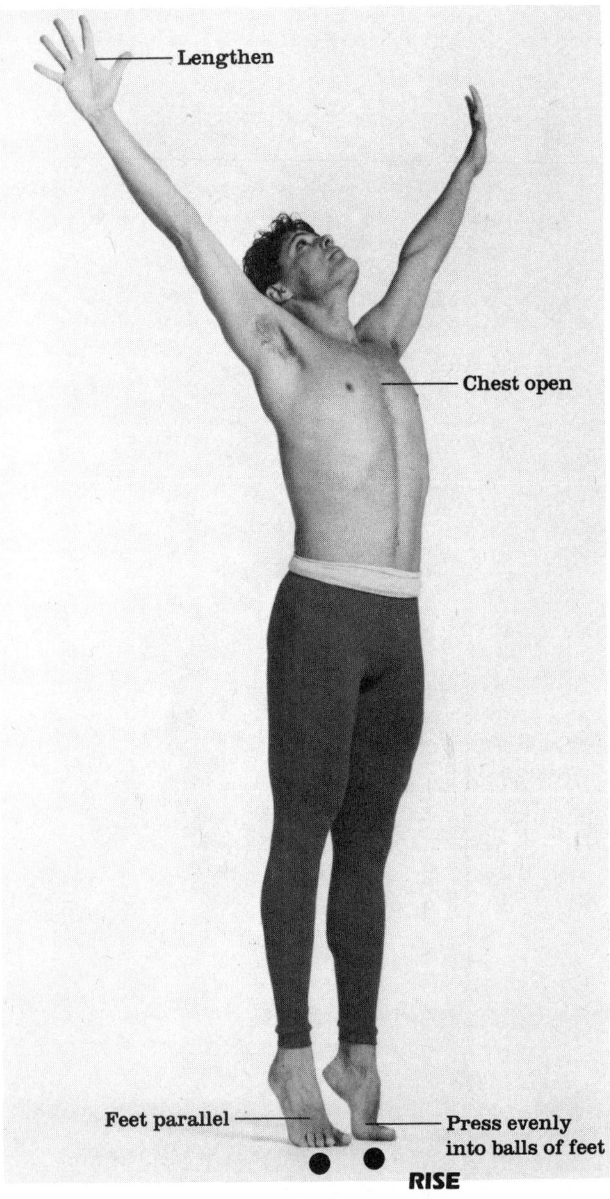

Standing in a closed stance, inhale and slowly rise up high onto the balls of your feet as though you're peeking over a fence. Feel the lengthening of your whole spine run up through your neck, the even strength of your legs surging down through your feet. As you rise, spread your arms up wide on a diagonal above your head as if you're reaching up and grabbing some sunlight. Pause and hold the lift for greater strength and balance.

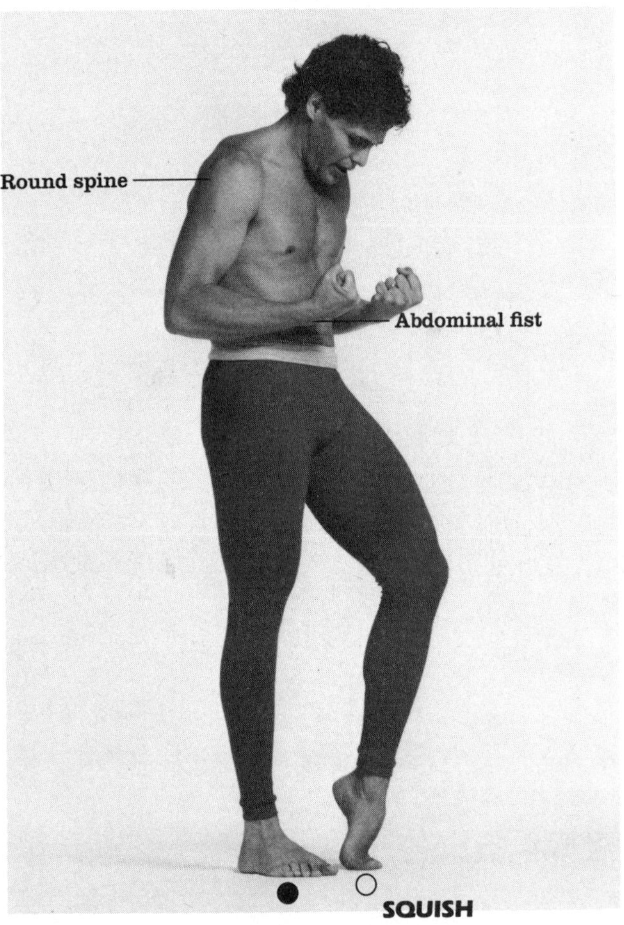

Now exhale and soften your right knee to the front as your left heel squishes into the floor and draw the sunlight into the core of your body, feeling the NIA Technique's kinetic sit-up. Rise and lower fluidly, evenly, alternating the heel squish. Let your hips follow the motion, being careful not to throw your hip out to the side but to let it sway slightly, softly toward the foot that's flat on the floor. Repeat 16 to 24 times, alternating left and right, up 2 beats and down 2 beats.

The Total-Body Boost

BENEFITS: To trim your inner and outer thighs, to tone your calves and hamstrings, to lift your buttocks, to increase your foot flexibility, to tone and define your upper body, to enhance your balance.

CUSTOMIZE: To work your inner thighs, turn your foot in. To work your outer thighs, turn your foot slightly out. To streamline the muscle down the center of your thigh, keep your toes pointing straight ahead.

Buttocks lower than heart
Lengthen neck
Knee aligned with second toe
Feet parallel

7:00 STEP BACK

Starting in your hip stance, shift your weight into your right leg and, with control, step back onto the ball of your left foot at 7:00, making sure your weight is evenly distributed in your feet. Now, keeping most of your weight on your front leg, slowly sink your back knee deeply toward the floor as you round your spine over your thigh by making an abdominal fist, your torso over a strong supporting leg. Pause and imagine picking up a ball from the floor.

Lengthen through crown
Strong legs
Press down through balls of feet

RISE & THROW

Now, pressing your front foot into the floor and exhaling, round up, stacking your vertebra one at a time, stepping back to center, and rising high onto the balls of your feet as you flick the ball straight up into the air as if you're shooting a basket.

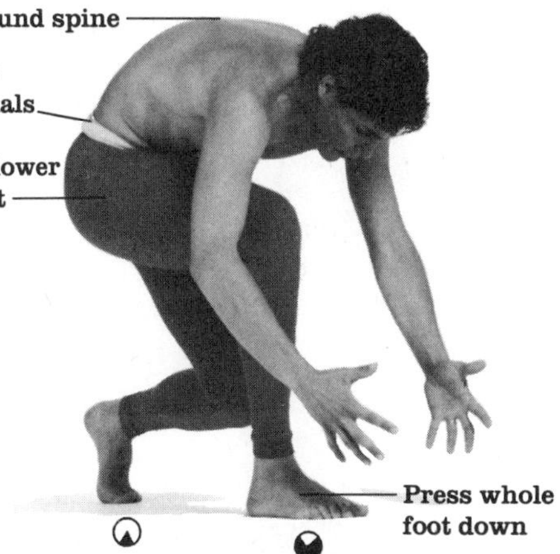

5:00 STEP BACK

Repeat on the other side, stepping back onto the ball of your foot. Repeat 16 to 24 times altogether.

The Whole-Body Stretch

BENEFITS: To increase back and abdominal strength, spine and hip flexibility, to tone your inner and outer thighs, to trim your buttocks.

CUSTOMIZE: For greater definition from calf to buttock, press firmly through the balls of your feet as you rise high, squeezing your buttocks tightly.

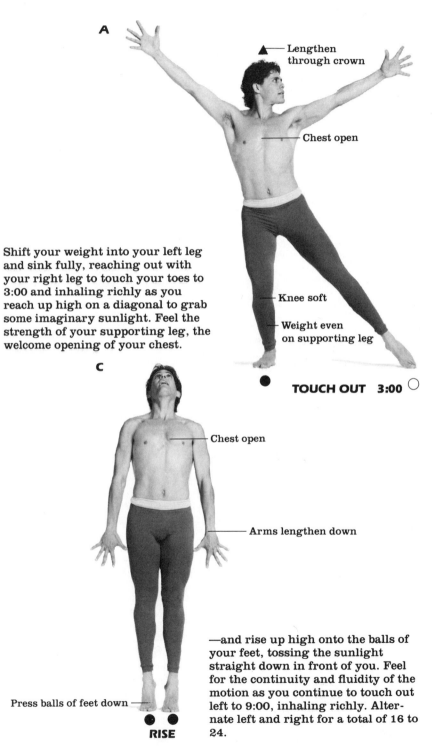

A

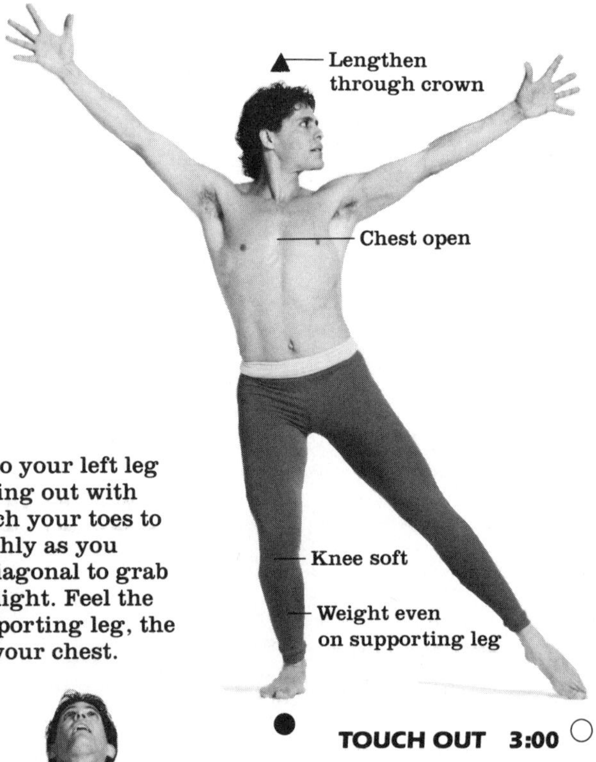

Lengthen through crown

Chest open

Knee soft

Weight even on supporting leg

TOUCH OUT 3:00

Shift your weight into your left leg and sink fully, reaching out with your right leg to touch your toes to 3:00 and inhaling richly as you reach up high on a diagonal to grab some imaginary sunlight. Feel the strength of your supporting leg, the welcome opening of your chest.

B

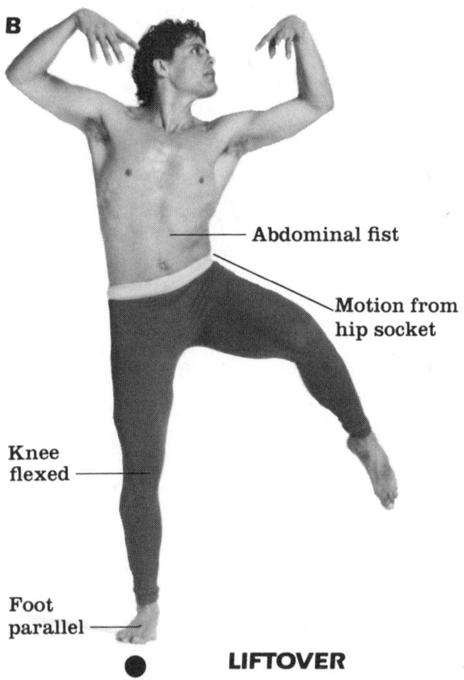

LIFTOVER

Then exhale as you step back to center, lifting your leg over a large imaginary rock—

C

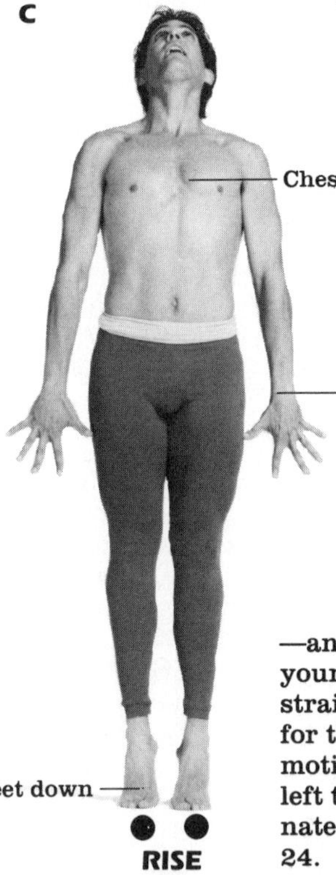

Chest open

Arms lengthen down

Press balls of feet down

RISE

—and rise up high onto the balls of your feet, tossing the sunlight straight down in front of you. Feel for the continuity and fluidity of the motion as you continue to touch out left to 9:00, inhaling richly. Alternate left and right for a total of 16 to 24.

The Speed Walk

BENEFITS: To increase arm and upper body strength and definition, to promote hip flexibility, to enhance coordination.

CUSTOMIZE: Sink low and pump your knees into your chest as you walk for hip, buttock, and thigh streamlining.

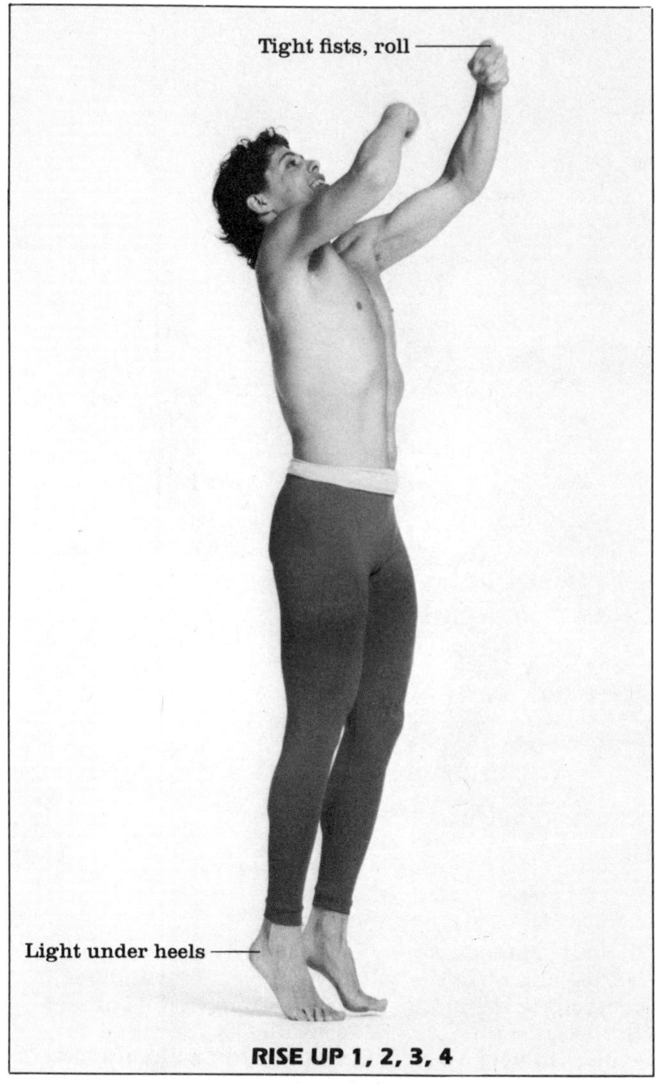

RISE UP 1, 2, 3, 4

Jazz walk lightly and loosely with your knees softened, letting your hips sway fluidly. Then, still jazz walking, inhale and rise high onto the balls of your feet as you rapidly circle your forearms comfortably above your head, punching an imaginary bag. Count 4 steps up.

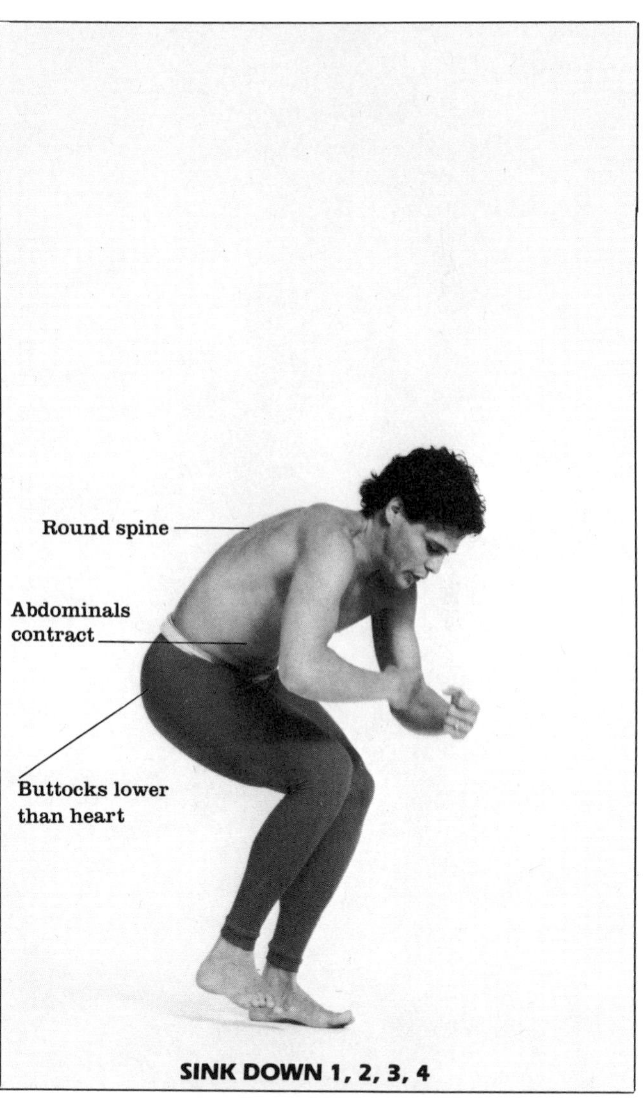

SINK DOWN 1, 2, 3, 4

Still jazzy, exhale and sink deeply toward the floor as you punch low and count 4 steps down. Repeat up 4 steps and down 4 steps until you've punched high 16 to 24 times.

Torso Trimmer

BENEFITS: To extend your range of motion through your hips, to increase your spine and torso flexibility, to tone your buttocks, inner and outer thighs, to create chest definition.

CUSTOMIZE: For firm abs, exhale strongly and scoop your abdomen as you rotate your chest.

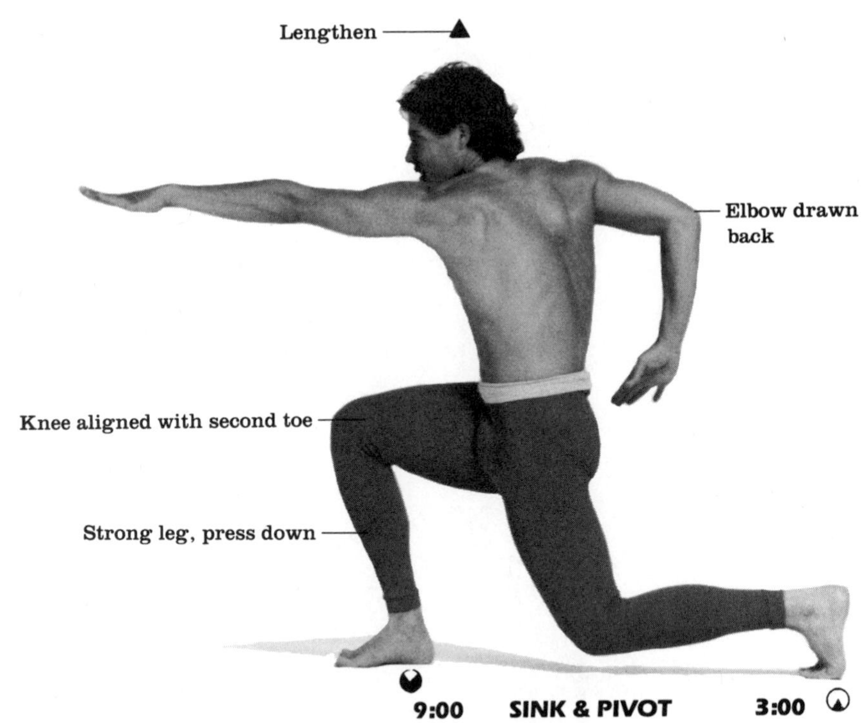
Lengthen
Elbow drawn back
Knee aligned with second toe
Strong leg, press down
9:00
SINK & PIVOT
3:00

In your *A* stance, sink your weight deeply into your left leg and pivot the ball of your right foot at 3:00, controlling the motion with the strength of your legs. At the same time, exhale forcefully as you reach out wide with your right arm and wipe off an imaginary table at chest level, wiping from right to left, your arm following the rotation of your torso. Pause.

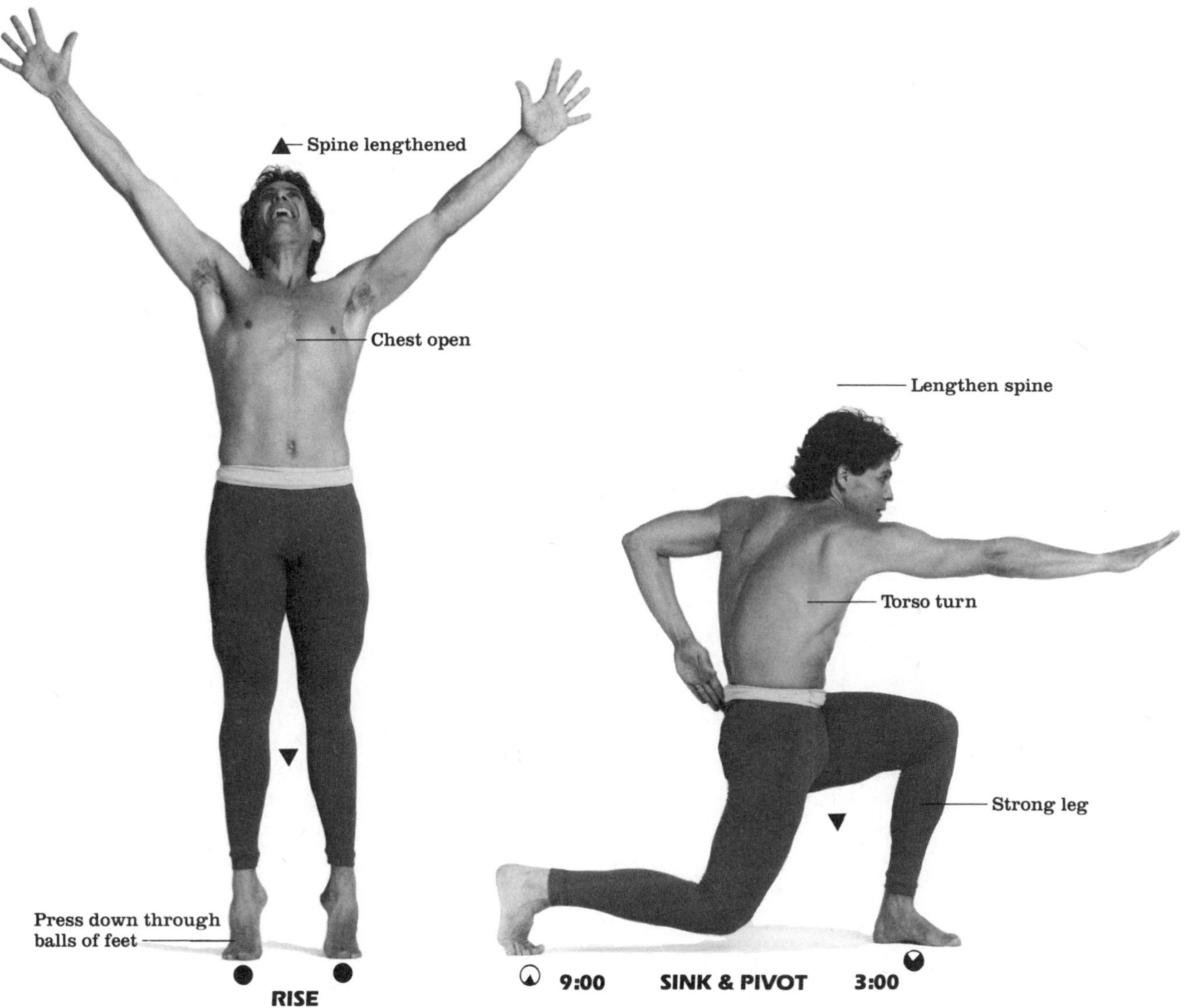

Pivot back to center, rising up high onto the balls of your feet, and inhale, your arms wide to either side, your feet parallel.

Repeat on the other side, pivoting at 9:00 and putting even more passion into your movement. As you pivot, be careful not to thrust your hip into your supporting leg or you might strain your knee. If you feel pressure in the knee of your supporting leg, let your foot turn out, decrease the pivot of your free leg, be sure to finish your pivot with both feet turned slightly out, and turn more with your torso, less with your hips. Never turn a leg that has weight on it. Empty first by shifting your weight off the leg and then rotate. Continue alternating left and right, 12 to 16 times on each side.

STICKY STEP-OUT/BUBBLE GUM

Tummy Tightener

BENEFITS: To tighten your abdominals, to tone your frontal thighs, to increase the strength and flexibility of your upper body, to trim your torso, to whittle your waist.

CUSTOMIZE: For faster results, contract your abdomen to generate your leg lift.

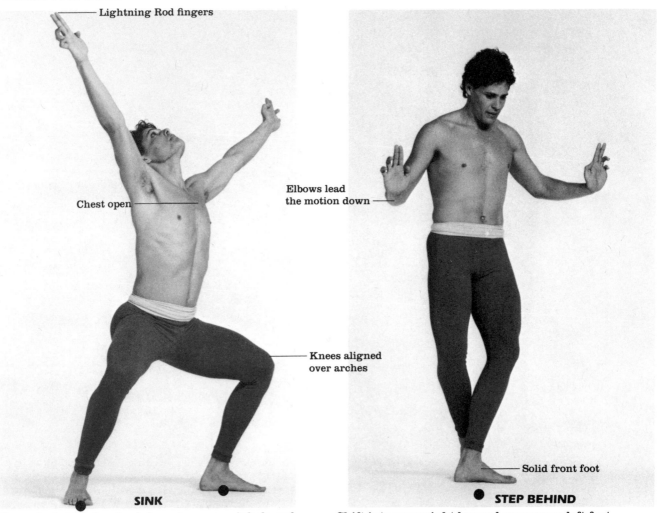

SINK

In an A stance, deeply sink center as you inhale and draw your arms up high.

STEP BEHIND

Shift into your right leg and cross your left foot behind, your arms beginning to float back down.

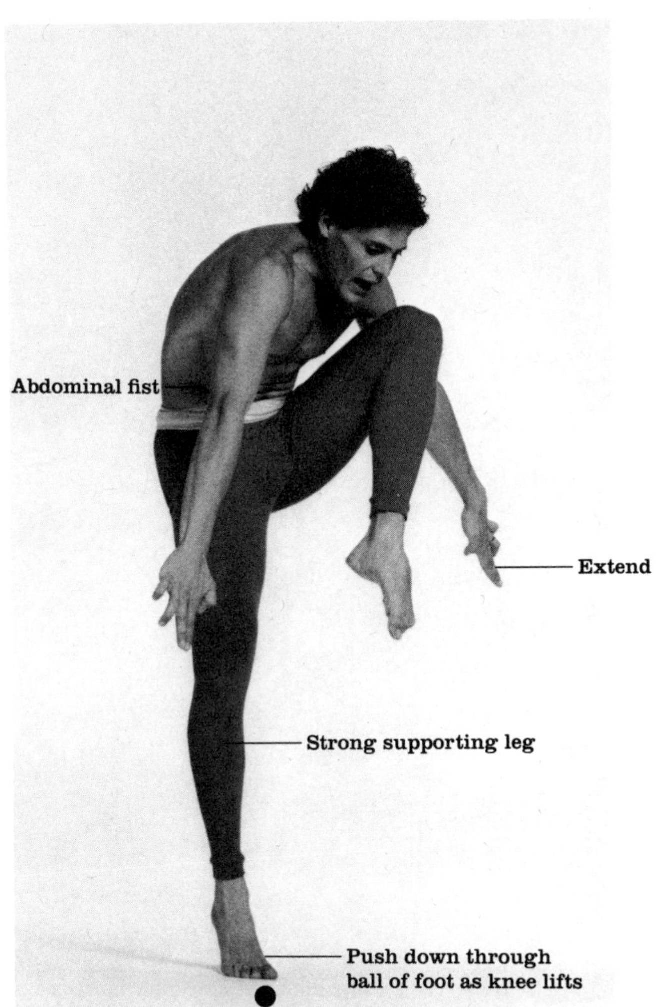

Rise up high onto the ball of your left foot as you exhale and draw your right thigh up in front of you, your arms coming fully down to your sides.

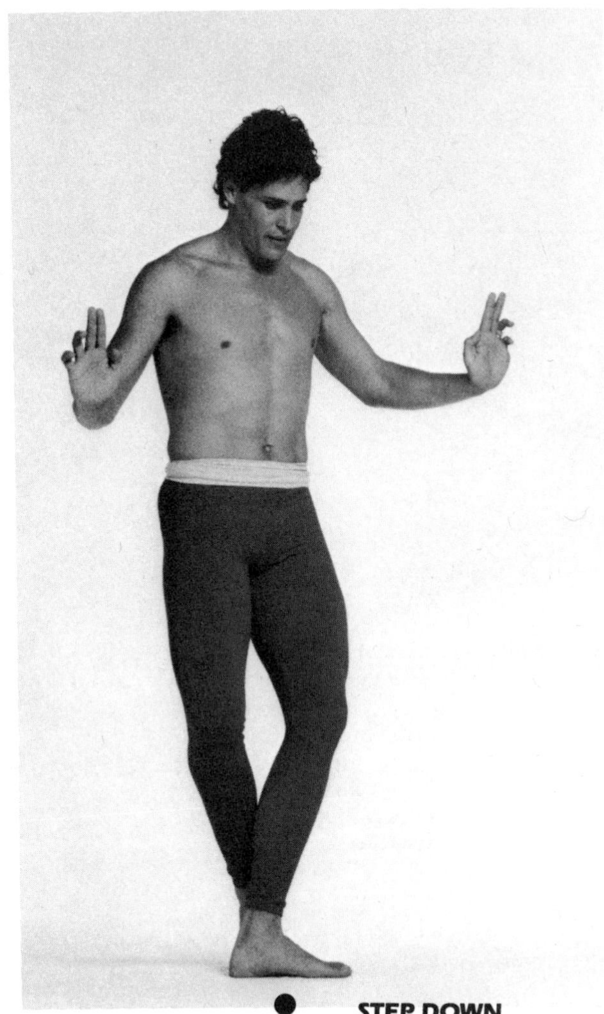

STEP DOWN

Step back down with your right foot, your arms rising, and sink back into your A stance, your arms high. Continue fluidly through to cross your right foot behind and rise high as your arms now sweep down, your left knee draws up. Counting 1–2 through center, 3 for the cross and lift, and 4 for the step back down, alternate for a total of 16 to 24 times on each side.

Thigh Trimmer

BENEFITS: To strengthen and tone your thighs, calves, hips, buttocks, and upper back, to define and stretch your chest, to firm your abdominals.

CUSTOMIZE: To really slim your inner thighs, turn the inside of your lifted leg up toward the ceiling.

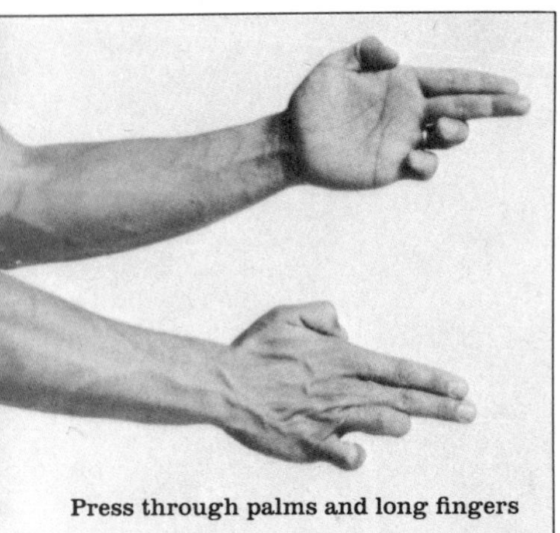

Press through palms and long fingers

To create resistance and greater arm defintion, use Lightning Rod fingers by pulling your thumb back, extending your first two fingers, cocking your last two fingers, and tensing your entire hand.

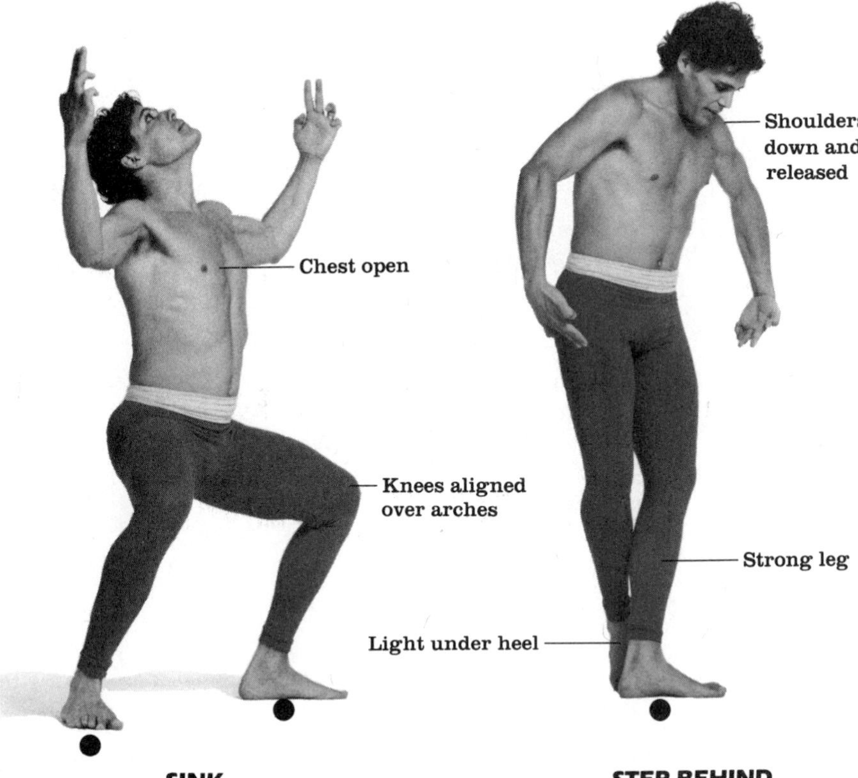

SINK

In your A stance, sink deeply center as you inhale and draw your elbows back, your chest wide.

STEP BEHIND

Shift onto your right leg and cross your left foot behind, drawing your arms down in front and crossing at the wrists.

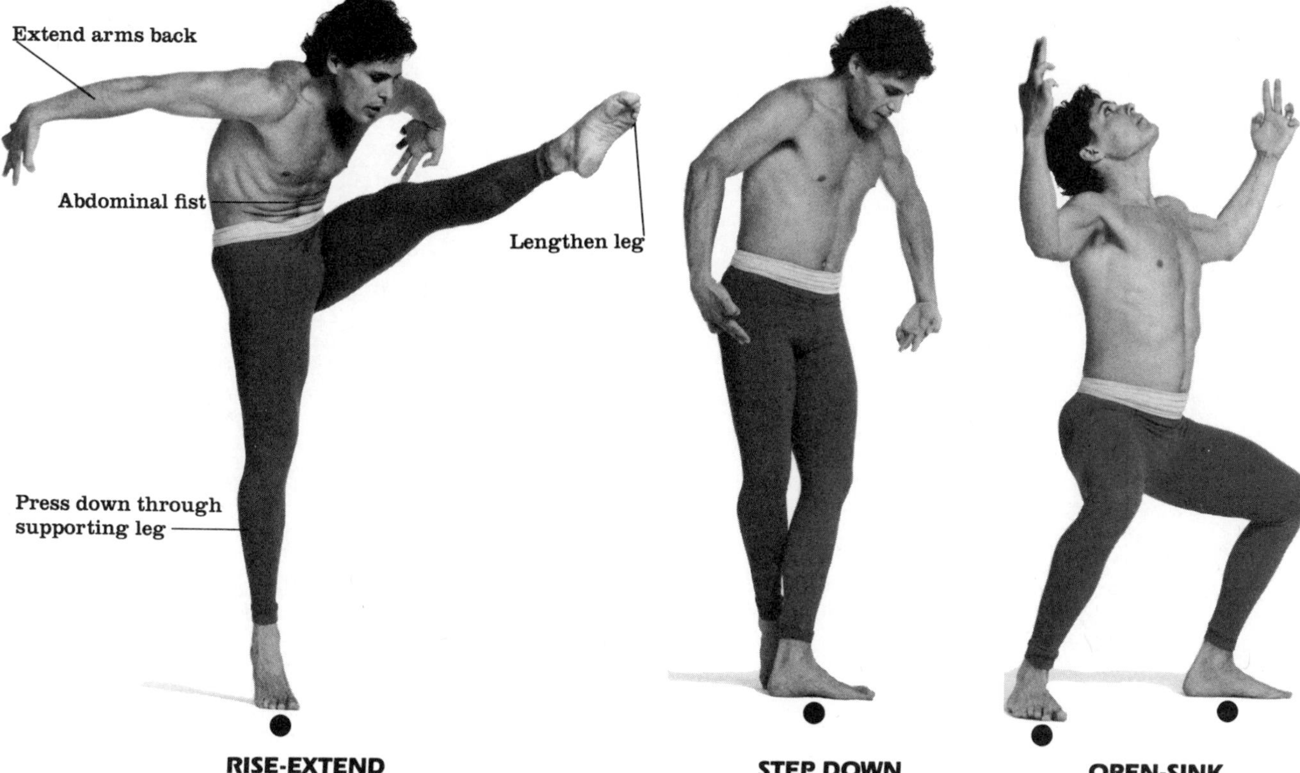
Extend arms back
Abdominal fist
Lengthen leg
Press down through supporting leg

RISE-EXTEND

Press into the whole ball of your left foot, exhale, and contract your abdomen to protect your lower back as you gracefully extend your right leg up high in front, squeezing your thigh bone with your muscles and using the support of your back leg to generate the movement. As your leg comes up, sweep your arms elegantly out and back.

STEP DOWN **OPEN-SINK**

Step back down with your right foot and sink deeply through your A stance to repeat on the other side. Continue for a total of 16 to 24 times on each side.

Leg Leaner

BENEFITS: To increase your ankle flexibility and strength, to tone your calves, to trim your thighs and buttocks, to define your shoulders, upper back, and chest, to enhance your coordination, to stretch your Achilles tendon.

CUSTOMIZE: To trim the back of your thigh and to lift your buttocks, lift your leg back on a slight diagonal with your heel pointing toward the ceiling.

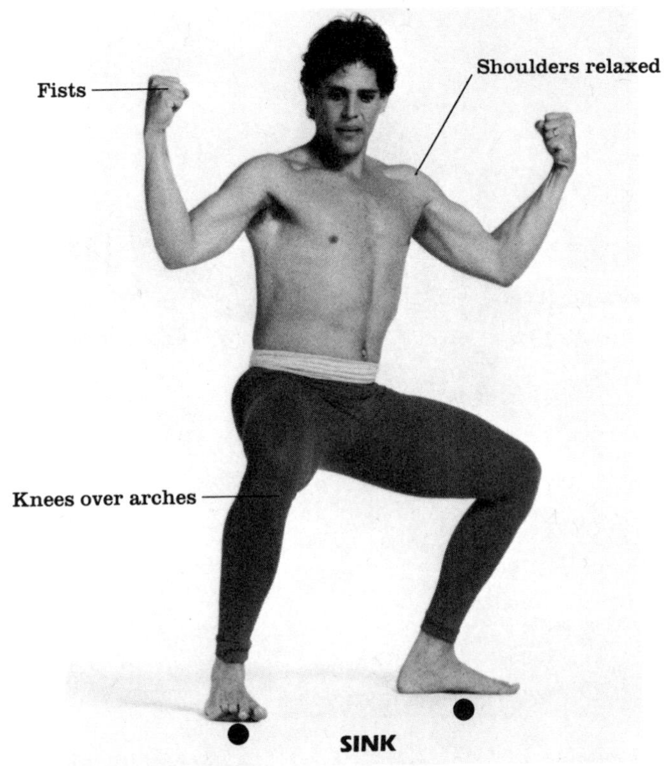

SINK

In a riding stance, sink deeply, your weight evenly distributed through your feet as you draw your elbows down as if pressing against tight springs.

RECHARGE
JAZZ WALK

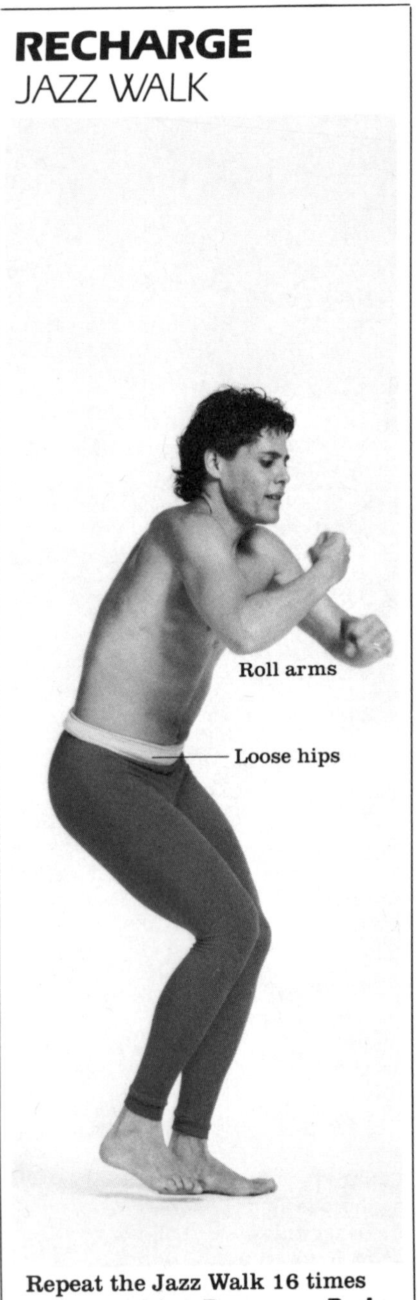

Repeat the Jazz Walk 16 times with Punching Bag arms. **Body Check:** Ease up or put more into your motion at this point. Breathe.

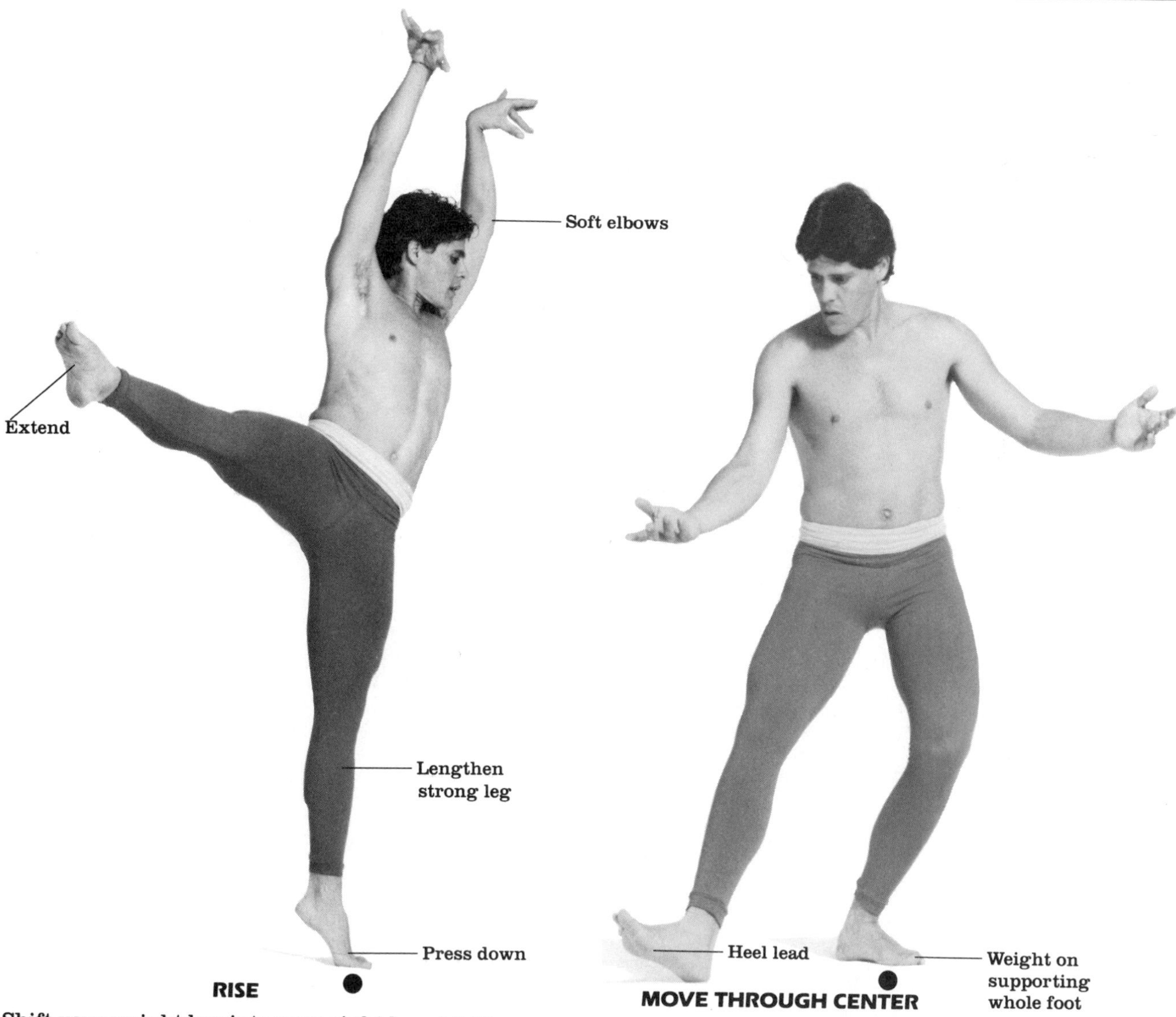

RISE

Shift your weight low into your right leg at 3:00. Press down through your foot and rise up high onto the ball as you inhale and lift your left leg up over 9:00, sweeping your arms out wide to either side and tapping your wrists high above your head. Let your arms be willowy and loose.

MOVE THROUGH CENTER

Exhale a rich sound as you sink deeply and shift back fully through center, pulling your arms down against the imaginary pressure of the springs.

Inhale as you rise up high onto the ball of your left foot at 9:00 and lengthen and lift your right leg over 3:00. When rising, don't jerk, but really use the power of your feet and legs to push away from the floor. Rise and sink at an even pace to ensure muscle balance. To keep your knees from thrusting forward when you sink, imagine sitting on a low stool and make sure you can lift your toes. The power of the motion starts in your feet and is generated by the strength of your thighs and buttocks; it should not be felt in your knees. Repeat 16 to 24 times, alternating left and right, counting 2 beats down and 2 beats up.

The Whole-Body Slimmer

BENEFITS: To stretch the sides of your body, to trim your waist, to tone your shoulders and chest, to tone and trim your calves, thighs, stomach, and buttocks, to strengthen and increase the flexibility of your feet and ankles, to enhance your balance.

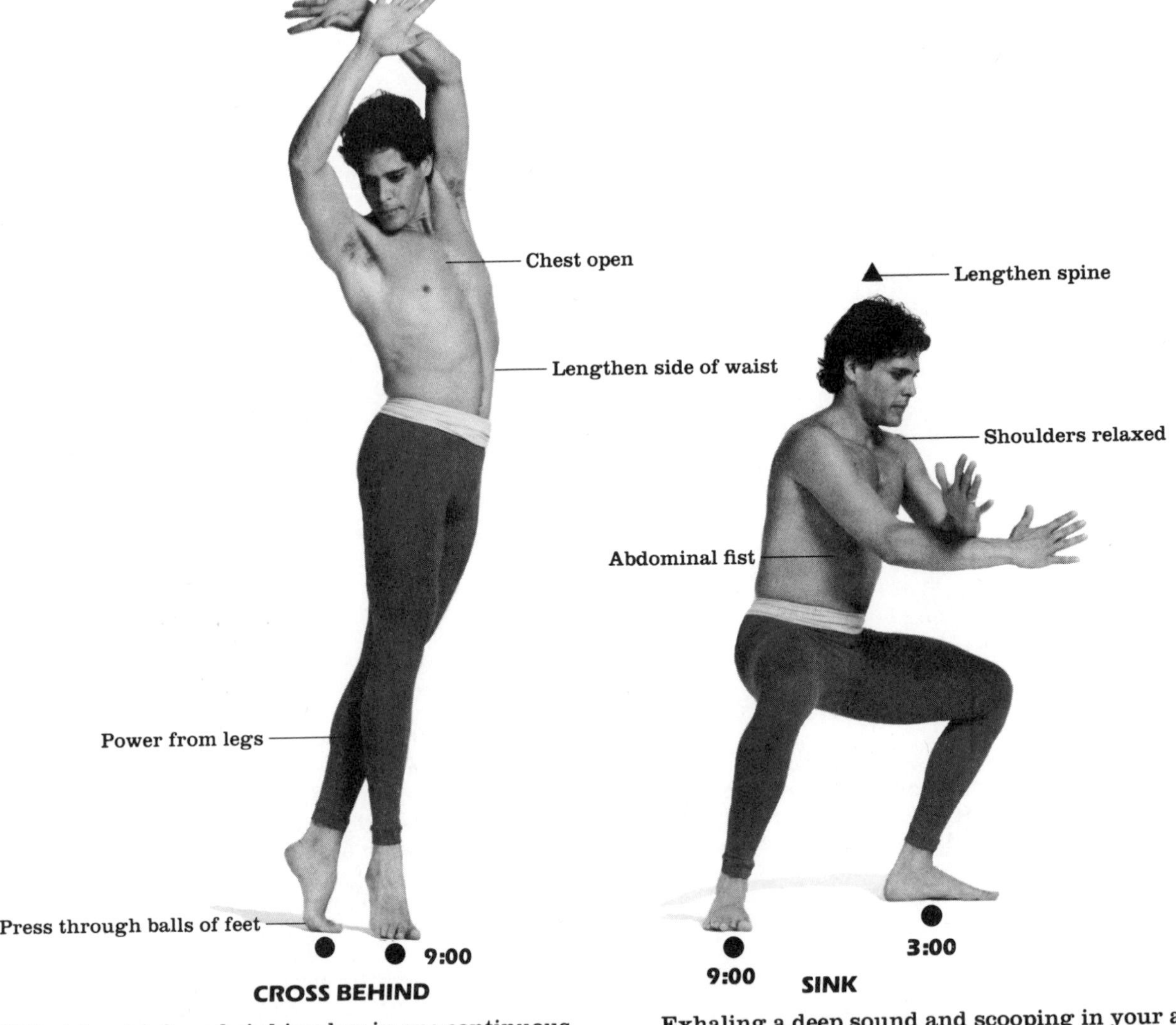

CROSS BEHIND

Still rising high and sinking low in one continuous, fluid motion, inhale, rise up at 9:00, press through the balls of your feet as you cross your right foot closely behind your left, and breaststroke high above your head, your elbows soft.

SINK

Exhaling a deep sound and scooping in your abdomen, sink deeply back through center, leading with your heel and stepping out to 3:00 as you breaststroke once at chest level.

RECHARGE
JAZZ WALK

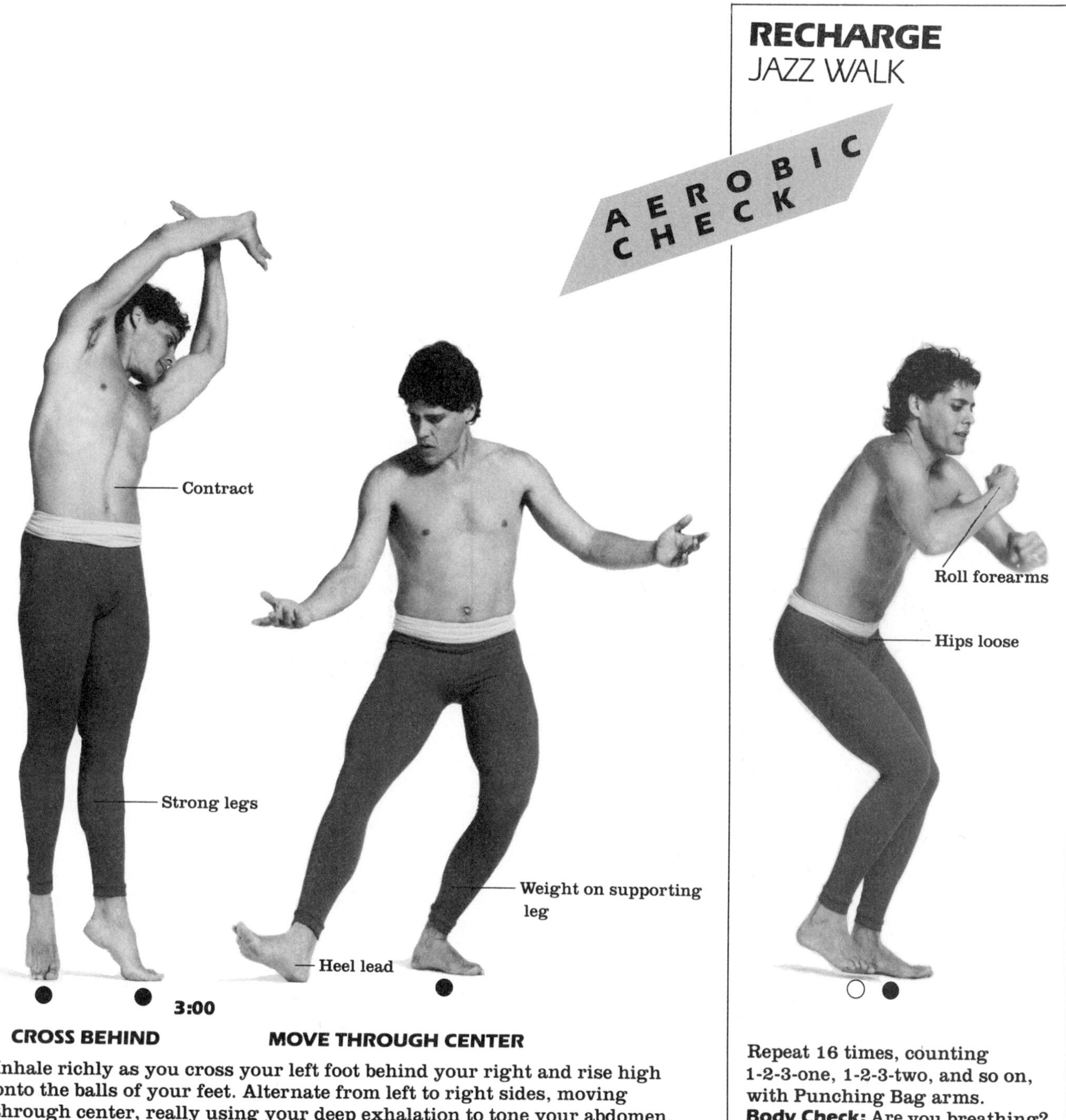

CROSS BEHIND **MOVE THROUGH CENTER**

Inhale richly as you cross your left foot behind your right and rise high onto the balls of your feet. Alternate from left to right sides, moving through center, really using your deep exhalation to tone your abdomen, your inhalation to recharge your body with oxygen. Repeat 16 to 24 times, alternating sides.

Repeat 16 times, counting 1-2-3-one, 1-2-3-two, and so on, with Punching Bag arms.
Body Check: Are you breathing? Breath is a wonderful recharge.

The Karate Dance

BENEFITS: To enhance your coordination, to stretch and strengthen your spine, to tighten your abdominals, to firm and stretch your buttocks and hamstrings.

CUSTOMIZE: To tone your frontal thigh, after drawing your knee into your chest, extend your leg into a full heel kick as you exhale "Yeet!"

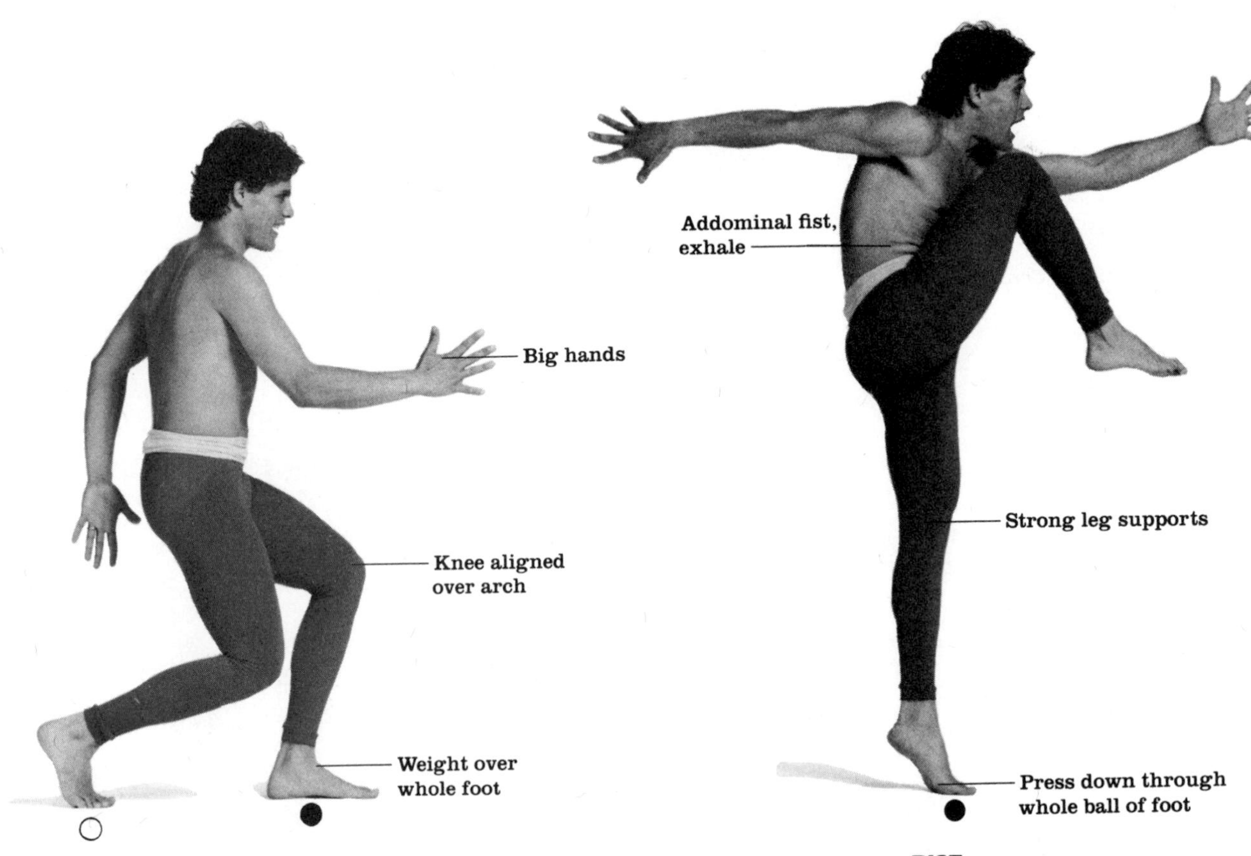
Big hands
Knee aligned over arch
Weight over whole foot
Addominal fist, exhale
Strong leg supports
Press down through whole ball of foot

STEP FORWARD

Step forward with your heel onto your left foot, extending your right arm forward, pushing through your palms, and spreading your fingers wide while your shoulders follow alluringly, your torso rotating slightly.

RISE

Rising up high onto the ball of your left foot, draw your right knee up toward your chest as you exhale "Yeet!" and sweep your left arm forward.

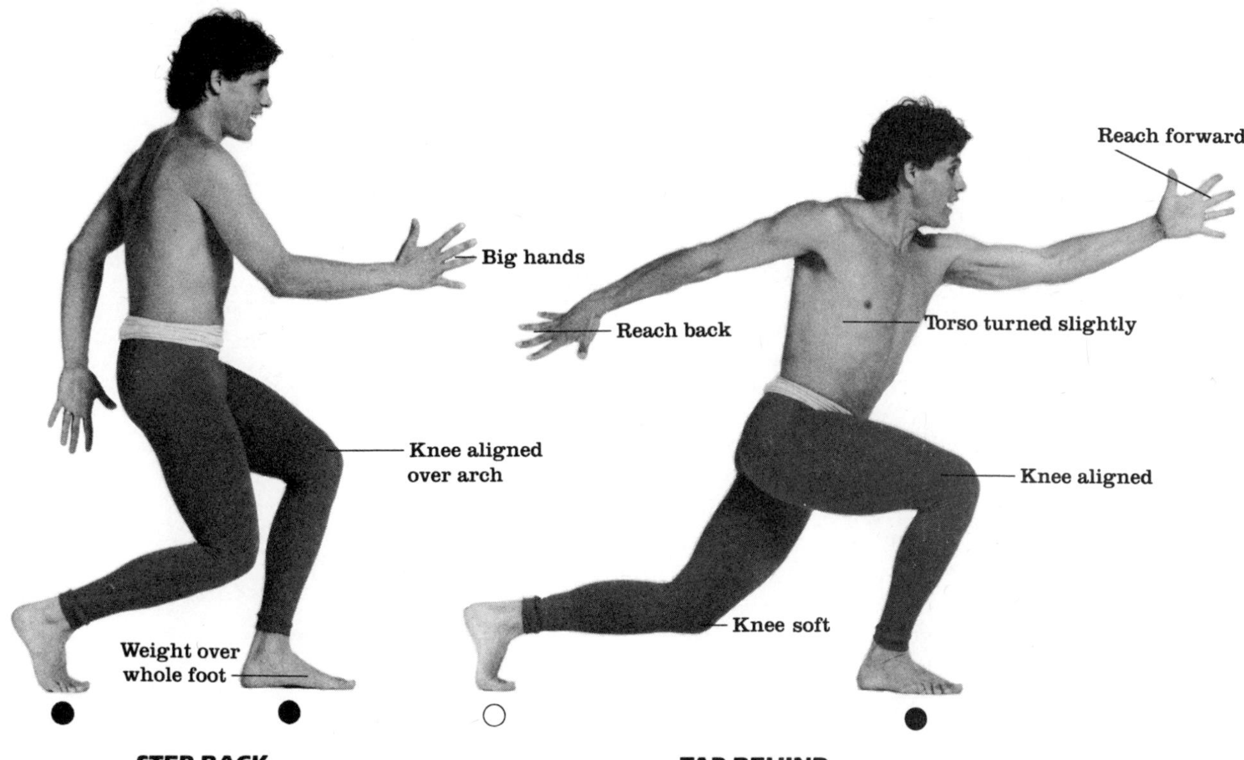

STEP BACK

Step back to center with your right leg, changing arms—

TAP BEHIND

—and, sinking deeply, tap behind with your left toes, reaching forward with your left arm.

Step forward again with your left foot, repeat the knee lift, and continue. Once you settle into the rhythm of the movement, let yourself dance back and powerhouse forward, your legs driving the motion. Repeat front and back for a total of 16 to 24 times, more if you feel snappy.

RECHARGE
CROSS BEHIND

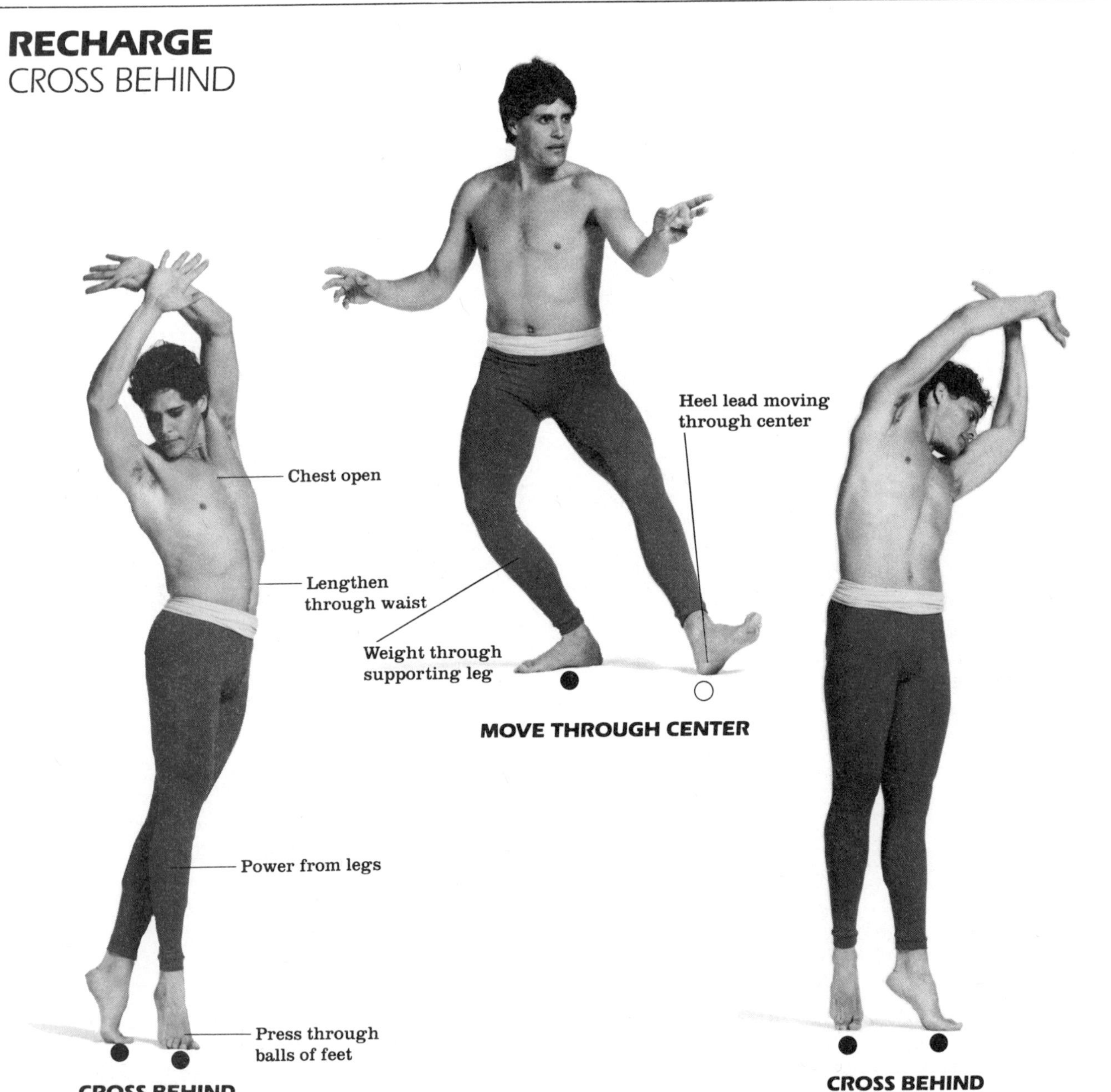

Repeat the Cross Behind, breathing rhythmically as you shift through left and right. Inhale as you cross one foot behind the other and breaststroke high above your head. Then exhale as you move through center, your arms relaxed down. **Body Check:** If your legs are tired, lighten up and put more into your arm and torso movement. Breathe. After 16 repetitions, alternating left and right, transit fluidly into the Charleston.

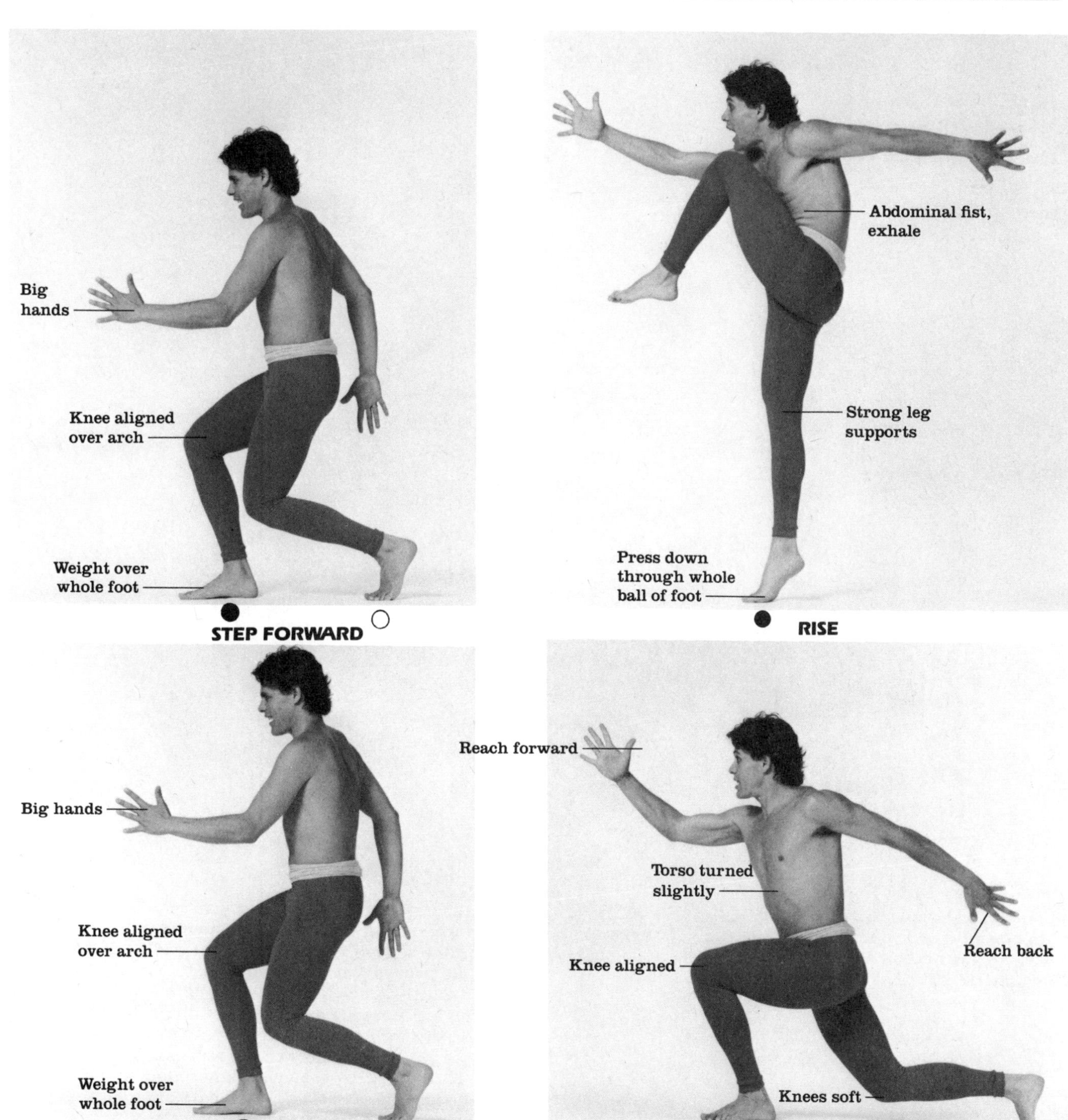

Repeat the Charleston on the opposite side, so that you begin stepping right, draw your left knee up, step back to center, and tap back with your right toe. Repeat 16 to 24 times.

Fun Firmer

BENEFITS: To tone your hips, buttocks, thighs, back, and chest, to increase your spine flexibility, to enhance your balance and coordination.

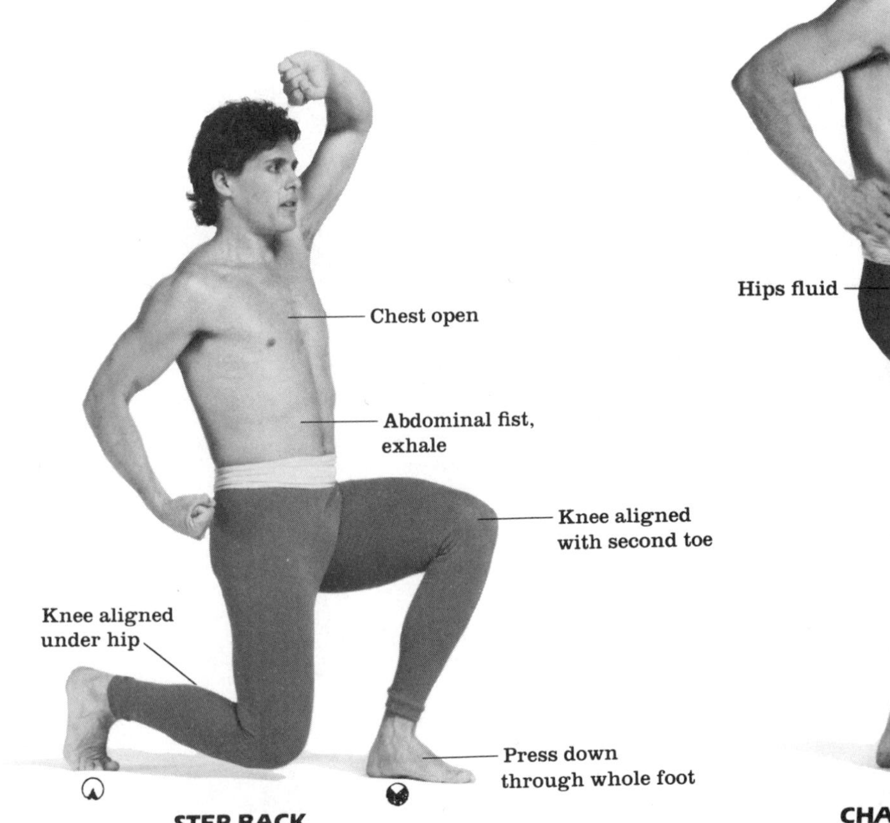
Chest open
Abdominal fist, exhale
Knee aligned with second toe
Knee aligned under hip
Press down through whole foot

STEP BACK

Step back onto the ball of your right foot to 5:00 and sink deeply over your left leg, scooping your arm up with an abrupt halt above your head accompanied by a forceful "Yeet!" exhalation and abdominal fist.

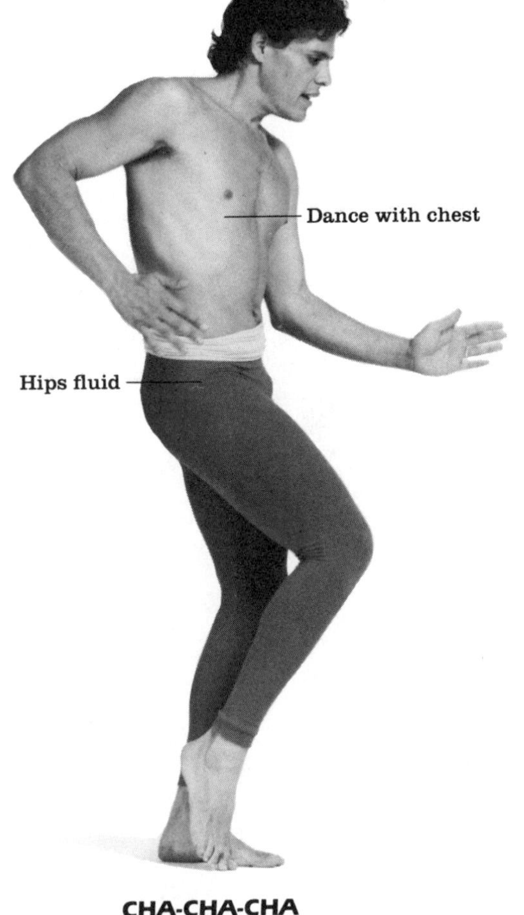
Dance with chest
Hips fluid

CHA-CHA-CHA

Then push away and scoop your arms down as you step back to center and then cha-cha-cha, walking high on the balls of your feet and imagining the floor is hot. As you walk in place, right, left, right, inhale and let your hips swish, your arms extend and sweep, your fingers tensed. Repeat on the other side, stepping out through your left heel to 11:00, sinking deeply as you scoop your arm up and exhale "Yeet!" again. Now push away, step back to center, and then cha-cha-cha, left, right, left, with passion. Repeat 8 times on each side and then repeat another 8 times, sinking right to 3:00, your toes pointing right, center to cha-cha-cha, sinking left to 9:00, your toes pointing left, and center to cha-cha-cha. Repeat again 8 times front and 8 times side.

RECHARGE
SINK 'N' RISE

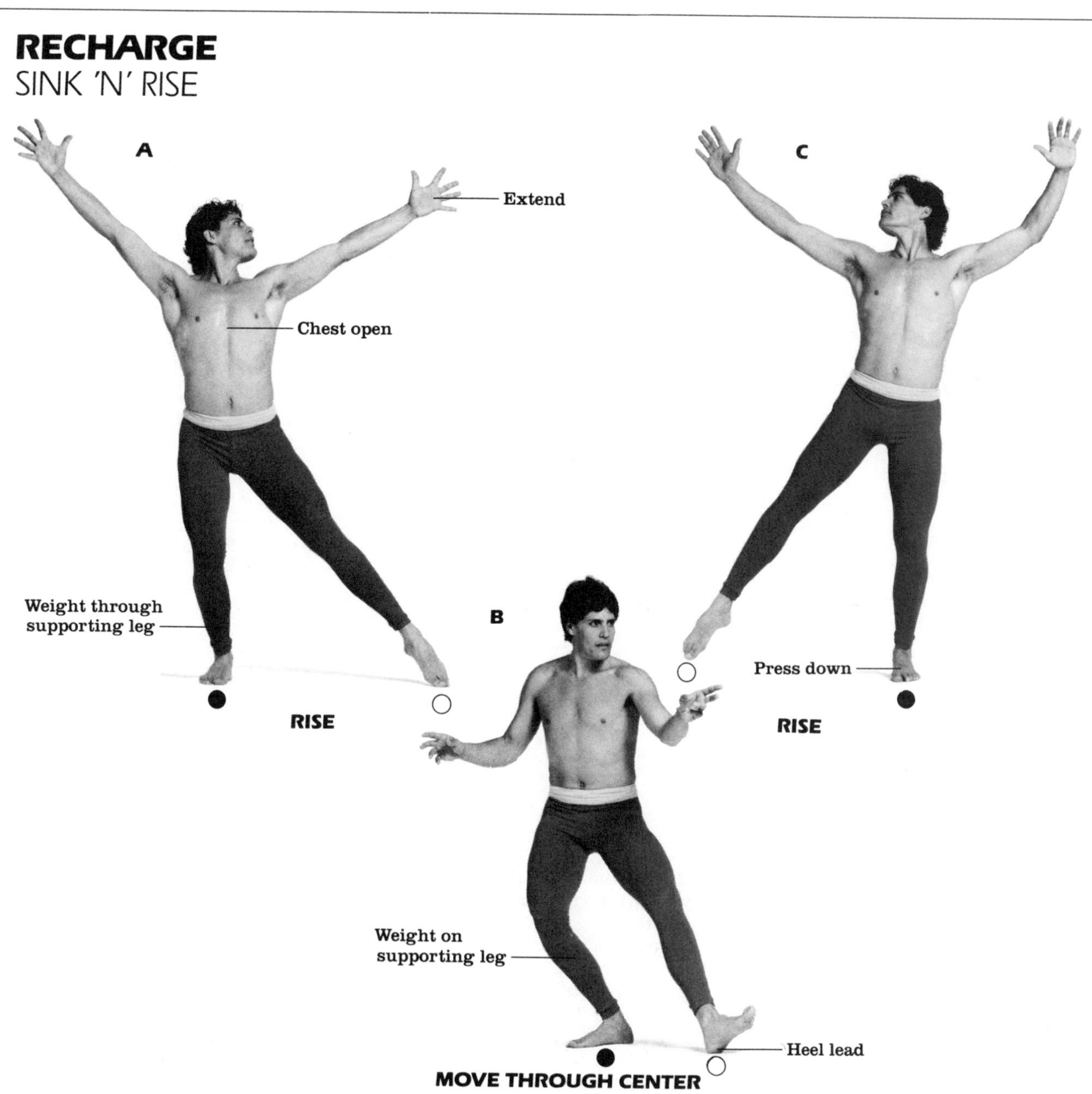

Shifting side to side and moving through center, lift your free leg back on a diagonal on the rise, pointing over 7:00 with your left toes and then over 5:00 with your right toes. Sweep up with your arms as you lift your leg back and sweep them down as you move through center. Inhale on the rise; exhale on the sink. Repeat 8 times on each side.

AEROBIC CHECK

Design Options

CONGRATULATIONS!
YOU'VE DONE A GREAT JOB!

- If you feel like you've done enough work for today, skip over to the Aerobic Check, page 169, and Ease-Out.
- If you want just a little more work, but not a whole lot, go back and repeat, starting with the Step-Back/Ball Throw. After the Charleston, go to the Aerobic Check, page 169, and Ease-Out. If you can, work a little deeper on the rerun, sinking a bit lower, rising a bit higher, reaching a bit farther.
- If you're still feeling pretty snappy, come along for the next part.
- If you feel like you're just getting started and have a whole lot left, go back to the Step-Back/Ball Throw and rework the first part as deeply as possible while still staying within your comfort zone. Then finish up by joining us for the next part.

Whatever your choice, give yourself a mental pat on the back for the work you've done. It makes all the difference in training your mind to want to come back tomorrow.

RECHARGE
CROSS BEHIND

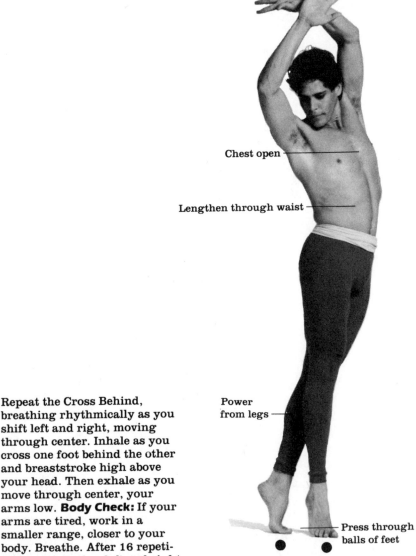

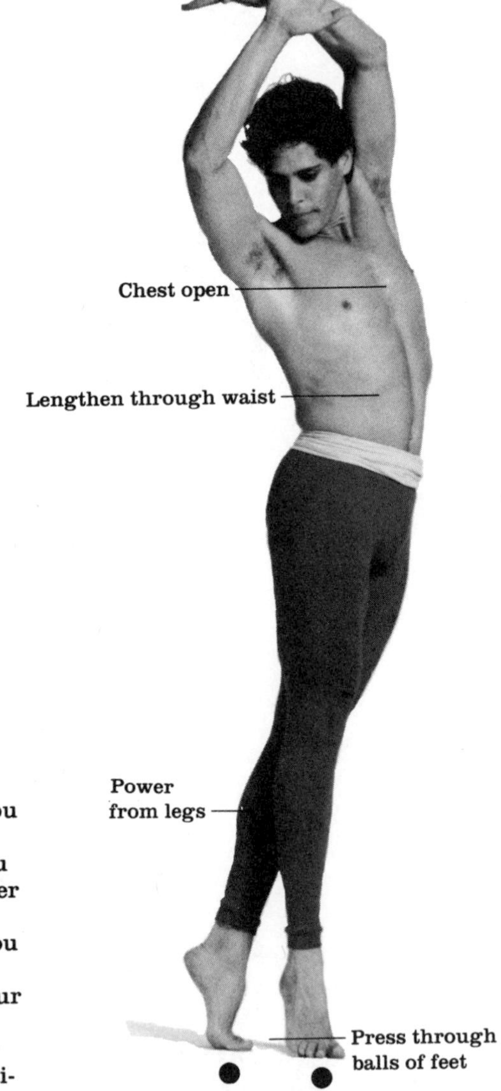

CROSS BEHIND

Repeat the Cross Behind, breathing rhythmically as you shift left and right, moving through center. Inhale as you cross one foot behind the other and breaststroke high above your head. Then exhale as you move through center, your arms low. Body Check: If your arms are tired, work in a smaller range, closer to your body. Breathe. After 16 repetitions, alternating left and right, transit fluidly into the Touch Front.

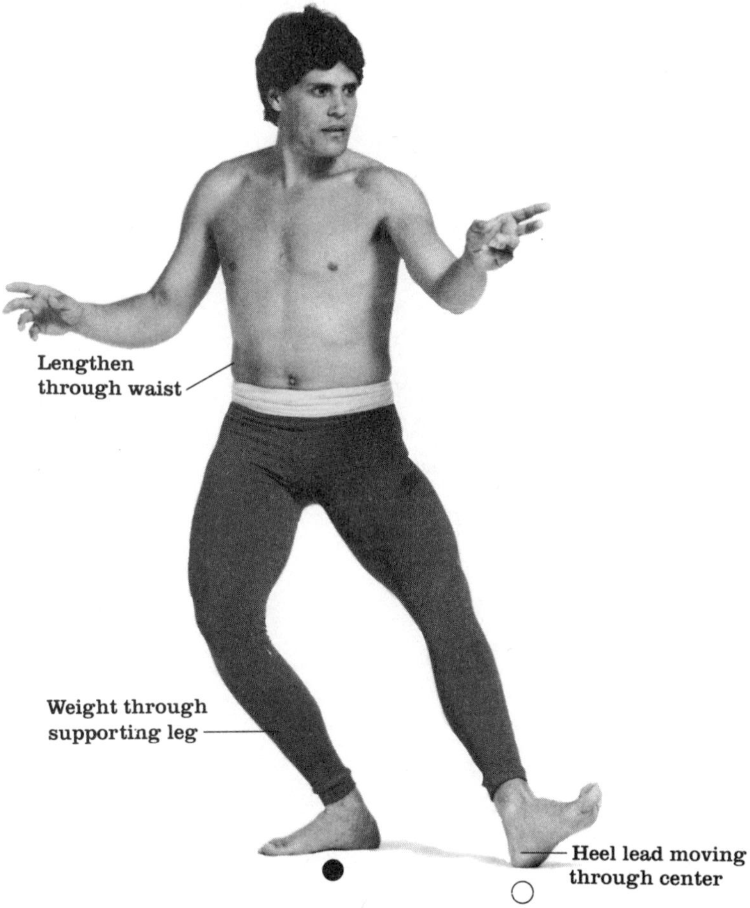

Lengthen through waist

Weight through supporting leg

Heel lead moving through center

MOVE THROUGH CENTER

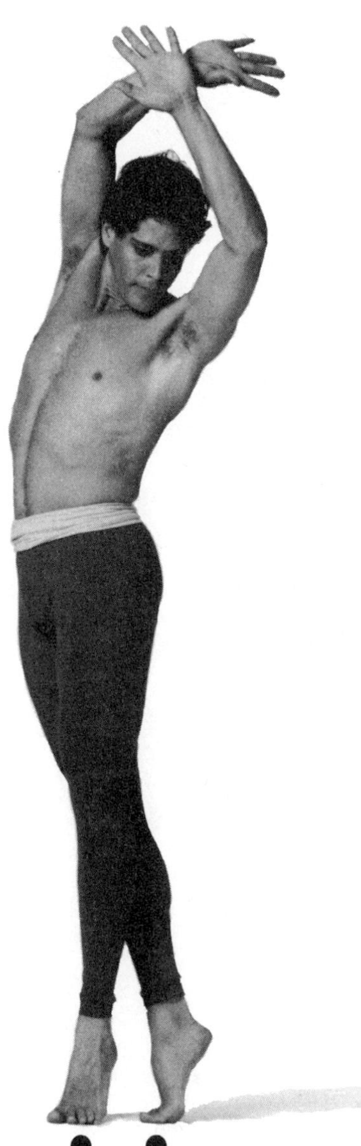

CROSS BEHIND

Abs Away

BENEFITS: To firm and flatten your abdominals, to tone your arms and chest, to strengthen and stretch your torso, to increase your spine flexibility, to trim and strengthen your thighs and buttocks, to stretch your calves and Achilles tendons, to strengthen your legs.

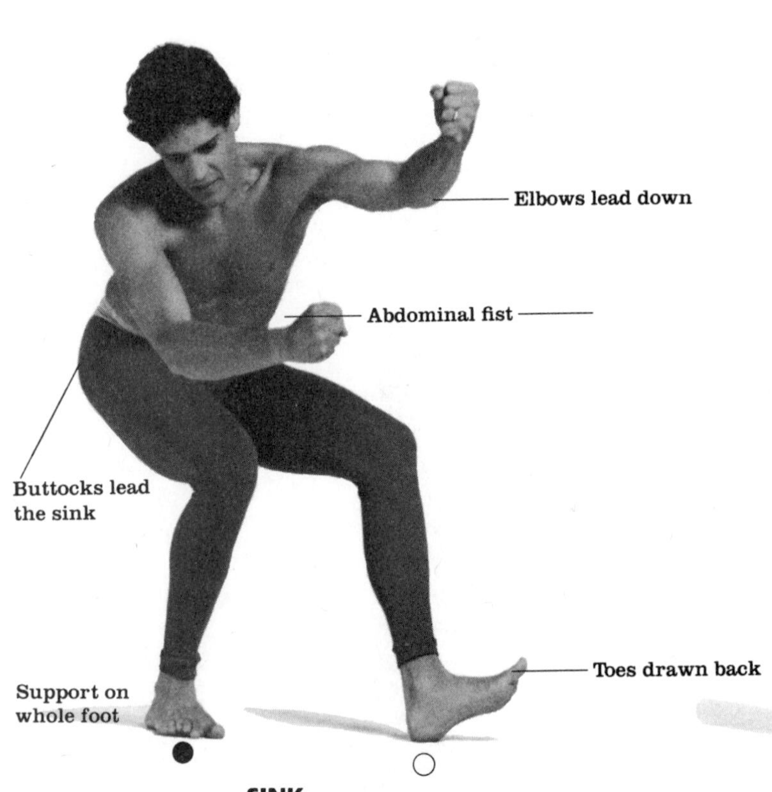

SINK

Still shifting lyrically side to side, alternately touch your left heel to 11:00 and your right heel to 1:00. Inhale and rise high onto the balls of your feet through center, exhale as you sink deeply and touch with your heel. Repeat, touching left and right, feeling the continuity of your movement, and when you've got the rhythm down, add the arms. Pretend that you're holding a long paddle and imagine tracing figure eights—

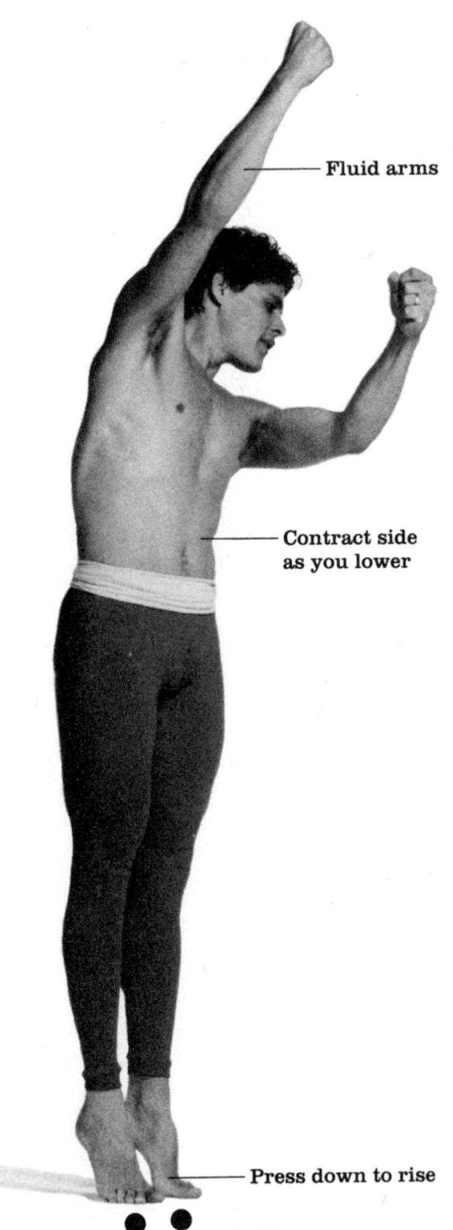

RISE

—as you sweep it up—

Torso rotates

Contract
as you exhale

Sink into whole foot

SINK

—and then scoop down so that it's next to your hip as you sink into your supporting leg. Pretend that you're paddling through thick glue and use the imaginary tension to more deeply work your muscles and demand more of your heart. Sinking and rising, travel 4 steps forward and 4 steps back for a total of 16 to 24 times on each side.

Let your torso follow the movement of your paddles, gently twisting at your waist (not your hips!). By keeping the rotation in your waist, you'll protect your knees from the torquing that can occur if you push through with your hips. Your right shoulder rotates forward as your foot touches front—and vice versa.

RECHARGE
JAZZ WALK

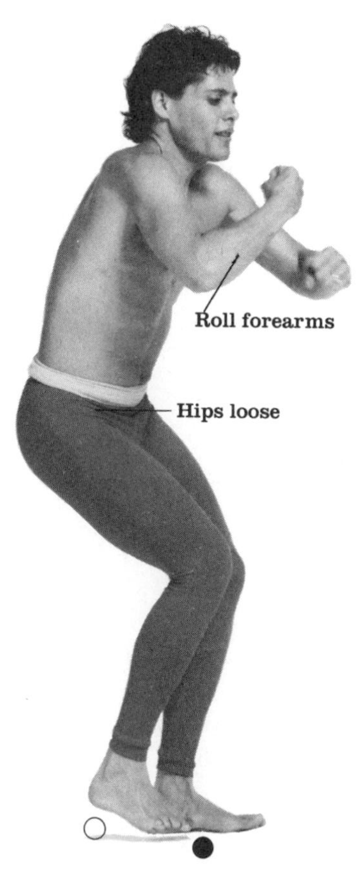

Repeat 16 times, counting 1-2-3-one, 1-2-3-two, and so on, with Punching Bag arms.

Body Check: If your lower back feels tight, breathe, use your abdominals, and feel the motion of your pelvis. Then transit fluidly into the 1-2-3 Curl Hide.

1-2-3-CURL HIDE

Definitely Definition

BENEFITS: To strengthen and define your abdominals, to stretch and tone your buttocks and thighs, to trim your waist, to enhance your balance.

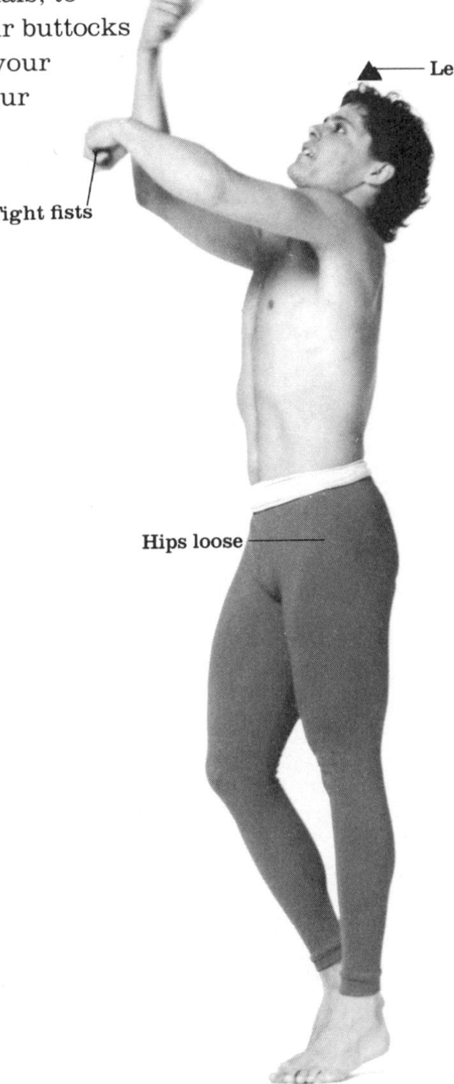

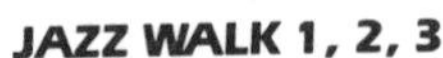

JAZZ WALK 1, 2, 3

Rolling your forearms tightly around one another, your arms high above your head, step lightly onto the ball of your feet as you jazz walk loosely, right, left, right, to the count of 3, and—

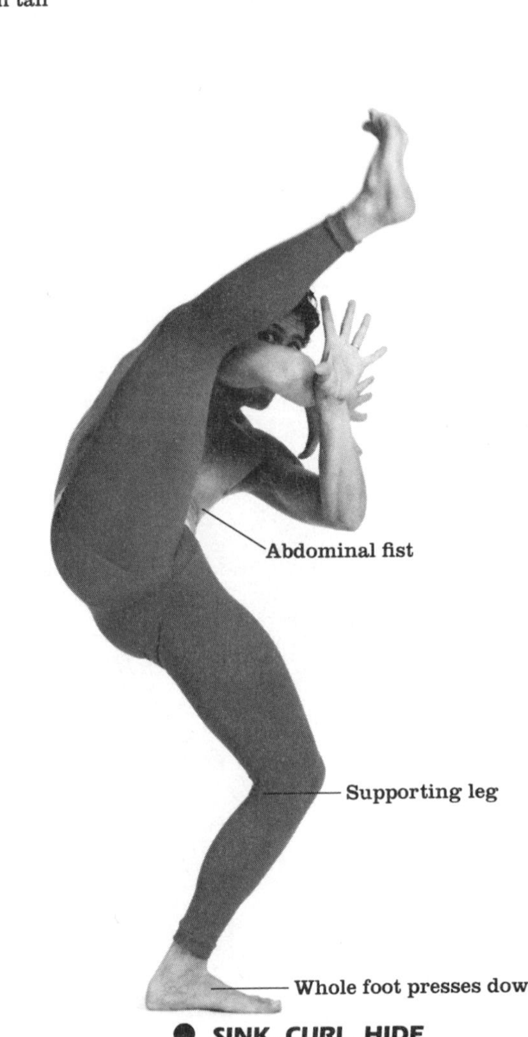

● **SINK, CURL, HIDE**

—on 4, sink deeply into your right leg as you draw your left knee up high toward your chest with a burst of *"Yeet!"* feeling the press on your abdominal muscles, the strength and balance in your supporting leg. At the same time, scoop your arms out and up in front of your face as if you're hiding and really stretch out through all five fingers for more definition in your forearm.

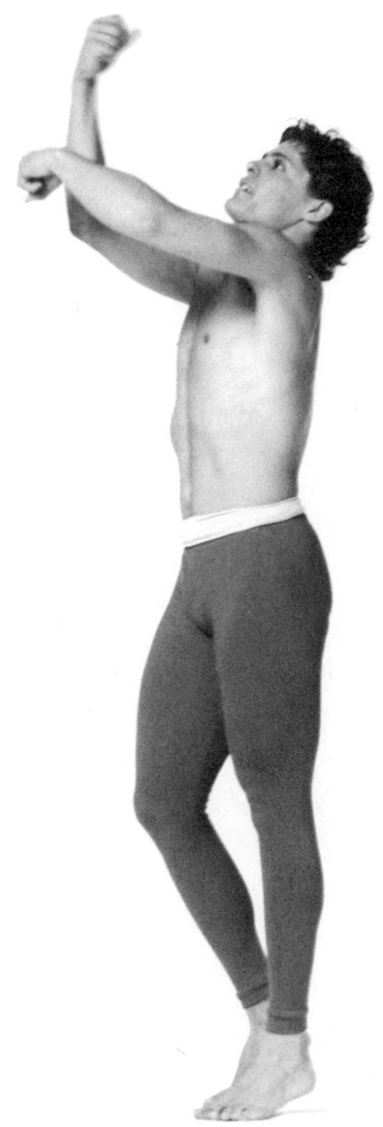

JAZZ WALK 1, 2, 3

Return to jazz walk high in place, left, right, left, inhaling richly and rolling your arms high, and then—

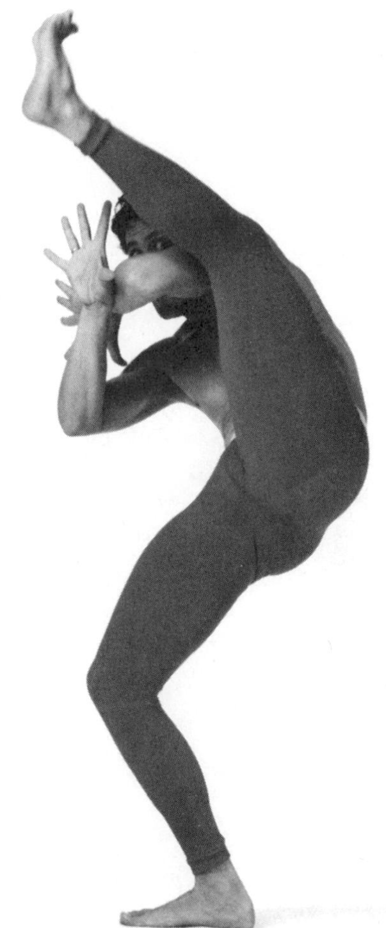

● **SINK, CURL, HIDE**

—on 4, sink deeply into your left leg as you scoop your arms and draw your right knee up high and exhale "Yeet!" with an abdominal fist. Repeat 8 to 16 times on each side. For more variation, as you jazz walk to the count of 3 in place, rotate turning left, then sink and hide; jazz walk rotating and turning right, sink and hide. Keep rotating left and right on the jazz walk. Repeat another 8 to 16 times on each side.

Tension Buster

BENEFITS: To strengthen and tone your thighs, buttocks, and abdomen, to stretch your hamstrings, to increase the strength and flexibility of your arms, to enhance your balance.

CUSTOMIZE: For stronger calves, rise high onto the ball of your foot as you kick.

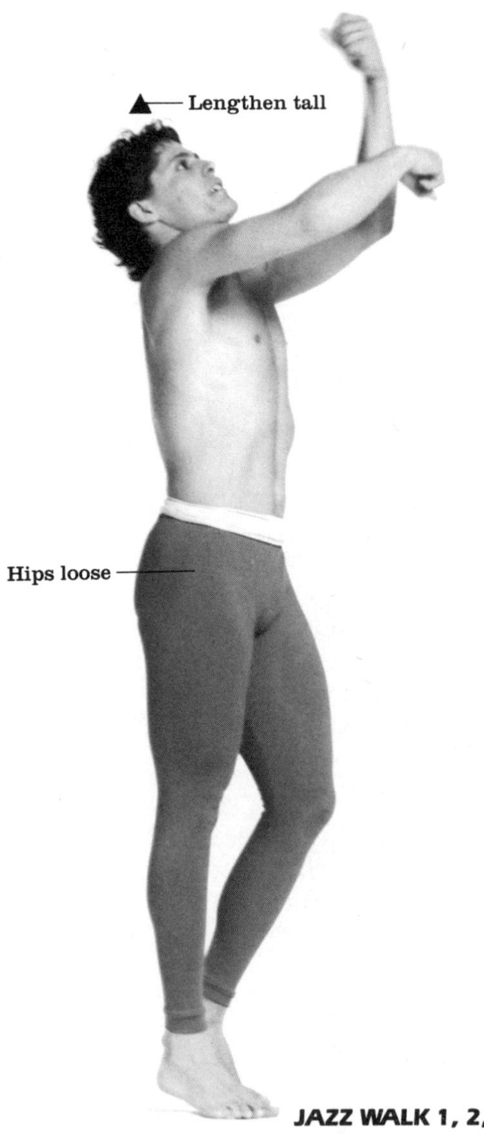

JAZZ WALK 1, 2, 3

Inhale and bathe your body with oxygen as you jazz walk in place, rising high onto the balls of your feet and rolling your forearms high above your head. On the count of 3, sink into your leg and—

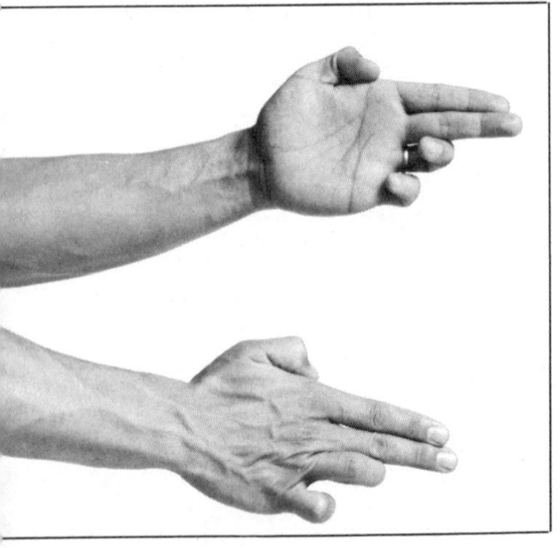

Tense your hand with Lightning Rod fingers.

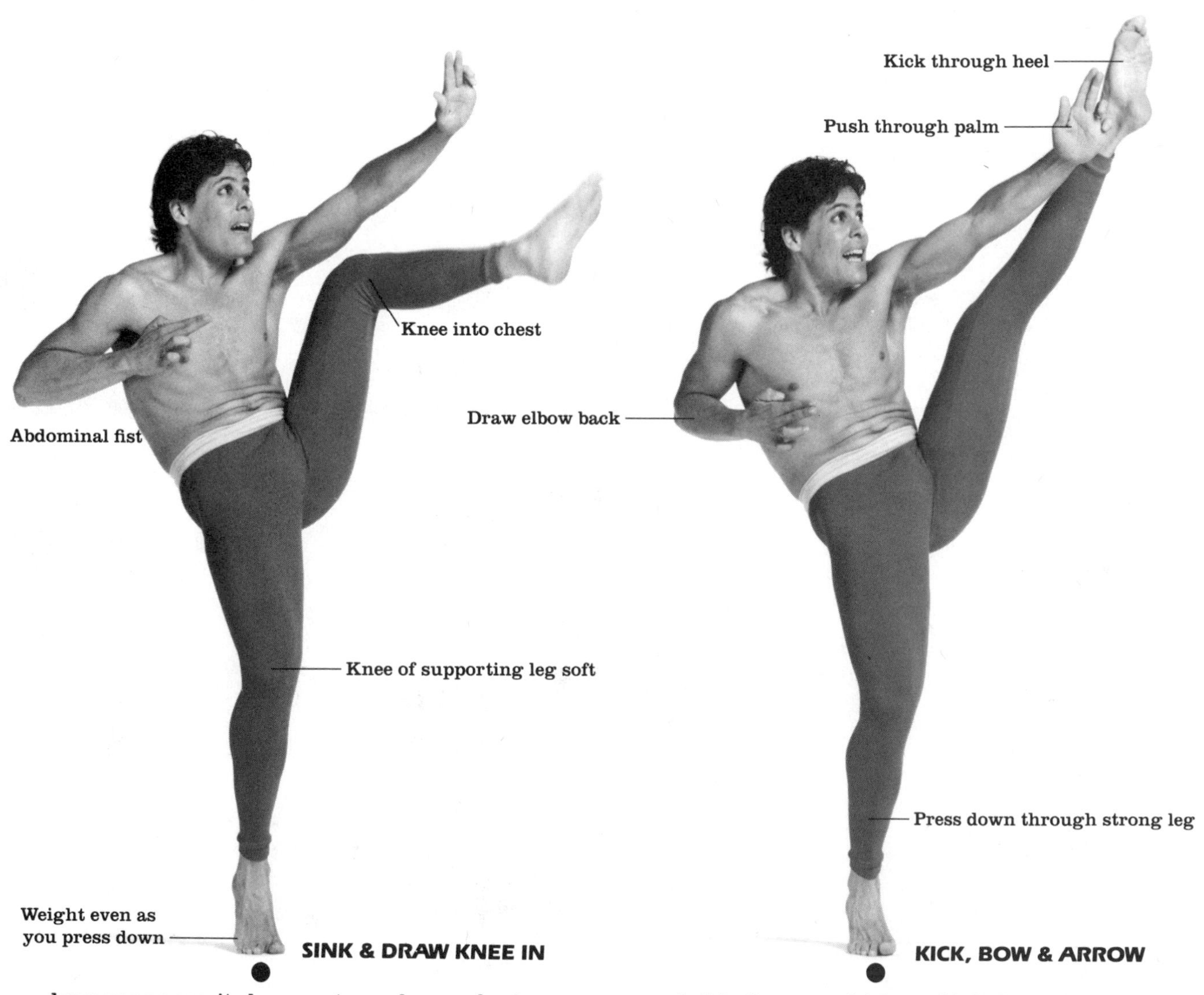
Knee into chest
Abdominal fist
Knee of supporting leg soft
Weight even as
you press down
Kick through heel
Push through palm
Draw elbow back
Press down through strong leg

SINK & DRAW KNEE IN

—draw your opposite knee up toward your chest—

KICK, BOW & ARROW

—and, this time on 4, kick out high through your heel, keeping your knee unlocked. This is your chance to really let loose with those *"Yeet!"* exhalations, sucking in your abdomen as if you've just been punched in the gut. You'll get a firm stomach in no time and save your lower back from strain. As you kick with *"Yeet!"* imagine that you're holding a bow and arrow, your right arm extending straight over your right leg, and pull back on the string, take aim, and fire passionately, letting a little more stress shoot out with each arrow. Repeat 8 to 16 times on each side, alternating left and right.

RECHARGE
PADDLE

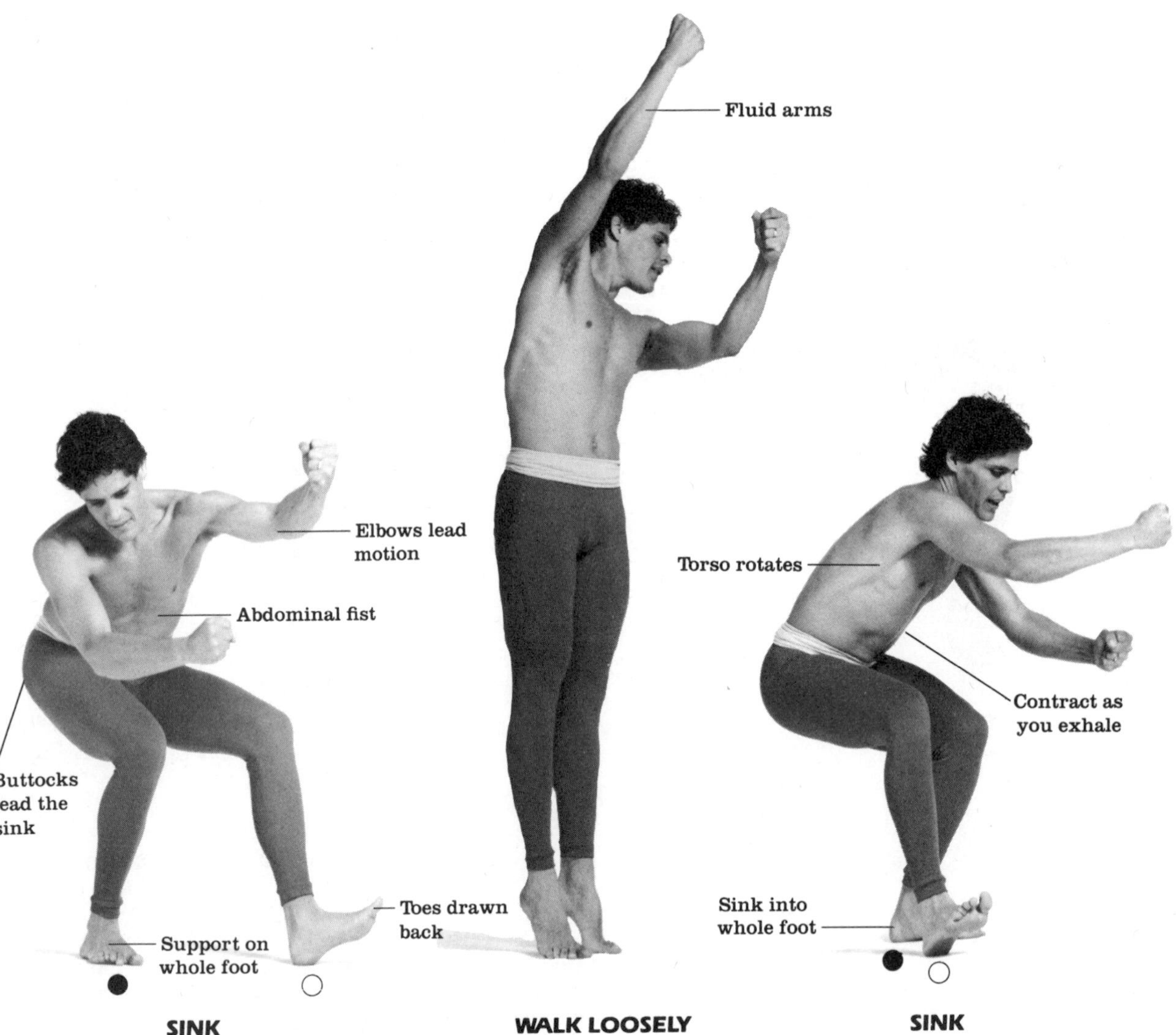

Fluid arms
Elbows lead motion
Abdominal fist
Buttocks lead the sink
Support on whole foot
Toes drawn back
Torso rotates
Contract as you exhale
Sink into whole foot
SINK
WALK LOOSELY
SINK

Walk loosely in place on the balls of your feet to the count of 3, then sink and touch front with your heel on 4, sweeping an imaginary paddle in broad horizontal figure eights from your left to your right side. Repeat 8 times on each side. **Body Check:** Listen to your body signals and adjust accordingly.

1-2-3-SWEEP/SLAP

Thigh Tamer

BENEFITS: To firm your inner and outer thighs, to increase flexibility of your hip socket, to tone your abdominal muscles, to enhance your balance and coordination.

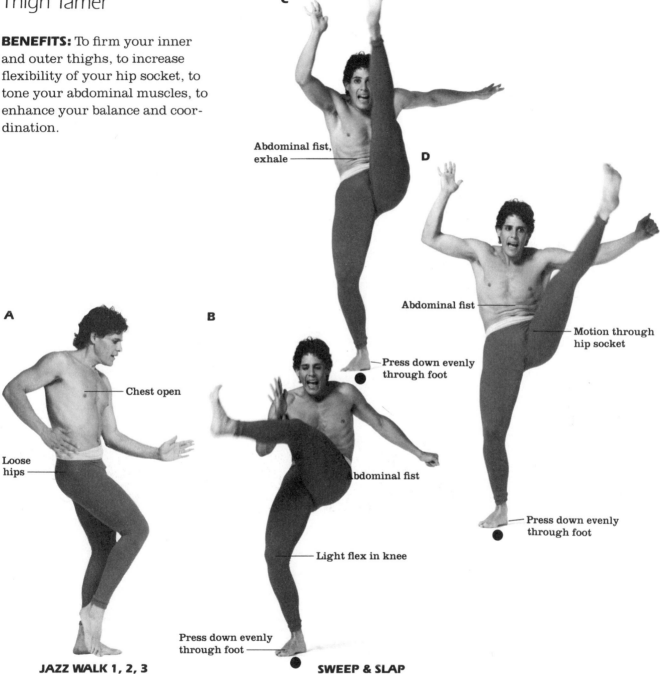

C

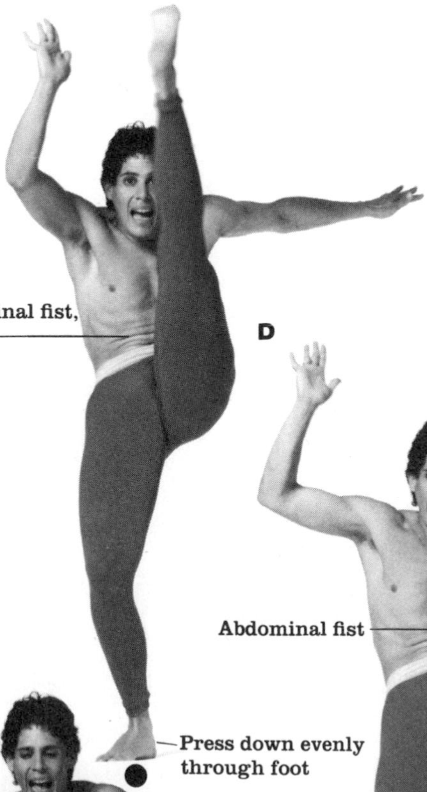

Abdominal fist, exhale

Press down evenly through foot

D

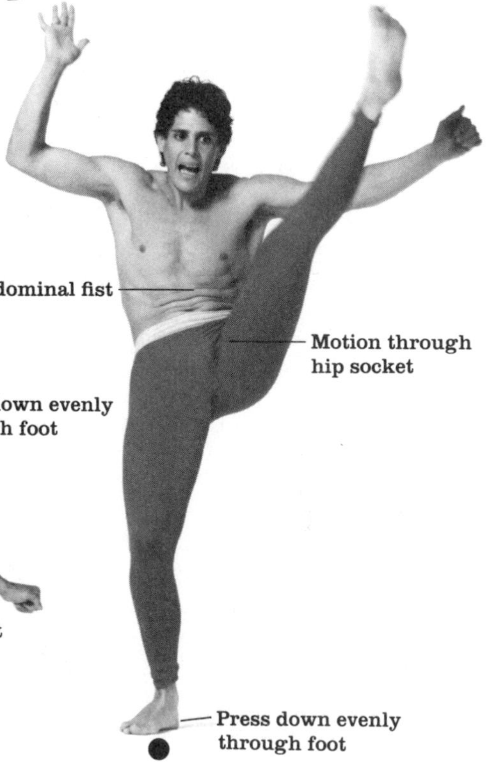

Abdominal fist

Motion through hip socket

Press down evenly through foot

A

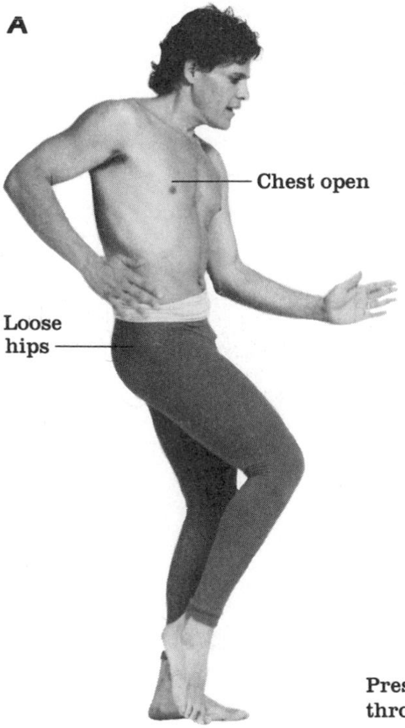

Chest open

Loose hips

B

Abdominal fist

Light flex in knee

Press down evenly through foot

JAZZ WALK 1, 2, 3

SWEEP & SLAP

Jazz walk left, right, left—

—and on 4, sweep your right knee up high and across your body to lightly slap your foot with your left hand before you sweep back out and down. Step to the side and pick up the count as you jazz walk right, left, right, and on 4, sweep your left knee up and slap your foot. The rhythm is shift, shift, shift, sweep. Be solid on your supporting leg and foot as you sweep. Repeat 8 to 16 times on each side.

The Power Pack

BENEFITS: To firm and trim your abdominals, buttocks, and thighs, to strengthen your calves, to increase your spine and torso flexibility, to define your upper arms.

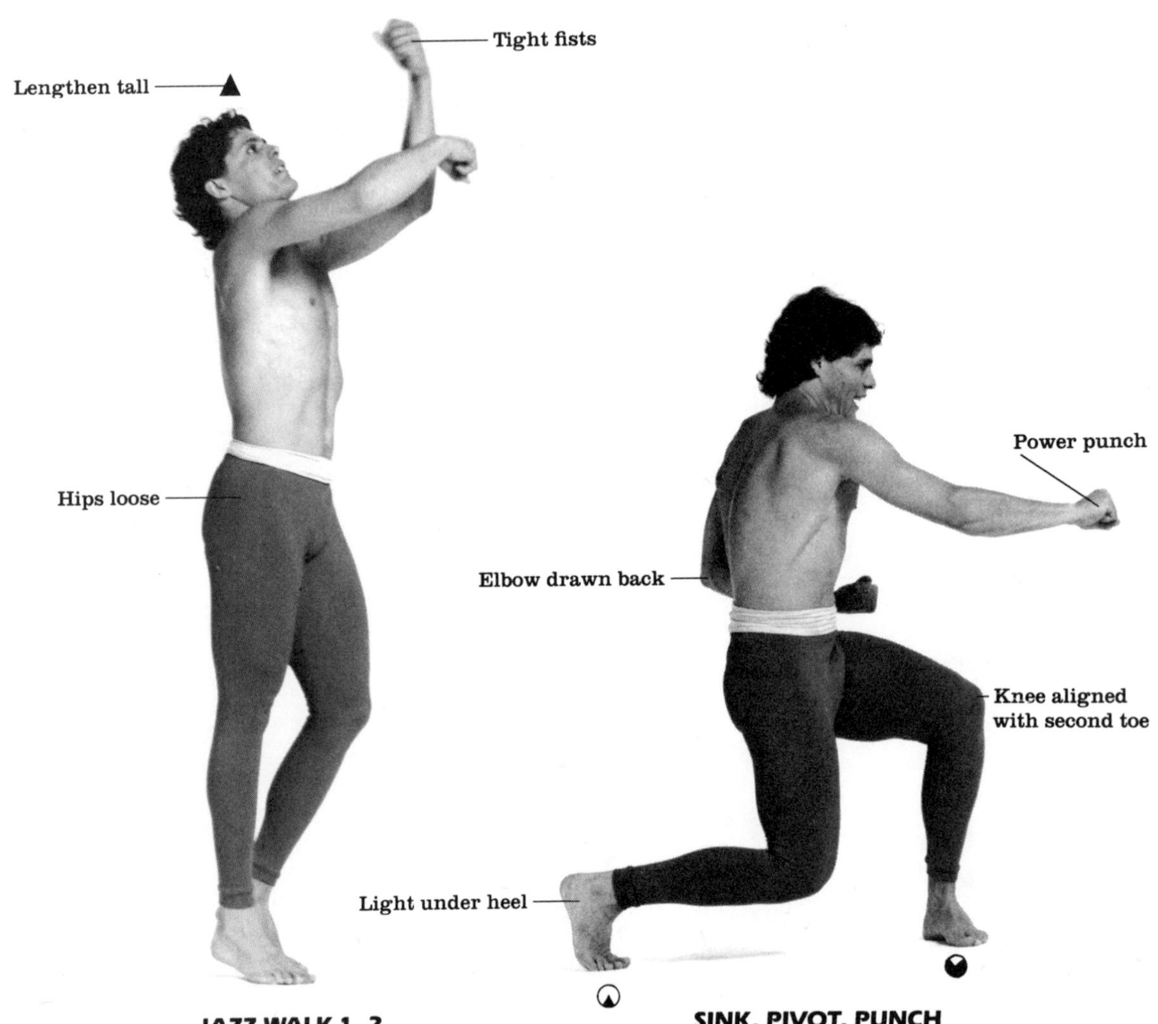

JAZZ WALK 1, 2

Inhale richly as you jazz walk in place, right and left, rising high onto the balls of your feet and rolling your forearms high above your head—

SINK, PIVOT, PUNCH

—on 3, sink deeply into your right leg, and on 4, rotate your left leg inward, placing the ball of your back foot firmly on the floor as you give a powerful karate punch right with your left arm, a forceful *"Yeet!"* and abdominal fist. Sink. Don't be thrown forward with your punch.

AEROBIC CHECK

Shifting easily side to side and keeping your legs in motion, check your heart rate now. (See page **35** for details.)

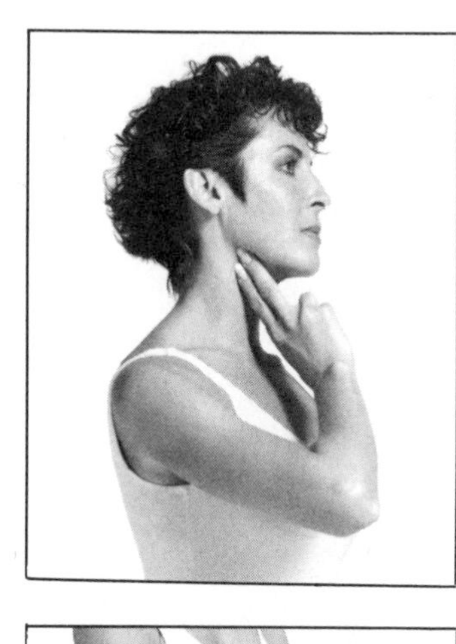

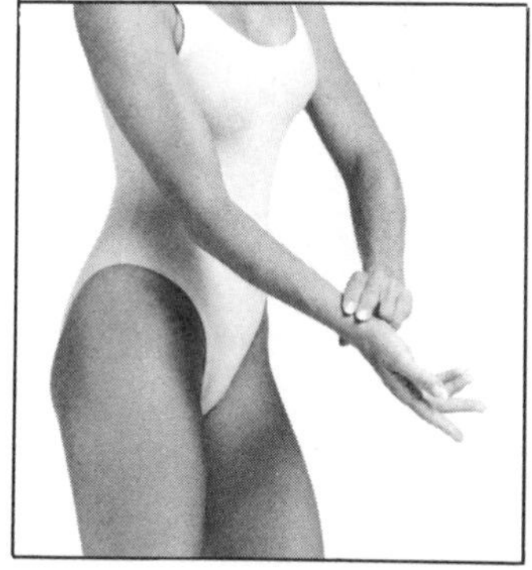

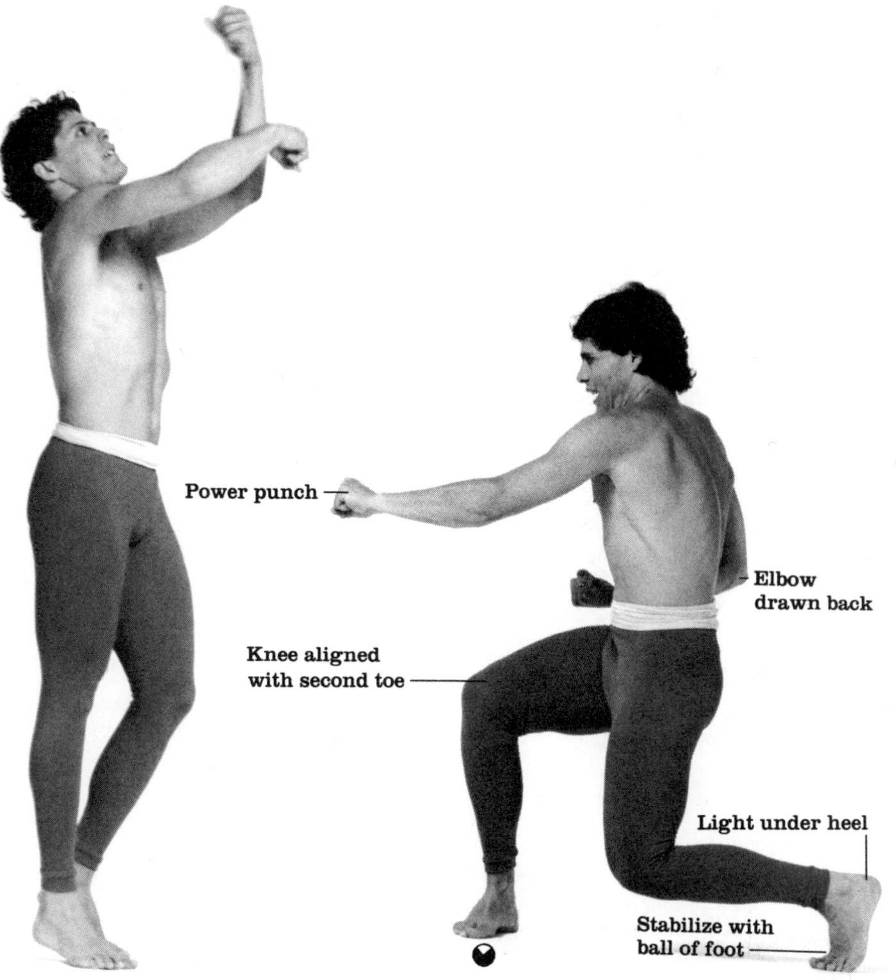

JAZZ WALK 1, 2

Inhaling and recharging in center, walk high, left and right, feeling your feet and calves working for you. Then—

SINK, PIVOT, PUNCH

—on 3, sink, and on 4, pivot your right leg and punch left with your right arm. Repeat 8 to 16 times on each side.

EASE-OUT

Your whole body should be surging with vibrant new energy. Now, let's ride that exhilaration through the Ease-Out to a sweet finale. Focus on and feel the smooth, velvety ease of your movements, the slow, sensual stretch in each motion. Breathe.

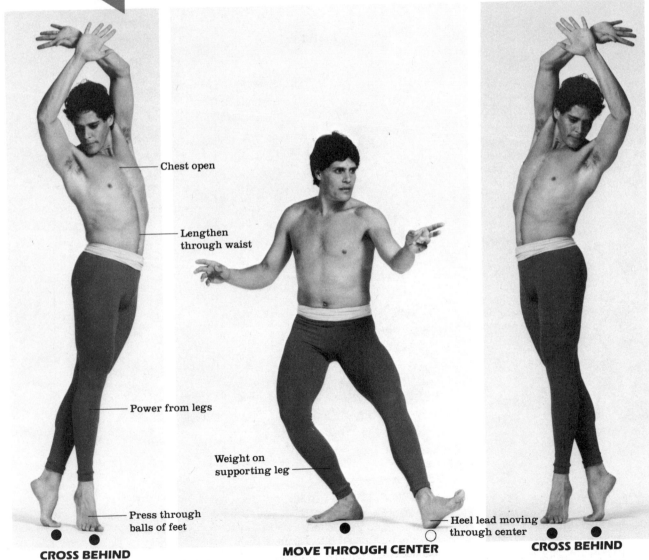

Easily cross one foot behind the other as you continue shifting side to side, your arms comfortably breaststroking above your head. Shift left and right 8 times. Feel the stretch along the sides of your torso.

A

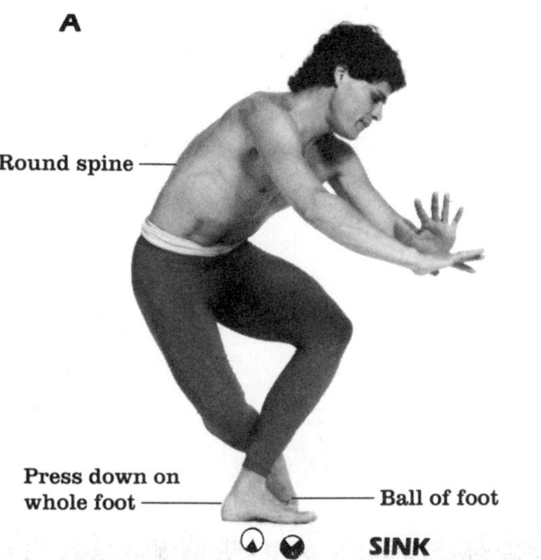

SINK

As you cross behind, slowly sink, exhaling fully as you breaststroke, feeling a warm stretch in your buttocks, along your spine, and through your hips.

B

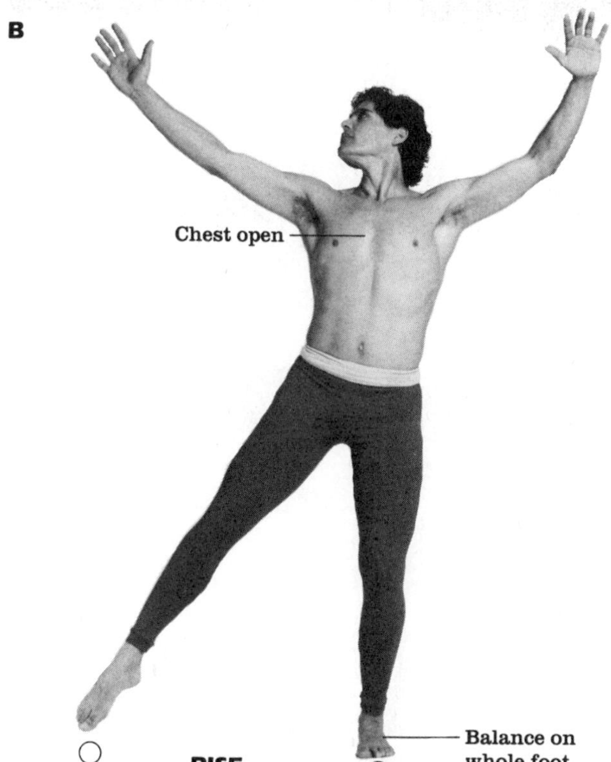

RISE

Inhale, using the strength of your legs to push away from the floor, feeling a catlike stretch along your spine as you open your arms, rising upright.

C

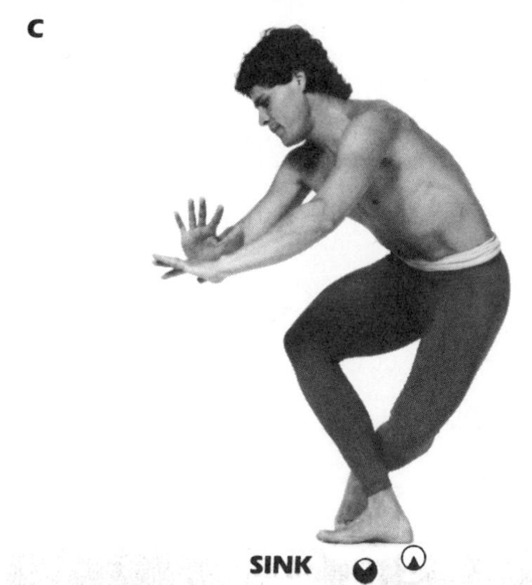

SINK

Shift through center and slowly sink, rounding down on the other side, letting your buttocks lower first. Exhale.

D

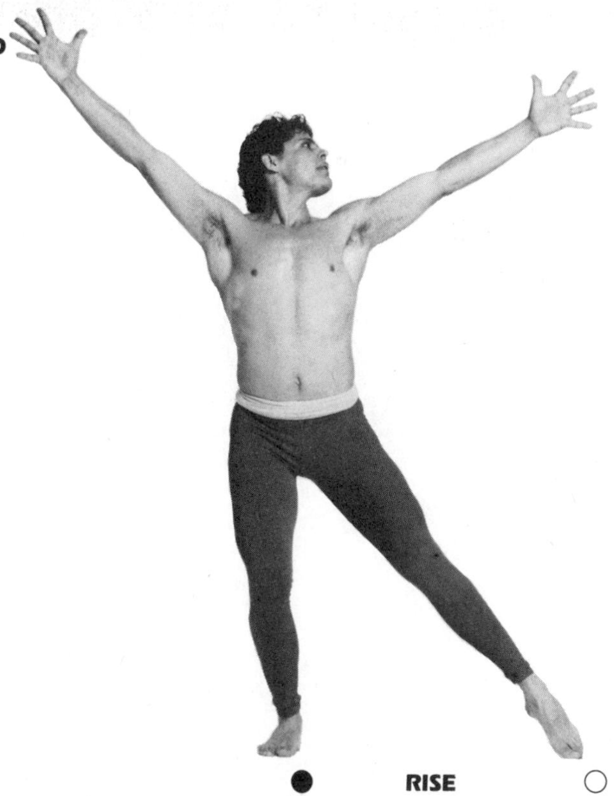

RISE

Come back through center, rising and inhaling deeply. Feel for a continuous, fluid motion as you rise and lower to stretch out. Repeat 8 times on each side.

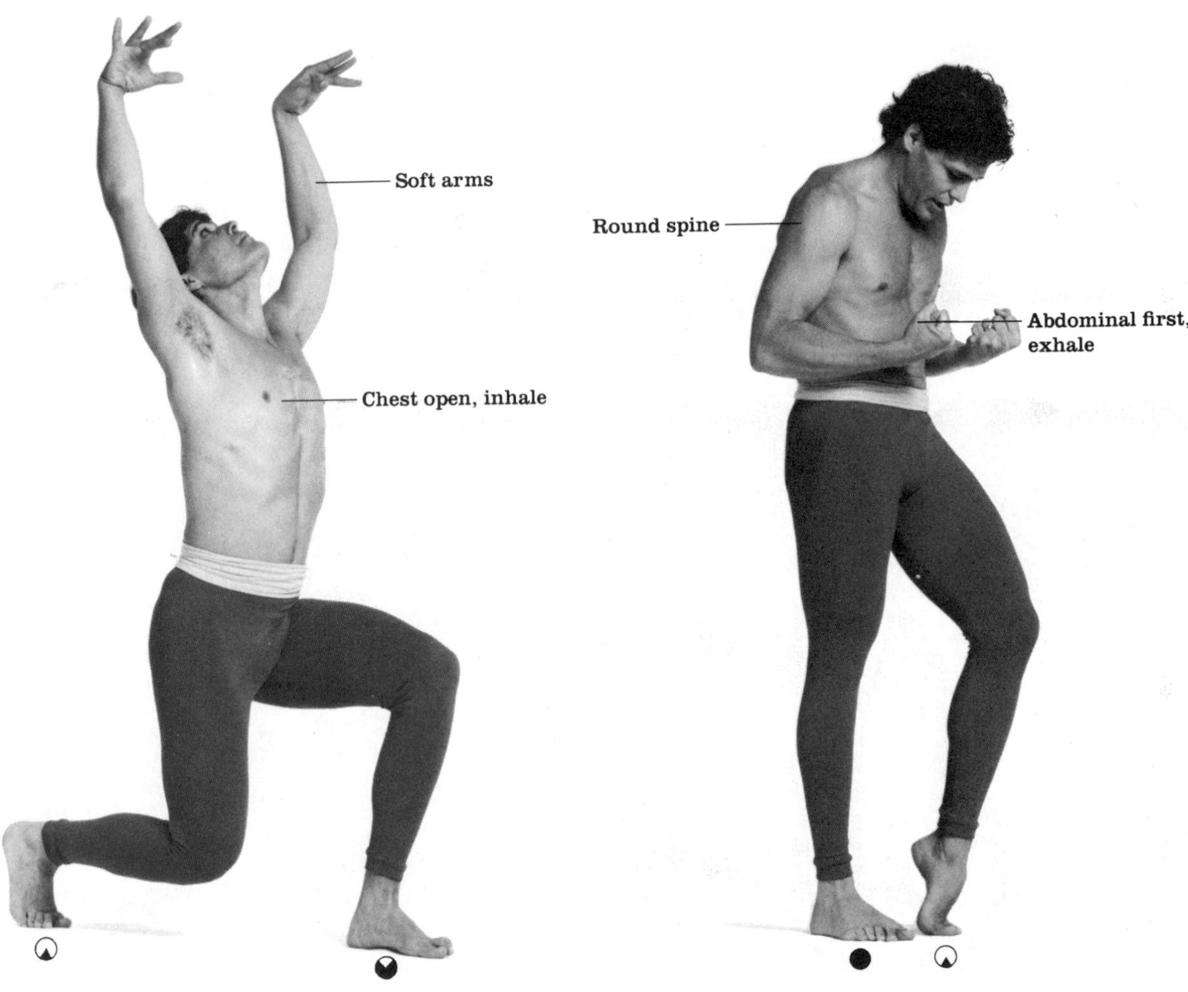

Step back onto the ball of your foot with your arms raised, inhaling richly, feeling the warm stretch through your thigh. Keep it comfortable. Feel your chest expand as you open up to your new flexibility.

Press down through your front foot to rise and step together, exhaling and feeling your abdominal tuck as you draw your elbows back. Repeat to the other side and continue alternating for a total of 8 times on each side. Feel a fluid lowering and rising. Take it slowly for more flexibility.

PIVOT/WIPE

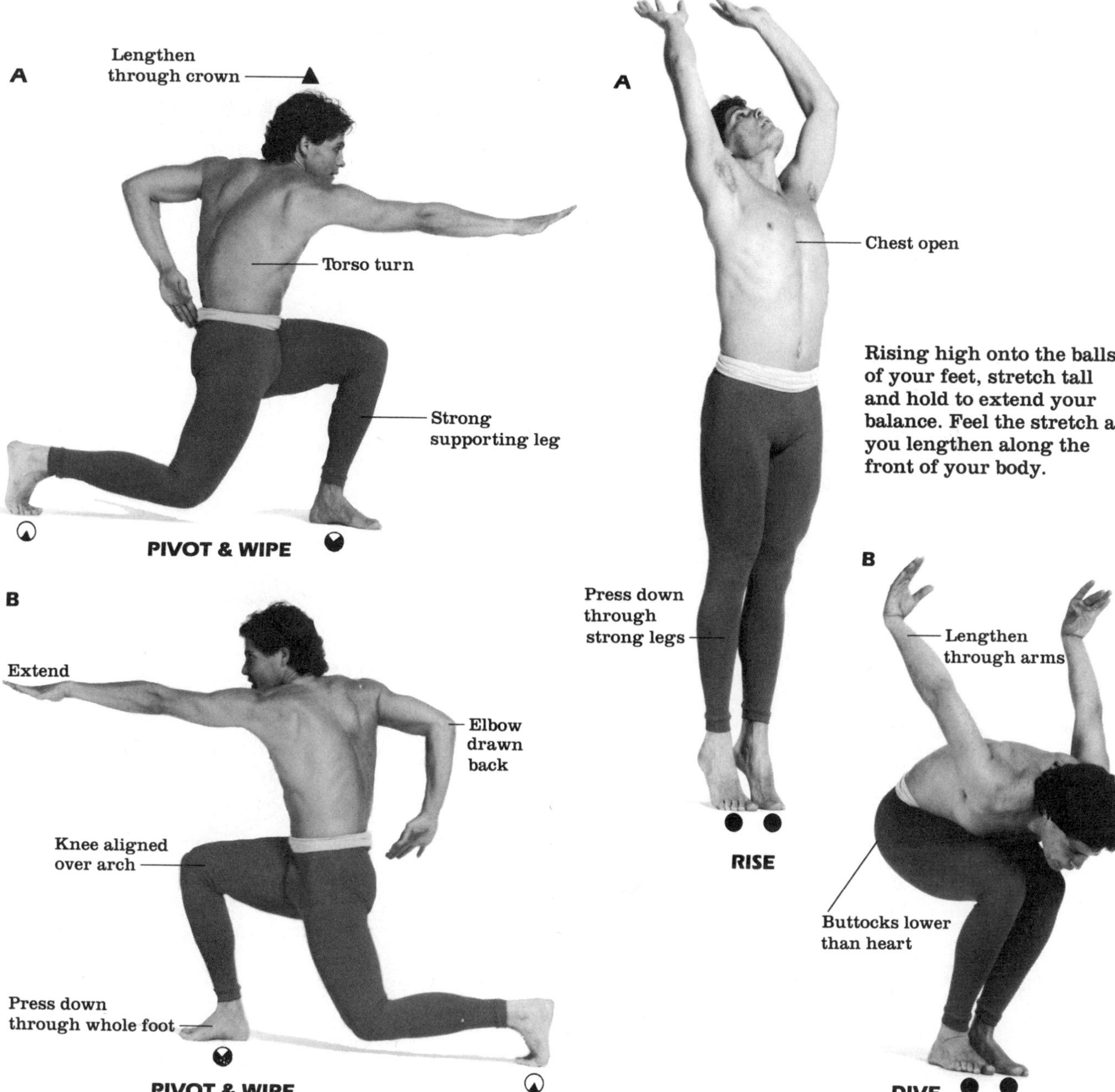

Shifting and pivoting side to side and purposefully lifting and placing the ball of your foot as you rotate, pretend to wipe your hand across a chest-level table, your arm following the rotation of your torso so that you get a nice stretch across your back as you exhale. Slow down and feel for balance and stretch. Move gently through center, inhaling. Repeat 8 times each side.

RISE 'N' DIVE

Rising high onto the balls of your feet, stretch tall and hold to extend your balance. Feel the stretch as you lengthen along the front of your body.

Sink down, firmly pressing through both feet, and keep lowering as you sweep your arms back behind you. Reach, extend, breathe, and stretch your shoulders and spine. Pause for 2 counts and lower your buttocks a bit farther to use the strength of your legs for pushing away from the floor and then rise high again for 2 counts. Repeat 8 times. Cool it down. Feel for control on the rise—stretch and lower—stretch.

SPINE ROLL

Standing in a hip or *A* stance, your feet parallel, inhale deeply as you place your hands softly on your thighs and, stretching your chest open, sink your buttocks, chest, and head, rounding over at a comfortable depth. You're coming out of your workout. Ebb gently and quietly.

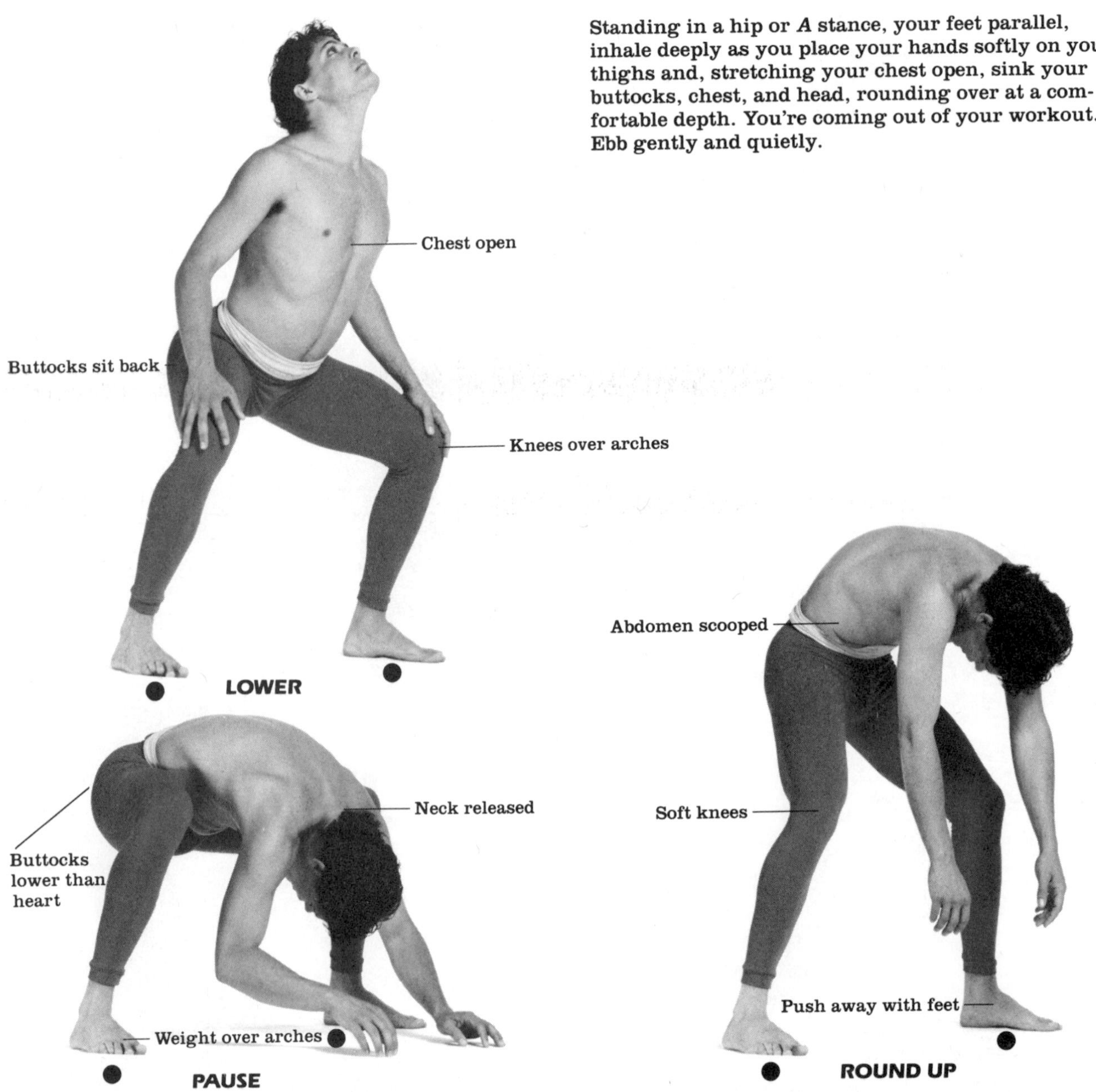

Pause and just hang for a moment, feeling that feline stretch along your spine. Acknowledge your good work, your healthier body.

Then, using the strength of your legs to push away, exhale fully and unroll your vertebrae, slowly, smoothly, one at a time, letting the weight of your body massage your back as you come upright. Come up very slowly, especially if you hang over for a while. Breathe in new energy. Repeat 4 times, ending rounded over.

ALL-FOURS CIRCLING

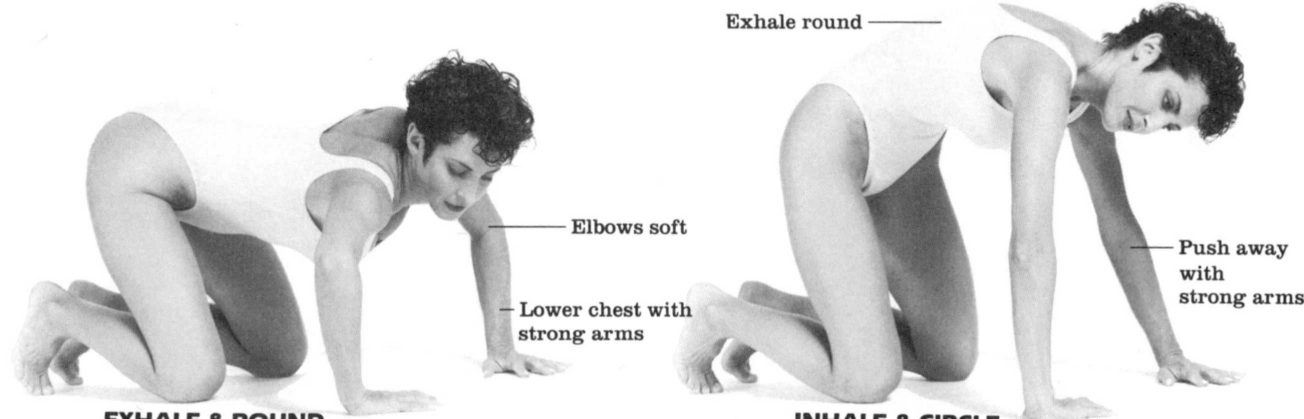

EXHALE & ROUND **INHALE & CIRCLE**

Reach down gently to the floor and slowly lower onto all fours. With your elbows soft, your hands below your shoulders, your knees under your hips, sensually circle your hips and torso 8 times in each direction, exhaling as your spine rounds to the ceiling. Feel a release in your entire spine, letting the muscle contractions massage you.

BACK STRETCH

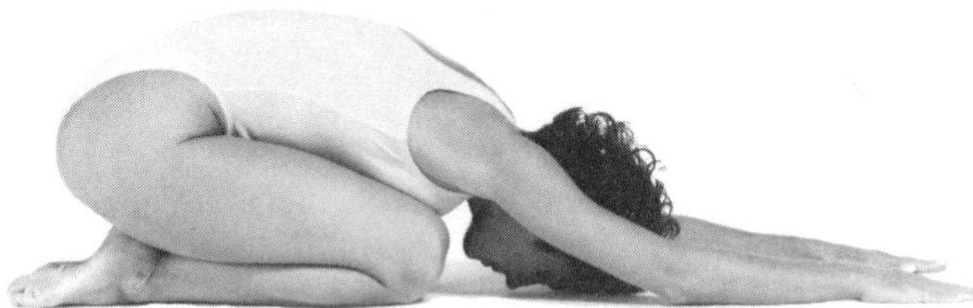

Without moving your hands, slowly lower your buttocks back onto your heels and feel the long stretch through your spine. Hold for 8 counts, breathing naturally. Rest. Feel at peace, calm.

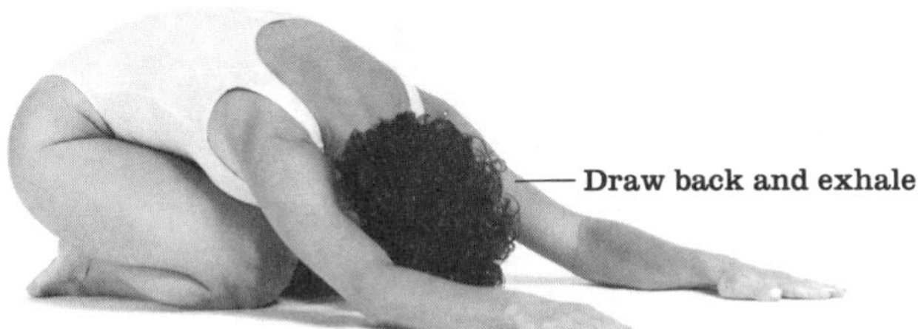

Then draw your elbows slightly back toward your body and exhale as you push your palms firmly into the floor. Without moving your hands, pull back, working against imagined tension, holding for a count of 4. Feel the contraction in your abdominals, the added stretch along your spine.

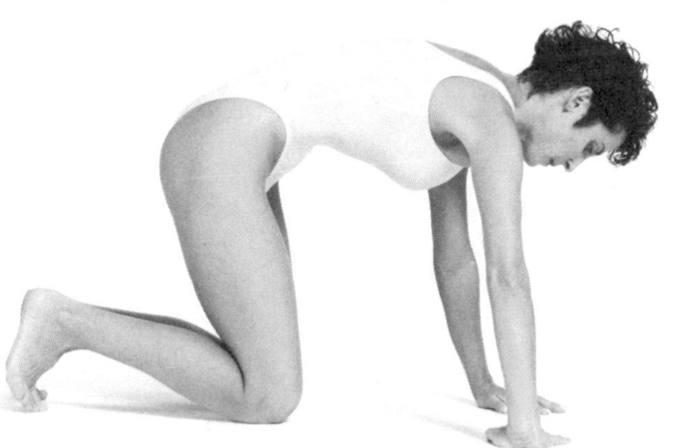

Inhale and rise back up onto all fours. Pause. Breathe.

HIP STRETCH

Now sit back on your heels slightly and, using your arm strength for support, lower yourself down to the left and slide your right hand out diagonally, reaching long through your right arm. Pause, hold for 8 counts, breathing naturally, and feel the stretch in your left hip. Imagine the floor responding to your touch with a smooth caress. Then gently push yourself back up to center and repeat on the other side.

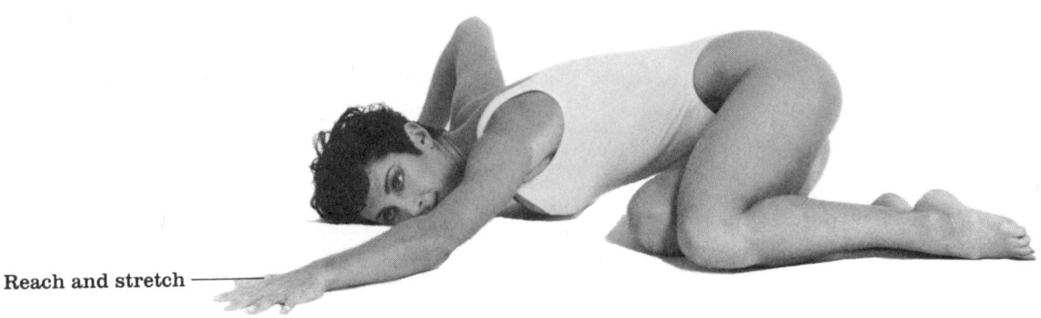

SPINAL TWIST

Using the strength of your arms, press your chest away from the floor, so you're sitting up tall over your right hip. Wrap your left leg over your right leg, your buttocks resting evenly on the floor. If your right side lifts up, extend your right leg out in front of you. Now lengthen upward and hug your left knee into your chest, turning your torso slightly and feeling the stretch through your hip and torso for a count of 8, breathing naturally. As you come back out of the twist, lead with your head first to release, your torso following. Pause. Breathe.

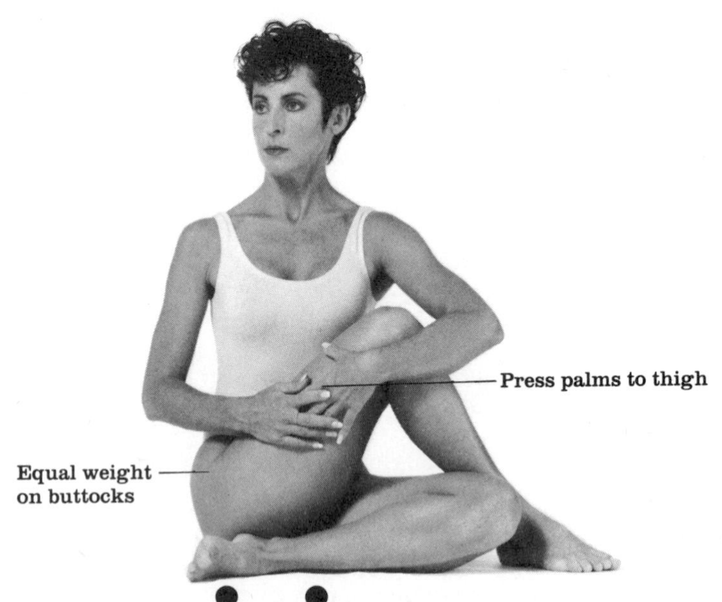

THIGH STRETCH

Your left leg still wrapped over your right, lower your torso down to the right and rest on your right elbow and forearm. Be sure your elbow is under your shoulder. With your left hand, take hold of your left ankle, and slowly draw your knee back, feeling a comfortable thigh stretch. If you feel pain in your knee, release your hold. Do not arch your back, but lengthen the front of your body. Hold for 8 counts, breathing naturally and release gently.

Press down through elbow under shoulder

SIDE STRETCH

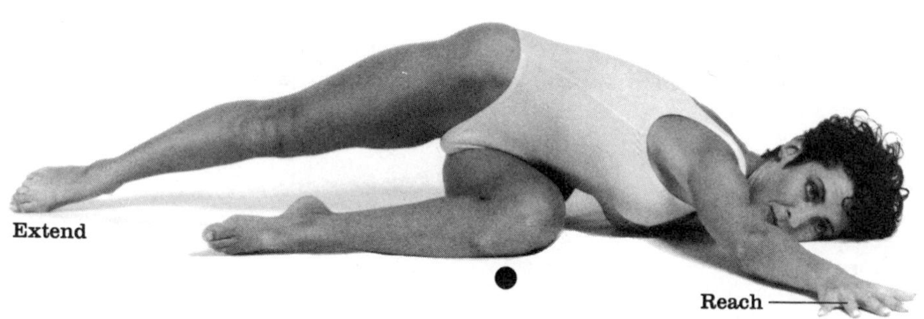

Extend your left leg back as you reach diagonally with your left arm, stretching into a full, long extension that ripples all along the left side of your body. Hold for 8 counts, breathing naturally and feeling your breath expand your chest to increase your spine flexibility. Then—

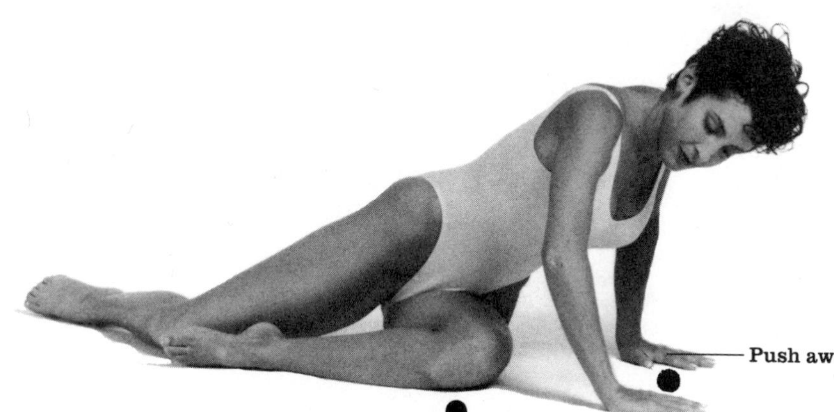

—soften both knees, drawing them closer to you, and bring your hands under your chest. Using the strength of your arms, exhale and push away from the floor to rise.

KNEE HUG

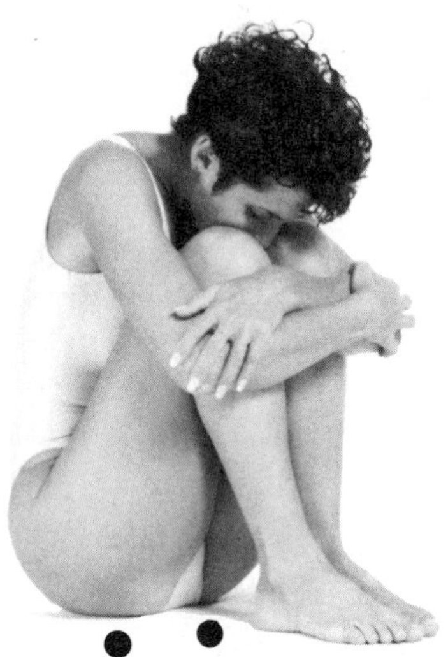

Sitting onto your buttocks, hug both knees into your chest. Pause and prepare to nourish the other side of your body with the stretches.

Muscle Balancer

Repeat the Spinal Twist, Thigh Stretch, and Side Stretch to the opposite side and end in a Knee Hug.

Then lower to the right and walk your hands out in front of you so that you're on all fours. Repeat All-Fours Circling.

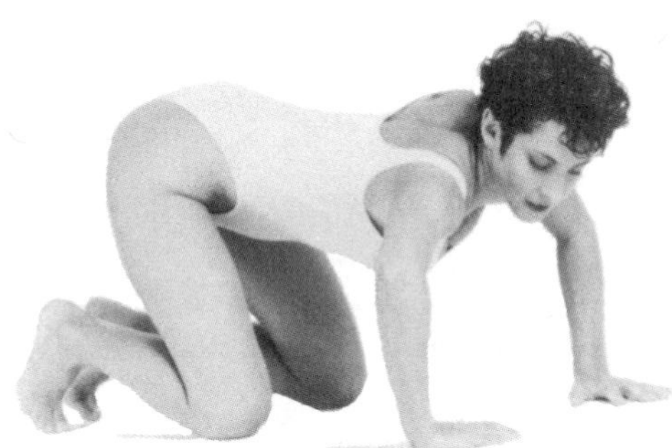

PUSH AWAY

With your toes curled under, your feet wider than your hips, and your hands below your shoulders, use the strength of your arms to push away from the floor, feeling your buttocks rise, your heels pressing into the floor. Now walk your hands back until you feel your pelvis above your arches. Pushing your fingertips forward, feel for a nice stretch through the back of your legs, your neck lengthened. Breathe naturally as you hold for 8 counts, adding new energy with each breath, new comfort with the stretch.

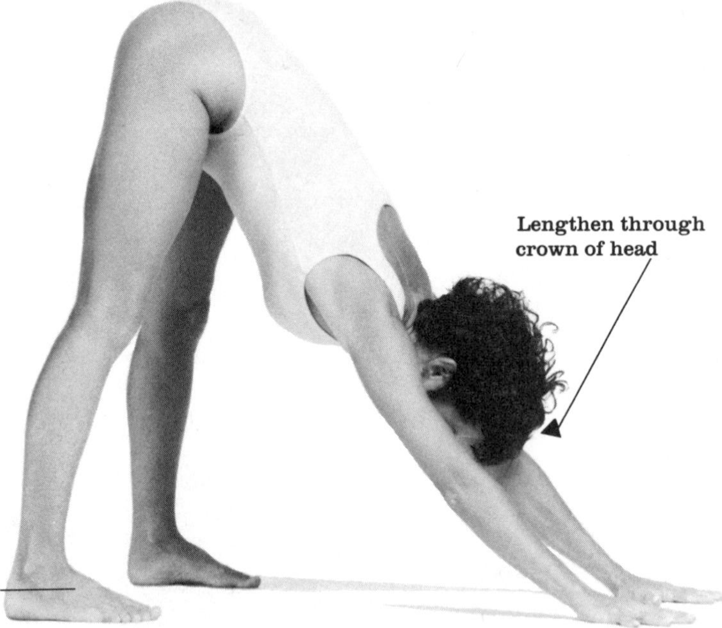

PUSH AWAY

ROUND-UP

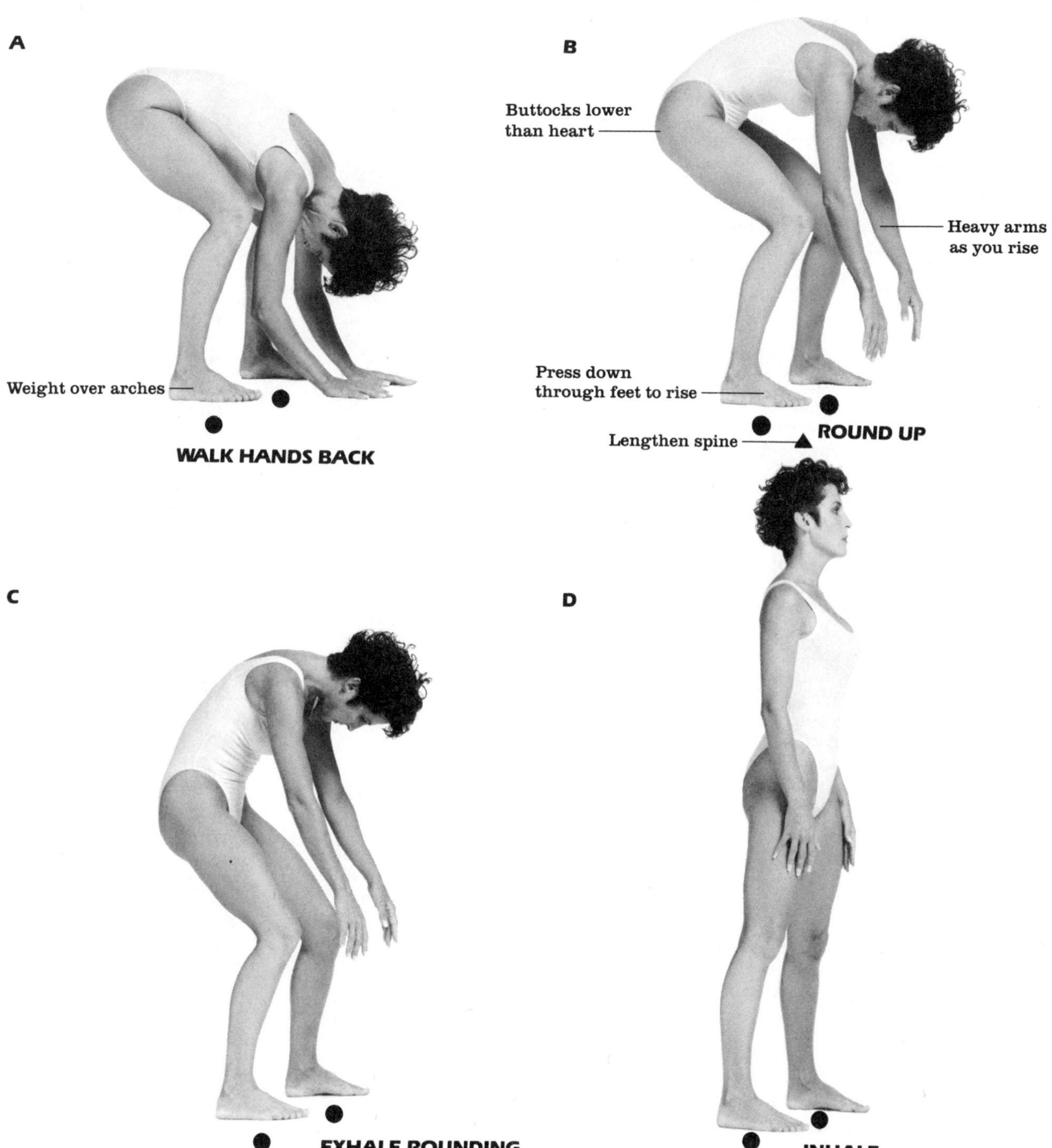

Walk your hands slowly back to your feet, lower your buttocks a few inches, and using the strength of your legs, exhale and slowly round up, stacking one vertebra at a time until your head is the last part of your body to come upright. Feel aligned. Breathe.

1. Inhale richly, feeling the new expanse of your lungs, and float your arms out to either side, drawing them up above your head. Now press your palms together and lift up through the crown of your head, lengthening your entire torso. Reach high, feeling the stretch run down from your fingertips through your arms, along the curve of your upper back and down your spine, imagining that you have roots growing out of the soles of your feet as the stretch pours down through your legs and out your feet.

2. With your palms pressed together, exhale, bend your elbows, and lower your thumbs to the nape of your neck, softening your knees. Feel the stretch along the underside of your upper arms. Inhale and reach high again, lengthening tall. Repeat 4 times, ending in a high reach.

3. Now exhale as you lower your arms straight down in front, slightly below shoulder level. Feel the stretch across your upper back. Open your hands so your palms face away from you, your thumbs and first fingers touching to form your Triangle. Pause. Breathe.

4. Inhale, breathing in new energy as you bend your elbows, and draw your Triangle toward your face so that your first fingers touch the tip of your nose. Then exhale, releasing and relaxing as you push your Triangle away, gazing through its center and feeling the relaxation take hold. Repeat 3 times.

5. Briskly rub your palms together, building up a good heat.

6. Open your palms, feeling that heat spread outward. Pause for a moment, feeling yourself at peace, in harmony with your life. Then close your hands and make a fist, keeping enough of that heat and energy for yourself today.

7. Inhale, drawing your elbows back by your sides and bringing that energy into your body. Open your chest and feel a wave of renewal course through every cell of your body.

8. Exhale and push your palms straight down by your sides, affirming that renewal. Jiggle, letting it reverberate through you.

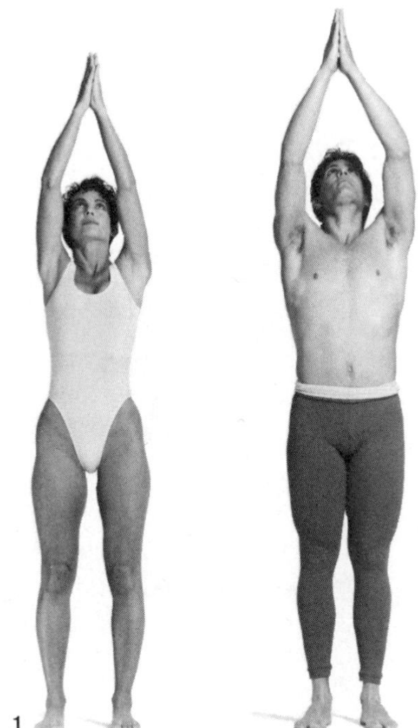

INHALE NEW ENERGY

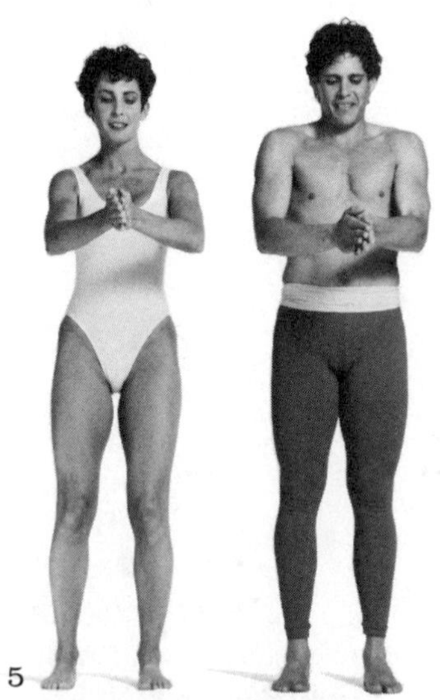

GENERATE WARMTH

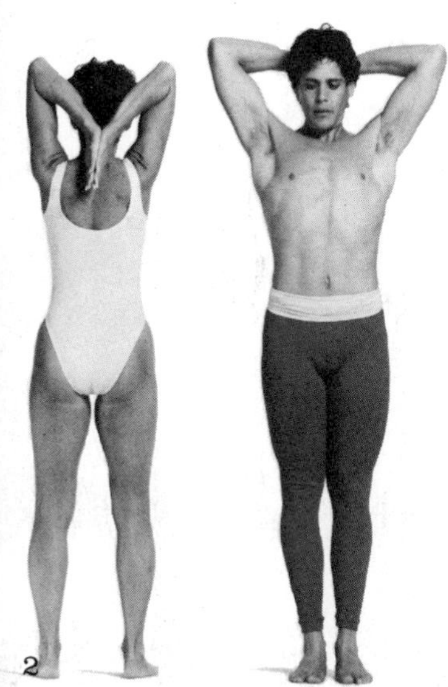

2

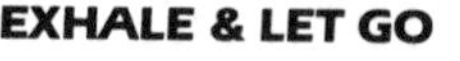

EXHALE & LET GO

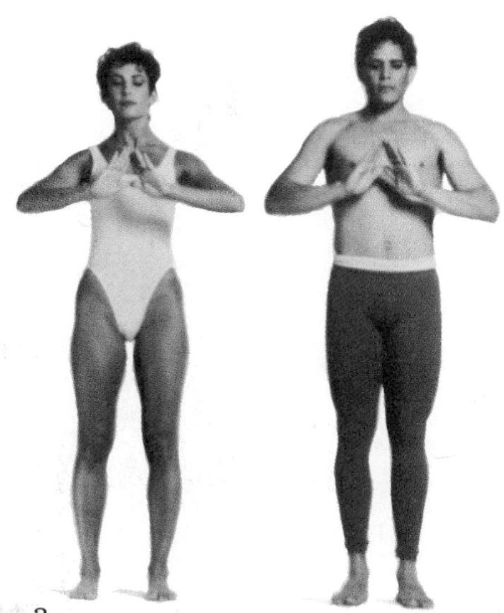

3

FOCUS & FEEL

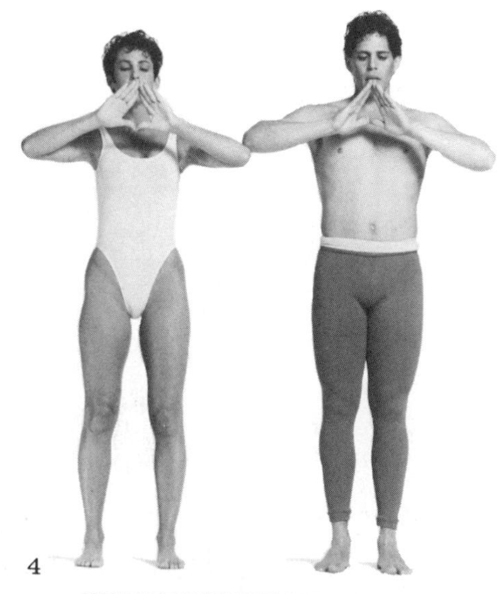

4

INHALE NEW ENERGY
EXHALE & RELEASE

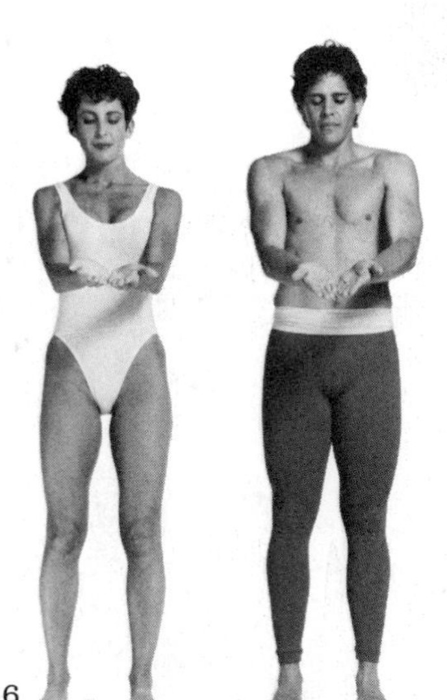

6

OPEN PALMS & FEEL

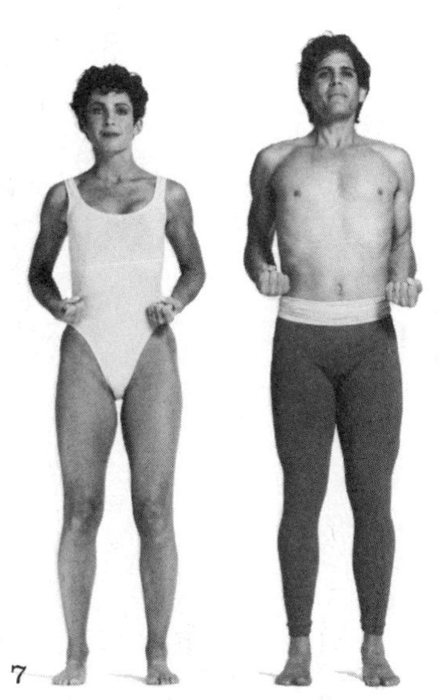

7

INHALE A NEW YOU

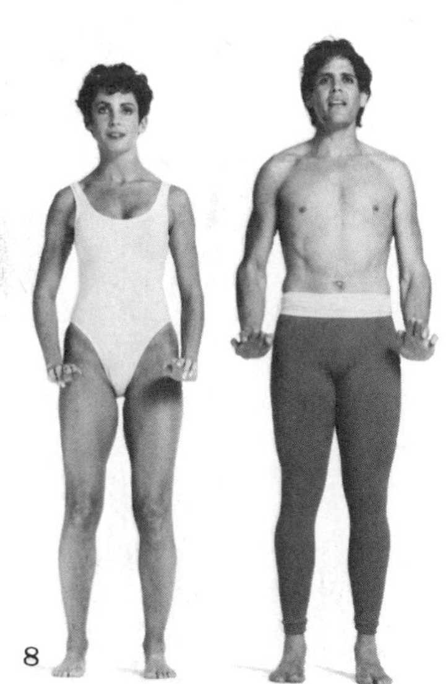

8

EXHALE WITH A NEW DAY

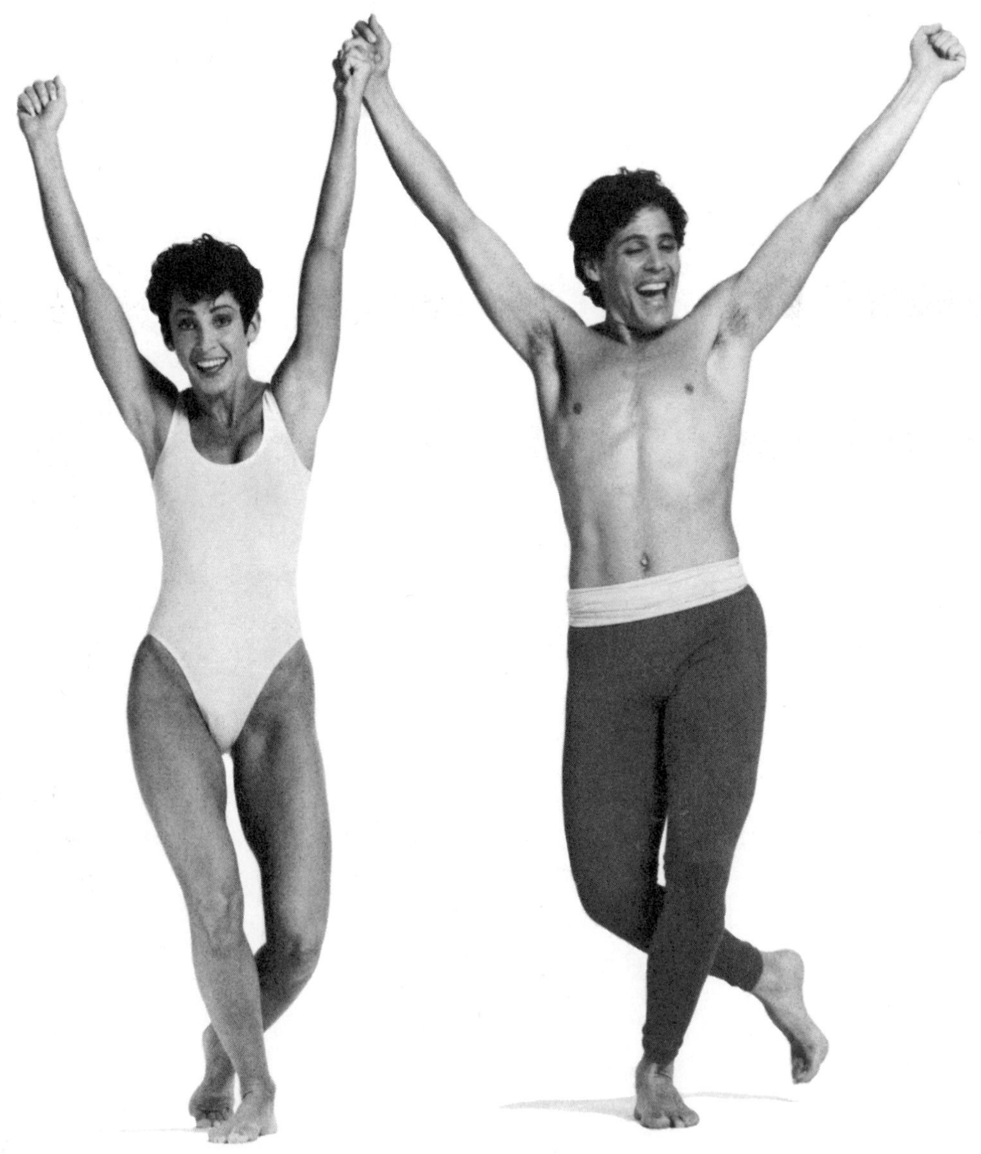

Take two purposeful steps gently back, stepping into a new body, a new you, a new day.

7/ EVERYDAY NON-IMPACT AEROBICS

Movement is the mother of fitness. Exercise is but one facet of fitness, one part of a day that is rich in possibility. Every day can be one systemic flow of movement, filling you with new energy, new vibrancy. It's not difficult to do. It simply means viewing your day with new eyes and an adventurous spirit, looking for little nuggets of movement in the most unlikely places. If you look for ways to tune up and stretch out all day, you'll discover your own private gold mine of movement to course new life through that magnificently intricate enterprise called your body. To spark your imagination about the latent possibilities in an ordinary day, read on. The following are ways to change an average day into a real energy pack by making the most out of what you do. Four times through is enough for each of the movements, but feel free to do as many as feels right for you in this new day of your life.

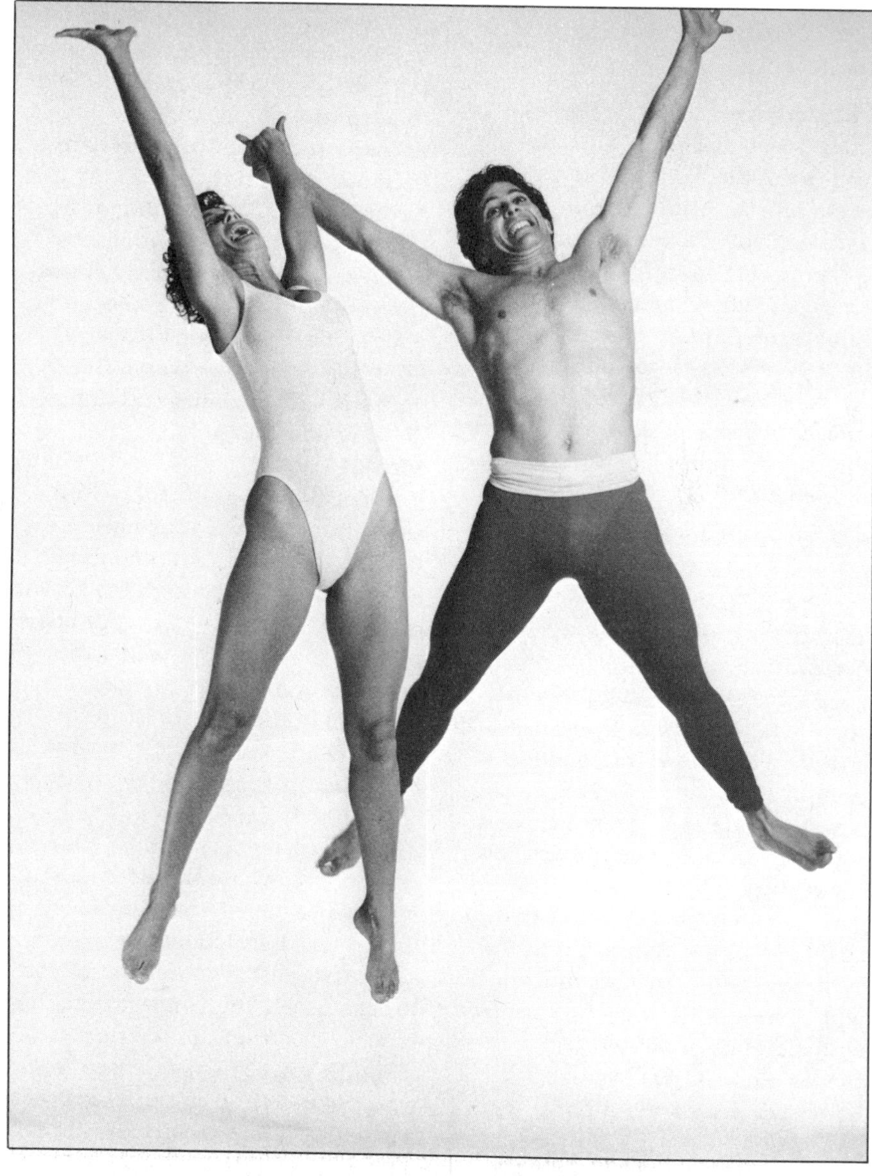

WAKE-UPS

When you wake up in the morning, before you even move an inch, bathe your body with rich oxygen. Lying still in bed, take a minute to breathe deeply, inhaling richly the newness of the day, exhaling and letting go of the night. Feel the feathery touch of your breath, the awakening of new life undulating like a wave through your whole body. Breath is the beginning of all movement.

The Bed Press

Next, roll over onto your back if you're not there already and simply press into the bed with your heels, and then your calves and thighs, working up through your buttocks, torso, shoulders, arms, hands, and fingers, and finally pushing your head back softly into your pillow. Release. Feel the light tension and release in every part of your body as it begins to come alive with tingling movement.

Stretch 'n' Shake

Just as we heat up for the workout with a Stretch 'n' Shake, you can heat up for the day ahead with a horizontal Stretch 'n' Shake. Sweep your arms out wide and up high above your head as if you're making angels in the snow. Stretch long and lean through the whole length of your body. Release and sweep your arms back down by your sides and shake, little jelly jiggles. Inhale your arms up, stretch, and exhale down and jiggle. Squinch up your eyes, squiggle your nose, munch with your mouth, wake up your face with all kinds of nonsensical shapes. Smile if you feel like it. Better yet, laugh. Set the tone for your day.

To do more in bed, refer back to the following Ease-Out movements which can be done as part of your Wake-Ups:

- All-Fours Circling (page 175)
- Back Stretch (page 175)
- Hip Stretch (page 176)
- Knee Hug (page 178)

Shimmy

Ease yourself out of bed and, with your feet comfortably at hip width, inhale as you sweep your arms out to the sides and up high above your head with a good yawn, stretching to touch the ceiling. Then whistle an exhalation as you float your arms back down and lightly shimmy like a rag doll, gently loosening every joint in your body. Lift your toes and feel your weight evenly spread through your feet, your knees soft, your spine fluid, your hips loose. Continue, inhaling up and filling yourself with vibrancy, exhaling down and letting go.

Step-in

Take two purposeful steps forward, leading with your heels, feeling your knees soft and fluid, lengthening tall through the crown of your head. Pause, feel your body relaxed and centered, your feet pressing evenly into the floor. Breathe. In the quiet of the morning, you are readying for the day, becoming in sync with the rhythm of your body.

Inhale deeply as you float your arms out slowly to the sides and up high above your head, your shoulders relaxed. Exhale, lowering your arms straight down in front of you to chest level, your fingers touching to form the Triangle. Looking through your Triangle, check in with yourself and run through the day ahead. What is the most important thing for you today? Whatever it is, visualize it in your Triangle, using your imagination to make it as vivid as you can, punching up the colors, listening to the sounds around it, touching, smelling, feeling all the tangibles and intangibles of this most important thing. Once you've got that image in full color and stereophonic sound, blow one single breath through your Triangle and imagine sending the image out to precede you. Then, close your Triangle, slowly draw your hands back toward your chest, and let them relax down the sides of your body.

Mime Walk

On your way to the bathroom, give your feet and ankles a light massage by taking baby steps and rolling up high onto the ball of each foot, listening for the crackle of your joints releasing.

BATHROOM BODY HEATS

Toothbrush Tango

While you're brushing your teeth, roll alternately onto the ball of each foot and imagine pulling bubble gum off the floor with your heels. If you're one of those people who can tap her head and rub her stomach at the same time, pick up your pace to tango tempo, letting your hips swish and lifting your elbows out to chest level while you polish those pearly whites.

Brush 'n' Roll

Instead of simply brushing your hair in a nonchalant fashion, do a Spine Roll at the same time. Brush in hand, your feet slightly beyond hip width, inhale deeply and gently slide your hands down your thighs toward your knees, easing your buttocks back like you're sinking into a beach chair and opening your chest to the warmth of the sun. Stop your hands at your knees (or higher up if that feels more comfortable) and pause to check for comfort, your knees aligned with the second toe of each foot and pressing no farther than your arches. Lift your toes once to refine your balance. Then continue inhaling, lowering your buttocks a little more and finally round over so that your neck releases, your head droops, and you feel a tingling stretch spill down your neck and back. Don't overdo. It's still early.

Now, while you're down there, brush your hair, counting to 30 and feeling the warmth of new circulation in your face, the tingling stimulation of your scalp. Then let your arms hang loosely toward the floor, release your neck, and very lightly circle your head in one direction and then the other. Hang loosely again. Then place one hand on the back of your head and very gently press your chin toward your chest just enough to feel a welcome stretch through your neck and spine. Release back and hang. Then, using the strength of your legs to push away from the floor, round slowly back up, stacking each vertebra until your head finally tops them all and you're back to an upright position. Inhale deeply.

Shower 'n' Shout

When you step out of the shower to dry off, put a little twist 'n shout into it. With your towel draped across your buttocks, lightly swish your hips back and forth. Then, sink slightly over your right leg, place the ball of your left foot out on a diagonal, and lightly bump left with your hips. Change and bump right, humming your favorite tune.

Towel Lifts

Replace your bath towel with a face towel and take hold of either end of it. Now, with your arms low, pull on either end as you slowly raise and lower your arms straight out in front of you, inhaling up and exhaling down. Still raising and lowering, dig your heels into the floor and alternately lift the front of your feet off the floor as high as possible. Don't let your knees snap back or your buttocks thrust behind, but stay soft and aligned.

Mirror Mirror on the Wall . . .

Standing with your back to the mirror, your towel in your right hand, rotate your torso right and look at yourself in the mirror. Pause, feeling the warm stretch through your spine. Then reach out with your right arm as though you're giving the towel to your reflection. Now, your head leading first, release front and switch the towel into your left hand. Continuing through with your torso, rotate left and extend the towel. Who *is* that wonderful person?

BREAKFAST PICK-ME-UPS

Sweet 'n' Roll

Still barefooted and cooking breakfast, rock forward onto the balls of your feet and backward onto your heels, feeling for the entire length of your feet as you rock back and forth several times. Then rock side to side, feeling the inside and outside edges and the warm massage across the balls of your feet. Finally, tie the movements together, making broad, full circles, your feet pressing into the floor all around the edges and your hips circling fluidly above. Keep your knees soft, your hips loose, your spine fluid, your shoulders relaxed.

Counter Tops

Standing tall at the kitchen counter, place your hands on top and press down as you soften your knees and, with your weight in your left leg, touch out with your right toes first to 3:00, then 4:00, 5:00, and 6:00, reversing back through each hour to 3:00. Then shift your weight over your right leg and touch left to 9:00, 8:00, 7:00, and 6:00 and back through to 9:00. Repeat the whole series, lifting your leg over each hour without touching the floor in between.

CAR-IDLE ISOMETRICS

While you're waiting for your car to warm up, exhale and scoop your abdomen in, pressing your lower back into the seat. Inhale as you release.

Then place your hands on the insides of your thighs and, exhaling, work opposing tensions by pressing your legs together while pulling them apart with your hands. The movement is all inside; your legs should barely budge. Reverse, placing your hands on the outsides of your thighs and pulling your legs apart while pressing them together with your hands.

Now place your hands on either side of the steering wheel and press in and release, press and release. Then hold tight to either side and pull and release, pull and release. To work different muscles in your chest, press and pull with your hands at 3:00 and 9:00, then 2:00 and 10:00, and finally 4:00 and 8:00.

DESKERCISES

Wing Stretch

Sitting tall in your chair, your feet firmly planted on the floor, float your arms out to either side and up high above your head so that they are on a slight forward diagonal. Press your palms together and reach high, lifting up through the crown of your head, lengthening your entire torso, and feeling the stretch pour down from your fingertips all the way through your spine. Your palms still pressed together, bend your elbows and, exhaling, lower your thumbs back to the nape of your neck. Inhale and reach high again; exhale and press back.

Shoulder Roll

When you've finished, float your arms down to your sides and just roll your shoulders back one at a time and then together. Reverse and roll alternate and then both shoulders forward.

Chair Press

Take hold of the bottom of your chair on either side and, bending your elbows, pull up, exhaling. Release and relax as you inhale. Then place your hands on top of the seat and press down, your elbows still bent. Release and relax and continue alternating the press and pull.

The Wrap

Ease forward on your chair a bit and, sitting tall with your left arm hanging down toward the floor, reach your right arm behind your back and grab hold of your left arm. Press forward with your chest just enough to feel a nice, easy stretch through your shoulders and chest. Then change arms and stretch again. As you stretch, wobble your head around a bit as though you had loose screws in your neck.

The Sit Roll

Next, push your chair away from your desk to do a sitting Spine Roll; make sure your thighs are parallel to the floor, your feet flat and parallel. Sitting tall, inhale deeply, opening your chest as you slide your hands down your thighs to your knees. Then, rounding your spine, ease your chest down toward your thighs, flexing forward as far as is comfortable and letting your arms hang loosely on either side of your chair. Release your neck so that your head falls softly forward and let the weight of your body gently stretch and lengthen your spine. Breathe naturally, letting the stretch take hold as you relax. While you're down there, make some wonderfully expressive faces to massage your face while the circulation pours down and brings new life to your skin. Then, using the strength of your legs and pressing through your feet, exhale, feeling the scoop in your abdomen, and slowly round back up, stacking each vertebra until your head finally tops them all and you're back to an upright position. Jiggle your shoulders, feeling a warm tingle spilling down your spine.

Jelly Jiggles

Finally, sitting tall and lengthened, sweep your arms out to the sides and up high above your head as you inhale deeply. Reach to touch the ceiling and then exhale and float your arms back down. With your arms hanging loosely on either side of your chair, shake out with little jelly jiggles. Inhale up, lengthen tall, exhale down, and jiggle.

LUNCH DANCE

Jazz Walk

Once everyone has cleared out of the office for lunch or when you've found a quiet midday moment at home, simply walk in place for a count of 30, shaking out your arms and rolling your shoulders to warm up a bit. If you've been in your shoes all day, now is the time to kick them off. Humming your favorite tune, sink into the rhythm of a Jazz Walk. With your feet at hip width, walk lightly and loosely, letting your hips be swishy, stepping first onto the ball of your foot and rolling down to your heel. Then, with your arms at shoulder level, imagine hitting a punching bag, making tight circles with your fists. Keep it easy, nothing too aggressive. As your body heat rises, increase the intensity a bit if you don't mind sweating. Sink slightly as you jazz walk and punch low, exhaling. Then, inhaling, rise up onto the balls of your feet and punch high above your head.

Cross Behind

Breathe rhythmically as you shift left and right, inhaling as you sink slightly through center, exhaling as you cross one foot behind the other and wipe your forearm across your forehead. Imagine plucking any tension from your morning off the top of your head and flicking it out to the side as you make full circles with each arm. Then transit fluidly into the next movement.

Sink 'n' Rise

Shift side to side and lift your free leg back on a diagonal, letting your arms follow the motion, reaching left and right smoothly, fluidly. Inhale as you lift; exhale as you sink. Keep your rhythm easy, your spine fluid. If you feel up to it, rise onto the ball of your supporting foot as you lift your opposite leg back on a diagonal.

4:00 SLUMP BUSTERS

Doorframe Miniseries

A door frame is a terrific spot for working out the kinks of tension that build up throughout the day.

Standing with your feet together in the center, reach straight out to either side and press your hands into the door frame for a count of 10. Release and press.

Then take a firm hold on either side and let your body fall gently forward, keeping your abdomen pressed back, your heels dug into the floor so you give yourself a light stretch through your torso, the backs of your legs, and Achilles tendons. Be careful not to press your hips forward or your lower back will overarch. Using the strength of your arms, pull yourself back to center, switch your hold to the opposite side of the frame, and let yourself fall gently backward onto your heels, scooping in your abdomen and feeling the gorgeous massage through your back.

Turn sideways, your feet together in the center. Reach back, place your hands on the frame, and gently ease yourself back against it. Lengthen tall so that your head and upper and lower back are pressed into the frame. Then, keeping that long, lean contact, sink as though you're sitting down into a chair until your knees are smack over your arches—no farther. Pause as long as is comfortable and then, digging your heels into the floor, slide slowly back up. Don't overdo. Even a slight sink may be just right.

This time reach forward with both hands and lean into the frame, your arms up on a comfortable angle, your buttocks still against the frame behind you. Take a firm hold of the frame, inhale, and drape your chest and head between your arms. Hold for a comfortable stretch. Then, bend your knees slightly before exhaling and rounding back up, scooping your abdomen in and pressing each vertebra into the frame while your fingers slide down the doorframe until just your fingertips are pushing away and finally your arms flop to your sides.

Turn around, snug the front of your body up against the frame, and take hold of it at shoulder level, crossing your hands so that your right hand grasps the left side and your left hand grasps the right side. Pull for a count of 10, release and pull.

Shoe Tie

Your feet parallel below your hips, shift your weight into your left leg and, with control, step back onto the ball of your right foot at 5:00 as you inhale. Then slowly exhale as you round over your left foot to tie an imaginary shoe, keeping your buttocks lower than your chest and sinking only as far as is comfortable. Pause for a moment and feel the warm stretch through your back, hips, and thighs, the even distribution of your weight in your feet. Lift your front toes once to refine your balance. Then, pressing into the floor with your left foot, exhale, scoop in your abdomen, and rise slowly, evenly, stacking each vertebra and letting your arms hang loosely at your sides as you rise. Repeat on the other side, stepping back onto the ball of your left foot at 7:00.

FROM HERE TO THERE

Elevator Tones

When you leave work, make the most of your elevator ride by simply softening your knees and pressing your heels into the floor, tightening your buttocks, thighs, and calves. Hold for a count of 10, release, and press again. With a nonchalant expression on your face, who's to know you're beautifying your buns and legs. Isometrics and isotonics like this are great whenever you're standing and waiting—for a bus, at a department store, in a theater line.

Grocery-Line Lifts

While you're waiting to check out your groceries, do the above isometric exercise and add this one: Place your hands on either side of your grocery cart handles and press in for a count of 10. Release and press. If you do it subtly, no one will be wise to the fact that you're firming your breasts.

Red-Light Relief

To take advantage of red stoplights or stopped-dead traffic, simply press your head back against your head rest, hold for a count of 10, and release. Press and release, feeling the tension melt from your neck.

Then, to release tension in your shoulders, press your hands up into the roof of your car, pause, then squeeze your shoulders up against your neck for a count of 10. Release your shoulders first and then your hands. Shimmy your shoulders. As you loosen and relax, walk your hands back a little farther each time you press up.

TELEPHONE TRIMMERS

Sink 'n' Chat

While you're catching up with friends on the telephone, step out to the side, leading with your heel and rolling through to the flat of your foot. Then lift your opposite leg slightly back on a diagonal. Sink through center, shift to the other side, and repeat the diagonal leg lift with the opposite leg. If you feel up to it, rise onto the ball of your foot as you lift your opposite leg.

Prone Phone

If the conversation is a long one, lie down on your back. Bend your knees and slide your feet toward your buttocks. Then, with even weight in your feet, press your lower back into the floor, hold for a count of 10 and then release. Press and release. This time, as you press, lift your buttocks just slightly off the floor, keeping an even press in your feet while you count to 10. Release down and then repeat.

Finally, pressing your lower back into the floor, bring your knees up toward your chest, feeling the warm relief in your lower back. Then extend one leg at a time straight up as you press your lower back into the floor. When you finish, bend your knees into your chest, roll onto one side, and just lie there luxuriously stretched until you're all talked out.

LANGUID LOUNGING

Couch Scoops

While you're snugged up on the couch watching television, sitting lengthwise, bring your knees up and slide your feet slightly in toward your buttocks. Holding onto your knees, inhale and lengthen tall through your spine; then release back and exhale as you scoop in your abdomen.

The Cat

Roll onto the floor and settle in on all fours, your hands below your shoulders, your knees below your hips. Slowly, sensually, circle your hips and torso in one direction and then the other, exhaling as your spine rounds toward the ceiling. Keep your elbows soft, the back of your neck lengthened.

Then, without moving your hands, lower back onto your heels and feel the long stretch through your spine, breathing naturally and letting the stretch take hold as you relax deeper. Press your palms into the floor, draw your elbows back just slightly closer toward your body, and exhale as you continue pressing and pulling backward, working with isometric tension. Release, press, and pull again. Finally, inhale and rise back up onto all fours.

With your knees and feet hip width apart, your hands below your shoulders, use the strength of your arms to push away from the floor, your buttocks rising, your heels pressing into the floor. Lengthen from the crown of your head to the tip of your tailbone as you exhale and press into the floor with your hands. If this is too difficult, bend your knees. Then walk your hands slowly back to your feet, lower your buttocks six inches, and using the strength of your legs, exhale and slowly round up, stacking your vertebrae one at a time until your head is the last part to come upright. Take a deep breath and let the warm relaxation cascade over your body.

Before slipping between your sheets, stand with your feet slightly beyond hip width, inhale richly and float your arms out to either side and up high above your head on a slight forward diagonal. Press your palms together and lift up through the crown of your head, lengthening your entire torso.

Now exhale as you lower your arms straight down in front of you, slightly below shoulder level. Open your hands so your palms face away from you, to form the Triangle. Inhale, breathing in the calm of the night, as you bend your elbows and draw the backs of your hands toward your face so your first fingers touch the tip of your nose. Exhale, releasing and letting go as you push your Triangle away, feeling the relaxation take hold. Then briskly rub your palms together, building up a good heat. Step together and open your palms, feeling that heat spread out into the night. Make a fist, keeping just enough of that heat for a deep sleep. Inhale, drawing your elbows back by your sides and filling yourself with soothing energy. Reach forward with your chest and feel a wave of sweet calm course through every cell of your body. Exhale and push your palms straight down by your sides, giving yourself over to the night. Gently step back, sinking into the soothing comfort of oncoming sleep.

Drift dreamily into bed and Stretch 'n' Shake just as you did this morning. Then do the Bed Press, this time filling each part of your body with deep relaxation as you let go of the last traces of tension. With your head sinking into your pillow, yawn wide and exhale, feeling the entire weight of your body growing heavier and heavier as you sink deeper, deeper toward sleep. The velvety curtain of night falls.

EPILOGUE

It's wonderful to want to look better, to begin a fitness program wanting to change the shape of your body. It's even more wonderful to experience all the unexpected benefits that fitness can bring into your life, to feel a new energy, a new vibrancy in your life, to move with greater ease and grace.

Through the NIA Technique we've found relaxation of mind and body. And that has allowed us to extend the range of our days so that we can go longer, do more, and not feel exhausted or stressed. The ease with which we go about our lives still astonishes us. The NIA Technique has given us energetic, agile bodies. We've become graceful and spirited in our motions, inside and outside the studio. The NIA Technique has helped us understand our bodies and respect them for the magnificent possibilities they allow. We want nothing less for you.

The NIA Technique, taken seriously but enjoyably, will enhance your life in ways maybe you don't even imagine now. Our greatest thrill is watching our students get a glimmer of something more, seeing them reap the unexpected gifts of The NIA Technique, hearing from them about ways that it has touched their lives.

The NIA Technique has much to give you if you do it consistently, efficiently, and with love. A lot of people talk a lot about motivation and self-discipline, as though exercise were a thing to conquer with sheer will power and ungodly drive. Through the NIA Technique we've discovered what it's like to feel that we'd have to discipline ourselves to *not* do it. We'd miss the wonderful massage, not just for our bodies but for our minds, our psyches, our souls. We'd miss the relaxation and release. We'd miss the fun of it all, the dance, the intoxicating movement we only dreamed of five years ago. For you we wish nothing less than that sweet taste of dreams come true, of a life filled not just with possibility, but probability and, yes, then reality.

THE NIA TECHNIQUE COMPANIONS

The best part about writing this book is sharing something we love passionately. The worst thing is not being with you in person to find out how you like the workout and whether you need any pointers. We may be coming to a city near you soon, however, to give guest workshops, and if you write us, we'll send you our schedule. To get a little closer, we've also made an audio cassette and a videotape and are working on lots of other ideas to bridge the gap between you and us.

Audio

"Get Ready"

One side is chock-full of basic NIA Technique movements, with plenty of detail about how to get the most out of them and plenty of energetic encouragement from both of us. You can do it gently or punch it up for a more vigorous 12-minute aerobic workout. The other side is a full-blown, get-down, 22-minute aerobic workout set to exciting, original music unlike anything you've heard on an exercise tape. You can use the workout to get ready for a dynamite day, a tennis match, a golf game, an important meeting—anything that you want to feel alert for, relaxed and unstressed. We love it as much as our friends do! Your local bookstore should have it. If not, call or write and we'll send one right away.

Videotape

You won't see another like it—original music for our unique way of moving; some of our students—not a hired cast—doing a knock-out workout at different levels, so you can pick and follow the one who seems closest to your level. As you progress, follow someone else. Eventually you'll work with us as we alternate moderate and advanced levels. Seeing the NIA Technique in motion, a room full of a collective, lyrical pulse, is a real thrill. Wait until you see it! You won't want to stop moving. Your local bookstore or video outlet should have it. If not, call or write.

Here's where to find us:

Debbie and Carlos Rosas
The NIA Technique, Inc.
110 Tiburon Blvd., Suite 5
Mill Valley, CA 94941
(415) 456-BODY